Materials for Medical Applications

This book discusses advanced knowledge about the synthesis and application of materials in the medical field for diagnostic and therapeutic conditions. These materials have been extensively used in various biological and medical applications, especially in drug delivery, tumor screening, bioimaging, diagnosis, and therapies. *Materials for Medical Applications* provides comprehensive but concise information about materials and their medical applications. The readers will get information about the trends in materials and their medical applications, as well as current material-based products that are used in the medical field. The book has 11 chapters, where shapes, sizes, and structural differences of materials and methods of synthesis have been described, and a few chapters are also dedicated to the characterization of materials and their medical applications. The book also discusses how materials are tested in research laboratories, preclinical (animal) trials, and clinical (human) trials, and how material-based products go through various regulatory and safety phases before reaching patients. It also discusses topics such as materials delivery, imaging, and treatments for various diseases. It includes a chapter dedicated to regulatory guidelines and policies in the application of nanomaterials and will include current clinical trial information on the materials. Finally, the book has topics such as health safety, toxicity, dosages, and long-term implications of materials. This book is intended for researchers, material scientists, and students in bioengineering, biomedical engineering, and biopharmaceuticals working on the development of biomaterials.

Firdos Alam Khan is Professor and Chairman, Department of Stem Cell Biology, Institute for Research and Medical Consultations (IRMC), Imam Abdulrahman Bin Faisal University, Dammam, Saudi Arabia. Currently, Professor Khan is studying the role of different nanomaterials and biomaterials in stem cell differentiation into neuronal cells and also in cancer treatment. Professor Khan has been elected as Fellow of the Royal Society of Biology (FRSB), UK.

Materials for Medical Applications

Principles and Practices

Edited by
Firdos Alam Khan

CRC Press
Taylor & Francis Group
Boca Raton London New York

CRC Press is an imprint of the
Taylor & Francis Group, an **informa** business

Designed cover image: Firdos Alam Khan

First edition published 2024
by CRC Press
6000 Broken Sound Parkway NW, Suite 300, Boca Raton, FL 33487–2742

and by CRC Press
4 Park Square, Milton Park, Abingdon, Oxon, OX14 4RN

CRC Press is an imprint of Taylor & Francis Group, LLC

ISBN: 978-1-032-32017-5 (hbk)
ISBN: 978-1-032-33007-5 (pbk)
ISBN: 978-1-003-31771-5 (ebk)

DOI: 10.1201/9781003317715

Typeset in Times
by Apex CoVantage, LLC

Contents

*Sundus Iftikhar, Hina Ashraf, Muhammad Ali Faridi, Maria
Khan, and Abdul Samad Khan*

Firdos Alam Khan

Chapter 11   Challenges of Materials Products Used in Medical Applications.... 199

V. Ravinayagam and B. Rabindran Jermy

Chapter 12   Research Trends in Materials Synthesis and Medical
Applications 217

*Muhammad Nawaz, Faiza Qureshi, Hira Fatima Abbas,
and Tooba Mahboob*

Acknowledgments

I am grateful to the Almighty Allah for the blessings and guidance. I am thankful to CRC Press, and Taylor & Francis Group, for showing trust in me and given me one more opportunity to edit this exciting book. I appreciate the support of Dr. Marc Gutierrez, Editor-CRC Press and Taylor and Francis Group. I am thankful to all the members of the production team of CRC Press and Taylor and Francis Group for their support and cooperation.

I am grateful to all the authors and corresponding authors for their immense contributions and cooperation. I want to thank the entire management team of the Institute for Research and Medical Consultations (IRMC), Imam Abdulrahman Bin Faisal University, Dammam, Saudi Arabia, for their support, especially to Professor Ebtesam Al-Suhaimi, Dean, IRMC, Imam Abdulrahman Bin Faisal University, Dammam, Saudi Arabia, for her constant encouragement.

I am grateful to all my teachers and mentors, especially Professor Nishikant Subhedar and Late Professor Obaid Siddiqi FRS, for their immense contributions to shaping my research career. I am also thankful to all my friends, well-wishers, and colleagues for their support and cooperation.

I am grateful to my entire family members, especially to my late father, Nayeemuddin Khan; late mother, Sarwari Begum; my brothers (Aftab Alam Khan, Javed Alam Khan, Intekhab Alam Khan, and Sarfaraz Alam Khan); my sisters (late Sayeeda Khanum, Faheemida Khanum, Kahkashan Khanum, and Ayesha Khanum); my wife, Samina Khan; my sons (Zuhayr Ahmad Khan, Zaid Ahmad Khan, and Zahid Ahmad Khan); my daughter (Azraa Khan); my father-in-law (Abdul Qayyum Siddiqi); and mother-in-law (Uzma Siddiqi) for their support.

Enjoy reading!

Firdos Alam Khan, PhD
Professor and Chairman
Department of Stem Cell Research
Institute for Research and Medical Consultations,
Imam Abdulrahman Bin Faisal University
P.O. Box No. 1982
Dammam 31441, Saudi Arabia
Email: fakhan@iau.edu.sa

About the Editor

Firdos Alam Khan is Professor and Chairman, Department of Stem Cell Biology, Institute for Research and Medical Consultations (IRMC), Imam Abdulrahman Bin Faisal University, Dammam, Saudi Arabia. In addition to his research work, he has been teaching (Cell Physiology, Biochemistry, Stem Cell Biology, and Regenerative Medicine) courses to MSc students. Professor Khan has completed his Ph.D. degree in zoology with a neuroscience specialization from Nagpur University, India. Over the past 25 years, Professor Khan has been involved in teaching various courses, such as Cell Biology, Pharmacology, Business of Biotechnology, Biomedicine, Cell and Tissue Engineering, and Bioethics-IPR, to undergraduate and postgraduate students. Professor Khan was associated with Manipal University (now Manipal Academy of Higher Education) Dubai Campus, United Arab Emirates. He was Professor and Chairperson, School of Life Sciences, and served as Chairman of the Research and Development Program. Professor Khan did his first postdoctoral fellowship at the National Centre for Biological Sciences (NCBS), Bangalore, India, and a second postdoctoral fellowship at Massachusetts Institute of Technology (MIT), Cambridge, USA. Professor Khan has also worked with the Reliance Life Sciences as Research Scientist in the Stem Cell Research Laboratory. Professor Khan has been granted four US patents and published five US patents. Professor Khan has authored two books; namely, *Biotechnology Fundamentals* (textbook) (first edition, 2009; second edition, 2014; third edition, 2020) and *Biotechnology in Medical Science* published by CRC Press, Taylor & Francis Group. He also edited one book, *Application of Nanomaterials in Human Health*, published in 2020 by Springer Nature, Singapore. Professor Khan was Associate Editor of the research journal *3 Biotech* from 2010 to 2020. Professor Khan has been a recognized reviewer in several scientific journals—*Nanomedicine, International Journal of Nanomedicine, Scientific Reports, International Journal Pharmaceutics, Pharmaceutics, IET Nanobiotechnology, Drug Design, Development, and Therapy, Journal of Nanostructure in Chemistry, Aging, Current Pharmaceutical Biotechnology, Tissue Engineering,* and *Nano Express*. Professor Khan is Fellow of Royal Society of Biology (FRSB), UK. He has more than 100 research publications. Professor Khan is currently studying the impact of different biomolecules, biomaterials, and nanomaterials on stem cell differentiation and cancer treatment.

Contributors

Hira Fatima Abbas
Department of Pharmacology
Faculty of Medicine
University of Malaya
Kuala Lumpur 50603, Malaysia

Faizan Ahmad
Department of Medical Elementology
   and Toxicology
Jamia Hamdard University
New Delhi, India

Hilal Ahmad
SRM Institute of Science and Technology
Kattankulathur, Chennai, India

Sultan Akhtar
Department of Biophysics
Institute for Research and Medical
   Consultations (IRMC)
Imam Abdulrahman Bin Faisal
   University (IAU), P.O. Box 1982
Dammam 31441, Saudi Arabia

Syed Ghazanfar Ali
Department of Microbiology
Jawaharlal Nehru Medical College
Aligarh Muslim University
Aligarh, U.P. India

Mohammad Azam Ansari
Epidemic Disease Research Department
Institute for Research & Medical
   Consultations (IRMC)
Imam Abdulrahman Bin Faisal
   University, P.O. Box 1982, 31441
Dammam, Saudi Arabia

Hina Ashraf
Department of Dental Materials
Ayub Medical College
Abbottabad 22040, Pakistan

Muhammad Ali Faridi
Department of Restorative Dental
   Sciences
College of Dental Sciences, College of
   Dentistry
Imam Abdulrahman Bin Faisal
   University
Dammam 31441, Saudi Arabia
Dammam, Saudi Arabia

Meghna Ghosal
Department of biosciences
Jamia Millia islamia
Jamia nagar, Okhla, New Delhi, India

Sundus Iftikhar
Department of Medical Education
Shalamar Medical and Dental
   College
Lahore 54000, Pakistan

B. Rabindran Jermy
Department of Nano-Medicine
   Research
Institute for Research and Medical
   Consultations
Imam Abdulrahman Bin Faisal
   University, P.O. Box 1982, 31441
Dammam/Saudi Arabia

Juweiriya
Department of Chemistry
Aligarh Muslim University
Aligarh, Uttar Pradesh, India

Abdul Samad Khan
Department of Restorative Dental
   Sciences
College of Dentistry
Imam Abdulrahman Bin Faisal
   University
Dammam 31441, Saudi Arabia

Firdos Alam Khan
Department of Stem Cell Research
Institute for Research and Medical
    Consultations (IRMC)
Imam Abdulrahman Bin Faisal
    University, P.O. Box 1982
Dammam, Saudi Arabia

Maria Khan
Dammam, Saudi Arabia

Manisha Lanka
Department of Biochemistry
Andhra University
Visakhapatnam, Andhra Pradesh, India

Tooba Mahboob
Faculty of Pharmaceutical Sciences
UCSI University
Kuala Lumpur Campus, Malaysia

Kamakshi Naik
Department of Microbiology and
    Molecular Biology
ICMR-NITM
Belagavi, Karnataka, India

Muhammad Nawaz
Department of Nano-Medicine Reserach
Institute for Research and Medical
    Consultations (IRMC)
Imam Abdulrahman Bin Faisal
    University, P.O. Box 1982
Dammam 31441, Saudi Arabia

Faiza Qureshi
Deanship of Scientific Research
Imam Abdulrahman Bin Faisal
    University, P.O. Box 1982
Dammam 31441, Saudi Arabia

V. Ravinayagam
Deanship of Scientific Research &
    Department of Nano-Medicine
    Research
Institute for Research and Medical
    Consultations
Imam Abdulrahman Bin Faisal
    University, P.O. Box 1982, 31441
Dammam/Saudi Arabia

Punya Sachdeva
Department of Neurosciences and
    Neuropsychology
Noida, Uttar Pradesh, India

Rashi Sharma
Department of Biotechnology
Delhi Technological University
Bawana, Delhi, India

Gagandeep Singh
Section of Microbiology
Central Ayurveda Research Institute,
    Jhansi
CCRAS Ministry of AYUSH, India
Kusuma School of Biological
    Sciences
India Institute of Technology
Delhi, India

Vidhya Sunil
Department of Life and Environmental
    Sciences
College of Natural and
    Health Sciences
Zayed University
Dubai, United Arab Emirates

1 Materials Types and Classifications— Materials Classification Is Based on the Sizes, Shapes, and Structural Differences

*Syed Ghazanfar Ali, Hilal Ahmad, Haris M Khan,
and Mohammad Azam Ansari*

1.1 INTRODUCTION

The primary domain of materials science is the focus on the relationship between the properties of the material and its microstructure, with the involvement of a combination of physics and chemistry. Solid materials have been classified into different groups, which include metals, ceramics, polymers, and composites. Solid materials (metals, ceramics, polymer, composite, etc.) possess some properties; for example, metals are hard, whereas ceramics are delicate. But when these solid materials are condensed into the nano form, their properties change from the bulk material. The science dealing with materials in the nano range is called nanotechnology, and the material is called nanomaterial or nanoparticle. Nanoparticles are minute particles with a size ranging from 1 to 100 nm, or in other words, a particle whose diameter is smaller than 100 nm is called a nanoparticle. The small size of particles, specifically in the nano range, provides some unique properties to the nanomaterials (Hasan, 2015). Nanomaterials have different properties from their bulk counterpart due to their large surface-to-volume ratio, providing many highly active uncoordinated sites for binding. Nanoparticles are materials wherein their bulk material has at least one dimension less than 100 nm (Laurent et al., 2010).

DOI: 10.1201/9781003317715-1

1.2 CLASSIFICATION OF NANOMATERIALS

1.2.1 CLASSIFICATION BASED ON THE SYNTHESIS

The synthesis of nanoparticles is classified under two categories:

1.2.1.1 Top-Down Synthesis

In top-down synthesis, larger molecules are converted into smaller units, and then these smaller units are further converted into nanoparticles. The top-down route was also used for the synthesis of colloidal carbon spherical particles with a control size (Garrigue et al., 2004). Some of the top-down synthesis methods are as follows.

1.2.1.1.1 Ball Milling

Benjamin et al. developed the process of ball milling in 1960. The ball mill is used by placing the powder and allowing the balls to collide with high energy. Inside the mill, the balls, which are made of tungsten carbide, silicon carbide, or hardened steel, rotate, and the pulling force on the material is provided by the magnet, which is placed outside the container. The presence of the magnet outside the container also increases the milling energy during the rotation of the mill. This kind of approach is also used to synthesize coconut shell nanoparticles (CS-NPs). The milling of CS powder using ceramic balls showed a decrease in particle size with different time intervals (Bello et al., 2015).

1.2.1.1.2 Photolithography

This technique exposes a layer of the radiation-sensitive polymer through a mask using UV light. The mask is an optically flat grass plate that contains the desired pattern. It is the most commonly used technique in an application that requires micron and submicron feature sizes, like electronic, integrated circuits, and micro-fluid devices. This technique can be used to transfer a design or pattern on the surface of the device by simply exposing it to light.

1.2.1.1.3 Dry Etching Technique

Semiconductor wafers are processed through this technique, and plasma or discharge containing etching species are used to immerse the material. Dry etching does not use an aqueous solution; instead, it is carried out in the gaseous phase to remove the material, and therefore, it has been named dry etching. The dry etching reaction takes place at an equal rate irrespective of a particular direction, and therefore, they are isotropic.

1.2.1.2 Bottom-Up Synthesis

This is a reverse approach to top-down synthesis. It is basically a building-up approach where the nanostructures are synthesized onto the substrate by stacking atoms one on top of the other, which results in crystal planes, and the stacking of crystal planes results in the synthesis of nanostructures. Bottom-up synthesis includes the following:

1.2.1.2.1 Hydrothermal Synthesis

Autoclaves are used for the hydrothermal route of synthesis in which the reaction takes place in water. The temperature inside the autoclave is increased above the boiling point of water until the pressure of the vapors is saturated. The hydrothermal route is most widely used for the synthesis of TiO_2 nanoparticles, which are obtained along with titanium precursor with water. The hydrothermal route is used to control the size and particle morphology by regulating the reaction temperature and pressure and by changing the solution composition.

1.2.1.2.2 Solvothermal Method

Hydrothermal and solvothermal methods of synthesis of nanoparticles are very much similar except for the difference in the solvent. In the solvothermal route, the solvent used is other than water. The solvothermal method is slightly advantageous since it has better control over size and shape, specifically with the organic solvents with a high boiling point.

1.2.1.2.3 Chemical Vapor Deposition (CVD) Method

In this method of nanoparticle synthesis, a substrate is used, which is then exposed to the volatile precursors. One or more volatile precursors could be used. The CVD method is mostly applied in industries where the deposition of thin films of different materials is required. The vaporized precursors are then introduced into the CVD reactor and are further allowed to be adsorbed onto a substance at an elevated temperature. The molecules that get adsorbed onto the surface react with the other molecules and produce the crystals.

1.2.1.2.4 Physical Vapor Deposition (PVD)

In this method, the material is evaporated to the vapor phase and then from the vapor phase back to the condensed state in the form of a thin film. PVD is mostly used at the industrial-scale level, where combining different methods to produce a coating with superior properties is required. This technique is quite useful for the fabrication of layers with desired microstructure and properties, as in the case of nanoscience.

1.2.1.2.5 Sol-Gel Method

This method involves the conversion of a solution, which is called a sol, into a gel-like system. The combination of the two is called sol-gel and is a biphasic system; that is, it has both the solid and liquid phases, which can range from discrete small particles to a large polymeric network. This method is mostly applied in the case of metal oxides, and the advantage of using the sol-gel method of synthesis of nanoparticles is that it has a greater yield, and the chemical composition of the product can also be easily controlled. Lastly, it is a cheap method.

1.2.1.2.6 Radio Frequency (RF) Plasma Method

In this method, RF heating coils are used, which generate plasma upon heating. The metal is initially placed in an evacuated chamber, and the RF heating coils, wrapped around the evacuated chamber, start heating. The heat provided by the RF coils is above the evaporation point of the metal. Helium gas is then passed into the system, and this gas forms the high-temperature plasma surrounding the coils. Further, the helium gas gets nucleated with the metal vapors, which get diffused to a cold collector rod. The nanoparticles are collected, which are then passivated by oxygen gas.

1.2.1.3 Green Synthesis

Green synthesis of nanoparticles, as the name indicates, involves plants, parts of plants, or microorganisms. The phytoconstituents in the plants act as a reducer and stabilizers. In the case of microorganisms, protein molecules act as reducers as well as stabilizers. The metal or metal oxide salts get reduced to the nano form by the phytoconstituents in the plants or by the protein from microorganisms. Examples: pods of *Butea monosperma* and leaves of *Crinum latifolium* for the synthesis of zinc oxide nanoparticles (Ali et al., 2021; Jalal, Ansari, Ali et al., 2018), bark of *Crataeva nurvala* (Buch.-Ham.), *Holarrhena pubescens*, and supernatant of *Candida glabrata* for the synthesis of silver nanoparticles (Ali et al., 2017, 2018; Jalal, Ansari, Alzohairy et al., 2018), and stem of *Tinospora cordifolia* for gold nanoparticles (Ali et al., 2020).

1.2.2 CLASSIFICATION BASED ON THE SIZES

Smaller-sized nanoparticles possess greater antimicrobial activity than larger-sized particles. Besides being antimicrobial in nature, there are other functions of nanoparticles that are dependent on the size of nanoparticles. Nanomaterials, due to their passive, active, and physical targeting properties, have shown a stimulating effect in biomedical detection. The size of nanoparticles, among all the properties of nanoparticles, is the main feature that affects tumor imaging; the small size of nanoparticles greatly enhance permeability and retention effects in tumors, which finally helps in providing a better view of contrast imaging in tumors (Oh et al., 2013). Nanoparticles have been used for the early detection and diagnosis of tumors since nanoparticles have a long circulation life in the blood and a good targeting mechanism (Bakhtiary et al., 2016). Mostly, the gold nanoparticles, which can range from 1 to 100 m, are used for the purpose of tumor detection, as they have a high fluorescence quenching efficiency (Meledandri et al., 2011; Sardar et al., 2011; Mesbahi et al., 2013).

When the function of nanoparticles is as a carrier of drugs then smaller-sized nanoparticles are preferred since, after loading the drug, the overall diameter would be enough to circulate through the blood. Iron nanoparticles of size 5 nm have good biocompatibility with breast and brain cancer cells and, therefore, can be used as a drug carrier (Ankamwar, 2012). Studies have shown that 75 nm AgNPs significantly inhibited Pgp efflux activity in drug-resistant breast cancer cells. It was also found that 75 nm AgNPs depleted endoplasmic reticulum calcium stores (Gopisetty et al., 2019).

Not only does the size of nanoparticles helpful in tumor detection, penetration, and drug carrier capability, but it significantly affects the blood circulation half-life and cellular uptake (Hoshyar et al., 2016). Since size is a key factor for determining the overall activity of nanoparticles, it has also been shown in the literature that nanoparticles with sizes ranging from 10 to 60 nm have enhanced cellular uptake (Hoshyar et al., 2016; Huang et al., 2012). As it is evident from the literature that the average renal filtration pore is 10 nm (Scott and Quaggin, 2015), therefore, the nanoparticles with less than 10 nm can be rapidly cleared by the renal excretory system (Longmire et al., 2008). Macrophages identify the nanoparticles whose size is more than 100 nm and accumulate in organs with the mononuclear phagocyte system (MPS) viz. lymph nodes, liver, spleen, and lungs (Zhou and Dai, 2018).

1.2.3 CLASSIFICATION BASED ON THE SHAPES

Nanoparticles are of different shapes, including spherical, triangular, cubic, hexagonal, oval, rod, helical, or prism-shaped (Gatoo et al., 2014). Studies have shown that the shape of nanoparticles affects the efficacy of nanoparticles. Different workers have interpreted their results in different ways considering different shapes, such as that triangular silver nanoparticles have shown better antibacterial efficacy than spherical and rod-shaped (Pal et al., 2007). Another study showed that sharp-edged and vertex triangular silver nanoprism showed better antiseptic properties than spherical ones (Dong et al., 2012). We are of the opinion that most of the nanoparticles, such as silver and zinc, possess antimicrobial properties, although the number of nanoparticles used for antimicrobial purposes may vary. The other application of nanoparticles is drug delivery, and workers have shown that drug delivery is dependent upon the shape of nanoparticles. Firstly, rod-shaped nanoparticles are better for drug delivery when compared with spherical nanoparticles since rod-shaped nanoparticles possess greater retention time inside the cells than spherical nanoparticles (Hao et al., 2012; Zhang et al., 2008). Secondly, rod-shaped nanoparticles that are less than 40 nm in width can pass through the nuclear envelope via the nuclear pore; therefore, they can carry a greater amount of drug (Hinde et al., 2017; Salem et al., 2003; Fan et al., 2014). Rod-shaped nanoparticles, after 1 hour of incubation, lead to the transformation of the plasma membrane to encapsulate the rods, but spherical nanoparticles are unable to do so (Han et al., 2012).

1.2.3.1 Classification of Nanomaterials Based on Size/Dimensions

Depending upon the shape or dimension, nanomaterials can be classified as 0D, 1D, 2D, or 3D (Tiwari et al., 2012).

1.2.3.1.1 *Zero-Dimensional (0D)*

When all the dimensions of the material are within the nano range, then it is considered a no-dimension or zero-dimensional material; sometimes, it is referred to as a quasi-zero-dimensional nanomaterial. These types of nanomaterials are very common. When analyzed, these particles seem to be point-like structures; for example, quantum dots, hollow spheres, and nanolenses (Jeevanandam et al., 2018).

1.2.3.1.2 *One-Dimensional (1D)*

When at least one dimension of the material is out of the nanoscale range and the rest are other dimensions within the nano range, then it is considered as one-dimensional or 1D; for example, nanotubes, nanorods, and nanofibers (Jeevanandam et al., 2018).

1.2.3.1.3 *Two-Dimensional (2D)*

When two dimensions of the material are larger than the nano range, then it is considered a 2D nanomaterial; for example, nanofilms and nanolayers. The plate-like structure is formed by these nanomaterial structures (Jeevanandam et al., 2018).

1.2.3.1.4 *Three-Dimensional (3D)*

When all three dimensions of the material are larger than 100 nm but component-wise are below 100 nm, they are referred to as three-dimensional or 3D. They are usually nonporous; for example, nanocomposites and nanofibers (Jeevanandam et al., 2018).

The particle size is the most important criterion for the nanoparticles to show their effect. The particle size also affects drug release and drug target. The surface morphology of nanoparticles may be amorphous or crystalline. The smaller the size of the nanoparticles, the greater the surface area covered. Therefore, smaller-sized nanoparticles, due to the large surface area, will load more drugs and will expose the particle's surface, leading to a fast drug release. The size of nanoparticles can be measured using scanning electron microscopy (SEM), transmission electron microscopy (TEM), dynamic light scattering (DLS), X-ray diffraction (XRD), or photon correlation spectroscopy (PCS). PCS measures the size of the nanoparticles based on DLS (DeAssis et al., 2008).

1.2.3.2 Classification of Nanomaterials Based on Shape and Materials

1.2.3.2.1 Carbon Family

The carbon family is of great interest to new technologies and modern challenges (Mauter and Eilmelech, 2008; Chen et al., 2020). The carbon-based family consists of mainly carbon nanotubes, fullerenes, graphene, and so on (Figure 1.1).

1.2.3.2.2 Fullerenes

Fullerenes were discovered in 1985. The carbon atoms in the case of fullerenes are specific, which are different from other allotropes. Fullerenes were the first

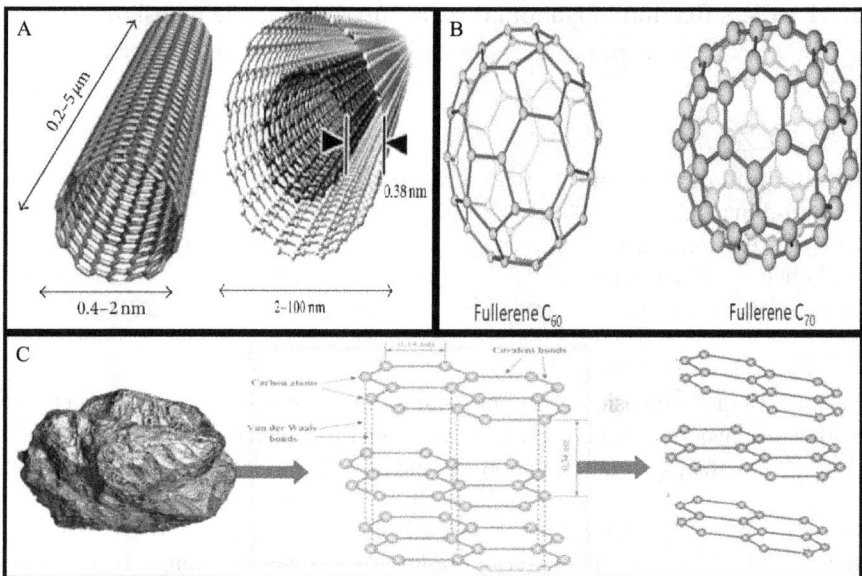

FIGURE 1.1 Image of (A) carbon nanotubes, SWCNT, and MWCNT; (B) fullerenes; and (C) graphene from graphite.

Source: (A) He et al., 2013; (B) Lim et al., 2021; and (C) Tiwari et al., 2020.

symmetric materials that opened a new perspective in the field of nanomaterials. The different sizes of fullerenes may be because of the different numbers of carbon atoms C60, C70, C72, C76, C84, and C100 (Mendes et al., 2013). The hollow structure of fullerene C60 has 12 pentagons and 20 hexagons, which are sp^2 hybridized. Due to its small size, spherical shape, and isotropic nature, it is considered an ideal zero-dimensional material (Fan et al., 2020). Fullerenes paved the way for the discovery of carbon nanotubes and graphene (Goodarzi et al., 2017). They have helped to develop an interest in nanocomposites due to the commercial applications of nanocomposites, such as fillers (Saeed and Khan, 2014, 2016) and gas absorbents as an approach for environmental remediation (Ngoy et al., 2014). The slightly soluble nature of fullerenes in different solvents makes them unique from other allotropes of carbon (Beck and Mandi, 1997).

1.2.3.2.3 Carbon Nanotubes

Carbon nanotubes were discovered by Iijima (1991). Carbon nanotubes are not only single-walled; they can be double- or multi-walled. The carbon in carbon nanotubes is sp^2 hybridized and arranged in hexagons (Zaporotskova et al., 2016). A one-atom-thick graphitic layer is present in single-walled carbon nanotubes, and the carbon atoms are connected through a strong covalent bond (Li, Hou et al., 2019). In double-walled carbon nanotubes, one single-walled carbon nanotube covers the other single-walled carbon nanotube, which makes it double-walled (Shen et al., 2011). Similarly, when multiple sheets of single-layered carbon atoms get rolled into one another, they are denoted as multi-walled carbon nanotubes. Therefore, one or more than one concentric carbon shell may be present in nanotubes.

1.2.3.2.4 Graphene

Graphene has emerged as an important material in the last couple of years. Graphene is very thin but possesses great mechanical strength (Geim AK, 2009). This property of graphene makes it very impressive since a thin material with high mechanical strength is required in many places (e.g., light panes and touch screens). Graphene possesses a honeycomb-like lattice with two-dimensional sp^2 hybridized carbon atom planar sheets that are tightly packed (Geim and Novoselov, 2007). Graphene and its derivatives are widely used in electrochemical sensors (Li, Xia et al., 2019). Due to the flat nature of graphene, each carbon becomes available; and due to the low diffusion resistance, the ion can easily access the surface, and this property makes it highly electrochemical (Lv et al., 2016). Graphene possesses higher sensitivity than carbon nanotubes and silicon nanowires (He et al., 2012). Since graphene is formed from graphite, therefore, it has some advantages; firstly, the main advantage is it is cost-effective, and secondly, it does not contain any metallic impurities present in carbon nanotubes, which makes graphene more valuable than other carbon-based materials. The pi-pi stacking interactions with the biomolecules and biocompatibility are another advantage during the development of biosensors and sensors (He et al., 2012).

1.2.3.2.5 Metals

This group is composed of mainly metallic elements, including Fe, Cu, and Au. They also have traces of nonmetallic elements mixed. Metals have non-localized electrons, which are not bound to any particular atoms. Metal nanoparticles have gained much importance nowadays due to their applications in different fields, including medicine, physics, and chemistry. The unique properties of nanoparticles are due to their small size (1–100 nm). Metal nanoparticles possess good thermal stability, optical properties, high mechanical strength, and high electrical properties (Khoshnevisan et al., 2019; Yaqoob et al., 2020). There are three categories of metal nanoparticles; the first category includes the pure form of metal only (e.g., Ag, Au, and Cu). The second type of nanoparticles includes metal oxide nanoparticles, such TiO_2 and ZnO_2. The third category comprises dope metal or metal oxide nanoparticles (Dar et al., 2011; Umar et al., 2013). Nanoparticles are of different shapes, as shown in Figure 1.2. Pabari (2022), through a theoretical model, showed that different properties, such as melting temperature, cohesive energy, and Debye temperature, are affected by changing the particle size and shape of different nano solids. A good texture at the surface, a greater number of binding sites, and a large surface are key characteristics of metals and metal oxides at the nanoscale level; this also favors the thermodynamics and kinetics of transportations required for heterogeneous reactions (Maduraiveeran et al., 2019). Scientists are focusing nowadays on the next generation of artificial enzyme production and the development of clean and renewable energy sources from metal and metal oxides. Hydrothermal route, solvothermal, sol-gel,

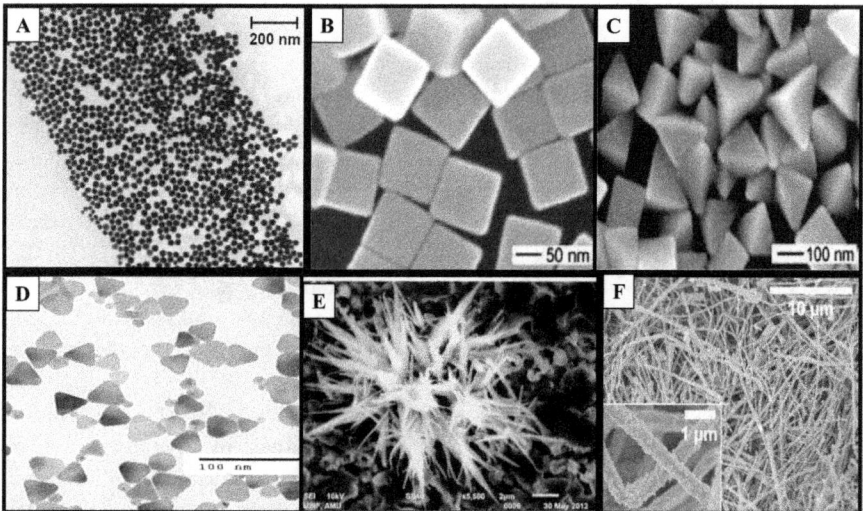

FIGURE 1.2   Different shapes of nanoparticles: (A) spherical shape, (B) cube shape, (C) pyramid shape, (D) prism shape, (E) flower shape, and (F) nanowires.

Source: (A) Maharaj and Bhushan, 2012; (B and C) Wiley et al., 2006; (D) Haber and Sokolov, 2017; (E) Khan et al., 2014; and (F) Maji and Chakraborty, 2019.

and green synthesis are some of the methods of synthesis of metal and metal oxide nanoparticles (Chen and Holt-Hindle, 2010).

1.2.3.2.6   Ceramic

Ceramics are those compounds that are neither metal nor nonmetal completely; instead, they are counted between metal and nonmetals. Ceramics are composed of mainly calcium phosphates, silica, alumina, zirconium, iron oxides, carbonates, and titanium dioxide, and due to their positive interaction, they are used with human tissues. For example, dentists typically use calcium phosphate and calcium hydroxide–based material for the filling, and alloys from metal-ceramic are used for crown formation (Whitters et al., 1999). Ceramics are also applied for different joints in bones and plastic surgery. The high mechanical strength with low biodegradability makes the ceramic material unique; it has a good body response also (Block and Thorn, 2000; Gladstone et al., 1995). The nanoparticles formed from inorganic compounds, such as silica, titania, and alumina, are called ceramic nanoparticles (Rawat et al., 2008). Proteins, enzymes, and drugs, which get entrapped due to these nanoparticles get protection from the denaturing effect of external pH and temperature since these nanoparticles do not involve any swelling or change in porosity due to the change in pH (Singh et al., 2013).

1.2.3.2.7   Semiconductors

Semiconductors are those materials that have electrical conductivity between a conductor and an insulator. There are two bands in the semiconductors; the one is valence band, which is completely filled with electrons, and the other one is the conduction band, which is empty in the ground state. The two bands are separated from each other by a gap, and the gap is called a band gap. Nowadays, researchers are developing an interest in the preparation of materials that have dimension/dimensions in the semiconductor nanocrystalline range (Henglein A, 1989; Steigerwald and Brus, 1990; Bawendi et al., 1990). The major reason behind the extensive research on the development of semiconductor nanoparticles may be the need for optical and electronic devices of miniature size (Stroscio and Eigler, 1991; Alivisatos AP, 1996). Extensive research on semiconductor nanomaterials is going on since they have shown promising applications in the field of solar cells, electronic devices, light emitting diodes, chemical and biosensors, packaging film, superabsorbent, parts of automobiles, and more. With the further advancement of nanotechnology, a significant change in the semiconductor industry would take place. High chemical and photobleaching stability, surface functionality with narrow and intensive emission spectra, and continuous absorption bands are some other properties that have attracted the researchers. In semiconductor materials, the spatial quantum confinement effect results in a change in optical properties. High surface-to-volume ratio also possesses some effect on optical properties. The H_2 production through photocatalysis shows an alternative for a sustainable energy system that can reduce the production of greenhouse gases causing global warming.

1.2.3.2.8   Polymer

A polymer is a combination of many smaller subunits that combine to form a macromolecule. Polymeric nanoparticles are organic-based nanoparticles that have

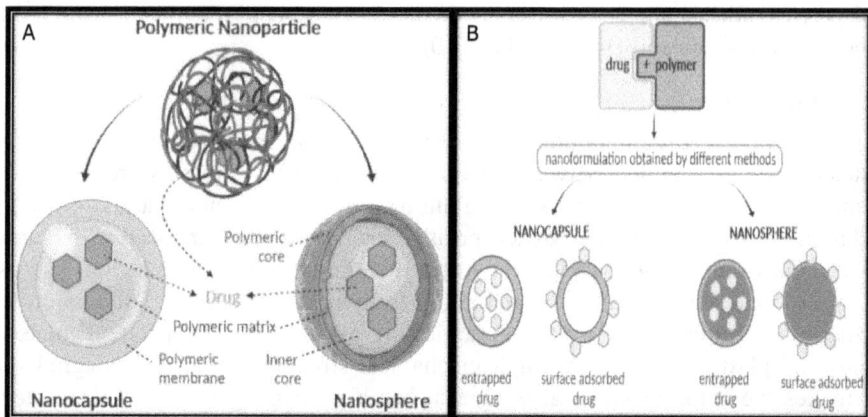

FIGURE 1.3 (A) Representation of a nanocapsule and nanosphere as carriers of drugs/bioactive compounds, and (B) a drug combined with a polymer.

Source: Zielinska et al., 2020.

natural or synthetic polymers. The polymeric nanoparticles can be nanospheres or nanocapsule-shaped (Mansha et al., 2017) (Figure 1.3). The nanosphere is spherical, with an overall solid mass, and on its surface, other molecules get adsorbed, whereas in the case of a nanocapsule, the solid mass gets encapsulated with the particle (Rao and Geckeler, 2011). Polymeric nanoparticles are mostly used as a carrier and are advantageous over other liposomes, micelles, and inorganic nanosystems. They have also scaled up themselves under good manufacturing practices (Van Vlerken et al., 2007). The availability of different types of polymers and the stability of polymeric nanoparticles in different biological fluids are some of the advantages of polymers. The polymeric nanoparticles have made their surface functionalize and have modulated the polymer degradation and the leakage of entrapped compounds, which is a function of specific stimuli (Venkatraman et al., 2010; Goodall et al., 2015; Sarcan et al., 2018). The functionalized nature of polymeric nanoparticles finds many applications; for example, the nanoporous polymers, which are superhydrophobic in nature, can be used as an organic contaminant and finds application in volatile organic compounds also (Zhang et al., 2009); the porous network in nanoporous polymers finds the way as good catalyst support. When fullerenes are combined with polymers, they act as good flame retardants (Pan et al., 2020).

1.3 CONCLUSION

Materials, when condensed to their nanoform, develop unique properties. The large surface area of nanomaterials allows greater material to attach to them. Since the nanomaterials are smaller in size (nano range), they can be used as a transporting agent. The drugs can be easily loaded on the nanoparticles and can be transported to the location where bulk material cannot reach. Some nanoparticles, like silver nanoparticles, possess good antibacterial activity and can be used against pathogenic microorganisms. The low biodegradation property of ceramic nanoparticles finds their application in protection against degradation. Similarly, the presence of a porous network in nanoporous polymers allows it to act as a good catalyst. Semiconductor nanomaterials are useful in nanoelectronics, solar cells, and so on. The high mechanical strength and rapid charge transfer properties of carbon nanotubes and graphene from the carbon family have attracted many workers to develop new materials composed of CNTs and graphene. Finally, it is concluded that size is an important factor in the classification of materials, and when material size is reduced to the nano range, then it becomes more functional compared with bulk material.

REFERENCES

Ali SG, Ansari MA, Alzohairy MA, Alomary MN, AlYahya S, Jalal M, Khan HM, Asiri SMM, Ahmad W, Mahdi AA, El-Sherbeeny AM, El-Meligy MA (2020). Biogenic gold nanoparticles as potent antibacterial and antibiofilm nano-antibiotics against *Pseudomonas aeruginosa*. *Antibiotics*. 9, 100.

Ali SG, Ansari MA, Jamal QMS, Almatroudi A, Alzohairy MA, Alomary MN, Rehman S et al. (2021). Butea monosperma seed extract mediated biosynthesis of ZnO NPs and their antibacterial, antibiofilm and anti-quorum sensing potentialities. *Arab. J. Chem.* 14(4), e103044.

Ali SG, Ansari MA, Khan HM, Jalal M, Mahdi AA, Cameotra SS (2017). *Crataeva nurvala* nanoparticles inhibit virulence factors and biofilm formation in clinical isolates of *pseudomonas aeruginosa*. *J. Basic Microbiol*. 57(3), 193–203.

Ali SG, Ansari MA, Khan HM, Jalal M, Mahdi AA, Cameotra SS (2018). Antibacterial and antibiofilm potential of green synthesized silver nanoparticles against imipenem resistant clinical isolates of *P. aeruginosa*. *Bionanoscience*. 8(2), 544–553.

Alivisatos AP (1996). Perspectives on the physical chemistry of semiconductor nanocrystals. *J. Phys. Chem*. 100, 13226–13239.

Ankamwar B (2012). Size and shape effect on biomedical applications of nanomaterials. In *Biomedical Engineering-Technical Applications in Medicine*; IntechOpen: London, pp. 93–114.

Bakhtiary Z, Saei AA, Hajipour MJ, Raoufi M, Vermesh O, Mahmoudi M (2016). Targeted superparamagnetic iron oxide nanoparticles for early detection of cancer: Possibilities and challenges. *Nanomedicine*. 12, 287–307.

Bawendi MG, Steigerwald ML, Brus LE (1990). The quantum-mechanics of larger semiconductor clusters (quantum dots)'. *Annu. Rev. Phy. Chem*. 41, 477–496.

Beck MT, Mandi G (1997). Solubility of C_{60}. *Fullerene Sci. Technol*. 5, 291–310.

Bello SA, Agunsoye JO, Hassan SB (2015). Synthesis of coconut shell nanoparticles via a top down approach: Assessment of milling duration on the particle sizes and morphologies of coconut shell nanoparticles. *Mater. Lett*. 159, 514–519.

Block JE, Thorn MR (2000). Clinical indications of calcium-phosphate biomaterials and related composites for orthopedic procedures. *Calcified Tissue Int*. 66, 234–238.

Chen A, Holt-Hindle P (2010). Platinum-based nanostructured materials: Synthesis, properties and applications. *Chem. Rev*. 110(6), 3767–3804.

Chen L, Zhao S, Hasi Q, Luo X, Zhang H, Li H, Li A (2020). Porous carbon nanofoam derived from pitch as solar receiver for efficient solar steam generation. *Global Chall*. 4, 1900098.

Dar AA, Umar K, Mir NA, Haque MM, Muneer M, Boxall C (2011). Photocatalysed degradation of herbicide derivative, Dinoterb, in aqueous suspension. *Res. Chem. Intermed*. 37, 567–578.

DeAssis DN, Mosqueira VC, Vilela JM, Andrade MS, Cardoso VN (2008). Release profiles and morphological characterization by atomic force microscopy and photon correlation spectroscopy of 99m Technetium—fluconazole nanocapsules. *Int. J. Pharm.* 349, 152–160.

Dong PV, Ha CH, Binh LT, Kasbohm J (2012). Chemical synthesis and antibacterial activity of novel-shaped silver nanoparticles. *Int. Nano Lett.* 2, 1–9.

Fan MM, Zhan WZ, Cheng C, Liu Y, Li BJ, Sun X, Zhang S (2014). Evaluation of rod-shaped nanoparticles as carriers for gene delivery. *Part. Part. Syst. Charact.* 31, 994–1000.

Fan X, Soin N, Li H, Li H, Xia X, Geng J (2020). Fullerene (C60) nanowires: The preparation, characterization, and potential applications. *Energy Environ. Matter.* 3, 469–491.

Garrigue P, Delville MH, Labrugere C, Cloutet E, Kulesza PJ, Morand JP, Kuhn A (2004). Top down approach for the preparation of colloidal carbon nanoparticles. *Chem. Mater.* 16, 2984–2986.

Gatoo MA, Naseem S, Arfat MY, Mahmood Dar A, Qasim K, Zubair S (2014). Physicochemical properties of nanomaterials: Implication in associated toxic manifestations. *Biomed Res. Int.* 1–8.

Geim AK (2009). Graphene: Status and prospects. *Science.* 324, 1530–1534.

Geim AK, Novoselov KS (2007). The rise of graphene. *Nat. Mater.* 6, 183–191.

Gladstone HB, Mc Dermott MW, Cooke DD (1995). Implants for cranioplasty, otolaryngol. *Clin. North Am.* 28, 381–400.

Goodall S, Jones ML, Mahler S (2015). Monoclonal antibody-targeted polymeric nanoparticles for cancer therapy-future prospects. *J. Chem. Technol. Biotechnol.* 90, 1169–1176.

Goodarzi S, Da Ros T, Conde J, Sefat F, Mozafari M (2017). Fullerene: Biomedical engineers get to revisit an old friend. *Mater. Today.* 20, 460–480.

Gopisetty K, Kovács D, Igaz N, Rónavári A, Bélteky P, Rázga Z, Venglovecz V, Csoboz B, Boros IM, Kónya Z et al. (2019). Endoplasmic reticulum stress: Major player in size-dependent inhibition of P-glycoprotein by silver nanoparticles in multidrug-resistant breast cancer cells. *J. Nanobiotechnol.* 17, 9.

Haber J, Sokolov K (2017). Synthesis of stable citrate-capped silver nanoprisms. *Langmuir.* 33, 10525–10530.

Han Y, Wang X, Dai H, Li S (2012). Nanosize and surface charge effects of hydroxyapatite nanoparticles on red blood cell suspensions. *ACS Appl. Mater. Interfaces.* 4, 4616–4622.

Hao N, Li L, Zhang Q, Huang X, Meng X, Zhang Y, Chen D, Tang F, Li L (2012). The shape effect of PEGylated mesoporous silica nanoparticles on cellular uptake pathway in Hela cells. *Microporous Mesoporous Mater.* 162, 14–23.

Hasan S (2015). A review on nanoparticles: Their synthesis and types. *Res. J. Recent Sci.* 4, 9–11.

He H, Pham-Huy LA, Dramou P, Xiao D, Zuo P, Pham-Huy C (2013). Carbon nanotubes: Applications in pharmacy and medicine. *Biomed Res. Int.* 578290. Doi:10.1155/2013/578290.

He Q, Wu S, Yin Z, Zhan H (2012). Graphene-based electronic sensors. *Chem. Sci.* 3, 1764–1772.

Henglein A (1989). Small-particle research: Physicochemical properties of extremely small colloidal metal and semiconductor particles. *Chem. Rev.* 89(8), 1861–1873.

Hinde E, Thammasiraphop K, Duong HT, Yeow J, Karagoz B, Boyer C, Gooding JJ, Gaus K (2017). Pair correlation microscopy reveals the role of nanoparticle shape in intracellular transport and site of drug release. *Nat. Nanotechnol.* 12, 81–89.

Hoshyar N, Gray S, Han H, Bao G (2016). The effect of nanoparticle size on in vivo pharmacokinetics and cellular interaction. *Nanomedicine (Lond).* 11, 673–692.

Huang Y, He S, Cao W, Cai K, Liang X-J (2012). Biomedical nanomaterials for imaging-guided cancer therapy. *Nanoscale.* 4, 6135–6149.

Iijima S (1991). Helical microtubules of graphitic carbon. *Nature,* 354, 6–58.

Jalal M, Ansari MA, Ali SG, Khan HM, Rehman S (2018). Anticandidal activity of bioinspired ZnO NPs: Effect on growth, cell morphology and key virulence attributes of Candida species. *Artif Cells Nanomed Biotechnol.* 46(sup1), 912–925.

Jalal M, Ansari MA, Alzohairy MA, Ali SG, Khan HM, Almatroudi A, Raees K (2018). Biosynthesis of silver nanoparticles from Oropharyngeal Candida glabrata isolates and their antimicrobial activity against clinical strains of bacteria and fungi. *Nanomaterials.* 8, 586.

Jeevanandam J, Barhoum A, Chan YS, Dufresne A, Danquah MK (2018). Review on nanoparticles and nanostructured materials: History, sources, toxicity and regulations. *Beilstein J. Nanotechnol.* 9, 1050–1074.

Khan MF, Hameedullah M, Ansari AH, Ahmad E, Lohani M, Khan RH, Alam MM, Khan W, Husain FM, Ahmad I (2014). Flower-shaped ZnO nanoparticles synthesized by a novel approach at near-room temperatures with antibacterial and antifungal properties. *Int. J. Nanomed.* 9, 853–864.

Khoshnevisan K, Maleki H, Honarvarfard E, Baharifar H, Gholami M, Faridbod F, Larijani B, Majidi RF, Khorramizadeh MR (2019). Nanomaterial based electrochemical sensing of the biomarker serotonin: A comprehensive review. *Microchimica Acta.* 186, 49–61.

Laurent S, Forge D, Port M, Roch A, Robic C, Vander Elst L, Muller RN (2010). Magnetic iron oxide nanoparticles: Synthesis, stabilization, vectorization, physicochemical characterizations, and biological applications. *Chem. Rev.* 110, 2574–2574. http://dx.doi.org/10.1021/cr900197g.

Li G, Xia Y, Tian Y, Wu Y, Liu J, He Q, Chen D (2019). Recent developments on graphene-based electrochemical sensors toward nitrite. *J. Electrochem. Soc.* 166, B881–B895.

Li X-Q, Hou P-X, Liu C, Cheng H-M (2019). Preparation of metallic single-wall carbon nanotubes. *Carbon.* 147, 187–198.

Lim JV, Bee ST, Tin Sin L, Ratnam CT, Abdul Hamid ZA (2021). A review on the synthesis, properties, and utilities of functionalized carbon nanoparticles for polymer nanocomposites. *Polymers.* 13, 3547.

Longmire M, Choyke PL, Kobayashi H (2008). Clearance properties of nano-sized particles and molecules as imaging agents: Considerations and caveats. *Nanomedicine (Lond).* 3, 703–717.

Lv W, Li Z, Deng Y, Yang Q-H, Kang F (2016). Graphene-based materials for electrochemical energy storage devices: Opportunities and challenges. *Energy Storage Mater.* 2, 107–138.

Maduraiveeran G, Sasidharan M, Jin W (2019). Earth-abundant transition metal and metal oxide nanomaterials: Synthesis and electrochemical applications. *Prog. Mater. Sci.* 106, 100574. https://doi.org/10.1016/j.pmatsci.2019.100574.

Maharaj D, Bhushan B (2012). Effect of spherical Au nanoparticles on nanofriction and wear reduction in dry and liquid environments. *Beilstein J. Nanotechnol.* 3, 759–772.

Maji CN, Chakraborty J (2019). Gram scale green synthesis of copper nanowire powder for nanofluid applications. *ACS Sustain. Chem. Eng.* 7(14), 12376–12388.

Mansha M, Khan I, Ullah N, Qurashi A (2017). Synthesis, characterization and visible-light-driven photoelectrochemical hydrogen evolution reaction of carbazole-containing conjugated polymers. *Int. J. Hydrog. Energy.* 42(16), 10952–10961.

Mauter MS, Eilmelech M (2008). Environmental applications of carbon based nanomaterials. *Environ. Sci. Technol.* 42(16), 5843–5859.

Meledandri CJ, Stolarczyk JK, Brougham DF (2011). Hierarchical gold-decorated magnetic nanoparticle clusters with controlled size. *ACS Nano.* 5, 1747–1755.

Mendes RG, Bachmatiuk A, Buchner B, Cuniberti G, Rummeli MH (2013). Carbon nanostructures as multi-functional drug delivery platforms. *J. Mater. Chem.* 1, 401–428.

Mesbahi A, Jamali F, Garehaghaji N (2013). Effect of photon beam energy, gold nanoparticle size and concentration on the dose enhancement in radiation therapy. *Bioimpacts.* 3(1), 29–35.

Ngoy JM, Wagner N, Riboldi L, Bolland O (2014). A CO2 capture technology using multi-walled carbon nanotubes with polyaspartamide surfactant. *Energy Procedia.* 63, 2230–2248.

Oh IH, Min HS, Li L, Tran TH, Lee YK, Kwon IC, Choi K, Kim K, Huh KM (2013). Cancer cell-specific photoactivity of pheophorbide a-glycol chitosan nanoparticles for photodynamic therapy in tumor-bearing mice. *Biomaterials.* 34, 6454–6463.

Pabari C (2022). Size dependent properties of metallic nanoparticles. *Mater. Today Proc.* 55, 98–101.

Pal S, Tak YK, Song JM (2007). Does the antibacterial activity of silver nanoparticles depend on the shape of the nanoparticle? A study of the gram-negative bacterium *Escherichia coli. Appl. Environ. Microbiol.* 73, 1712–1720.

Pan Y, Guo Z, Ran S, Fang Z (2020). Influence of fullerenes on the thermal and flame-retardant properties of polymeric materials. *J. Appl. Polym. Sci.* 137, 47538.

Rao JP, Geckeler KE (2011). Polymer nanoparticles: Preparation technique and size-control parameters. *Prog. Polym. Sci.* 36(7), 887–913.

Rawat M, Singh D, Saraf S, Saraf S (2008). Development and in vitro evaluation of alginate gel-encapsulated, chitosan-coated ceramic nanocores for oral delivery of enzyme. *Drug Dev Ind Pharm.* 34, 181–188.

Saeed K, Khan I (2014). Preparation and properties of single-walled carbon nanotubes/poly (butylenes terephthalate) nanocomposites. *Iran. Polym. J.* 23, 53–58.

Saeed K, Khan I (2016). Preparation and characterization of single walled carbon nanotubes/nylon 6,6 nanocomposites. *Instrum. Sci. Technol.* 44, 435–444.

Salem AK, Searson PC, Leong KW (2003). Multifunctional nanorods for gene delivery. *Nat. Mater.* 2, 668–671.

Sarcan ET, Silindir-Gunav M, Ozer AY (2018). Theranostic polymeric nanoparticles for NIR imaging and photodynamic therapy. *Int. J. Phar.* 551, 329–338.

Sardar R, Shumaker-Parry JS (2011). Spectroscopic and microscopic investigation of gold nanoparticle formation: Ligand and temperature effects on rate and particle size. *J Am. Chem. Soc.* 133, 8179–8190.

Scott RP, Quaggin SE (2015). Review series: The cell biology of renal filtration. *J. Cell Biol.* 209, 199–210.

Shen C, Brozena AH, Wang Y (2011). Double—walled carbon nanotubes: Challenges and opportunities. *Nanoscale.* 3, 503–518.

Singh D, Dubey P, Pradhan M, Rawat M (2013). Ceramic nanocarriers: Versatile nanosystem for protein and peptide delivery. *Expert Opin Drug Deliv.* 10, 241–259.

Steigerwald ML, Brus LE (1990). Semiconductor crystallites: A class of large molecules. *Acc. Chem. Res.* 23(6), 183–188.

Stroscio JA, Eigler DM (1991). Atomic and molecular manipulation with the scanning tunneling microscope. *Science.* 254, 1319–1326.

Tiwari JN, Tiwari RN, Kim KS (2012). Zero-dimensional, one dimensional, two-dimensional and three-dimensional nanostructured materials for advanced electrochemical energy devices. *Prog. Mater Sci.* 57, 724–803. http://dx.doi.org/10.1016/j. pmatsci.2011.08.003.

Tiwari SK, Sahoo S, Wang N, Huczko A (2020). Graphene research and their outputs: Status and prospects. *J. Sci. Adv. Mater. Dev.* 5, 10–29.

Umar K, Haque MM, Mir NA, Muneer M, Farooqi IH (2013). Titanium dioxide-mediated photocatalysed mineralization of two selected organic pollutants in aqueous suspensions. *J. Adv. Oxid. Technol.* 16, 252–260.

Van Vlerken LE, Vyas TK, Amiji MM (2007). Poly(ethylene glycol)-modified nanocarriers for tumor-targeted and intracellular delivery. *Pharm. Res.* 24, 1405–1414.

Venkatraman SS, Ma LL, Natarajan JV, Chattopadhyay S (2010). Polymer-and liposome-based nanoparticles in targeted drug delivery. *Front. Biosci. (Schol Ed).* 2, 801–814.

Whitters CJ, Strang R, Brown D, Clarke RL, Curtis RV, Hatton PV, Ireland AJ, Lloyd CH, McCabe JF, Nicholson JW, Scrimgeous SN, Setcos JC, Sherriff M, Noort RV, Watts DC, Wood D (1999). Dental materials: 1997 literature review. *J. Dent.* 27, 401–435.

Wiley BJ, Im SH, Li ZY, McLellan J, Siekkinen A, Xia Y (2006). Maneuvering the surface Plasmon resonance of silver nanostructures through shape-controlled synthesis. *J. Phys. Chem. B.* 110(32), 15666–15675.

Yaqoob AA, Parveen T, Umar K, Ibrahim MNM (2020). Role of nanomaterials in the treatment of wastewater: A review. *Water.* 12, 495.

Zaporotskova IV, Boroznina NP, Parkhomenko YN, Kozhitov LV (2016). Carbon nanotubes: Sensor properties. A review. *Mod. Electron Mater.* 2, 95–105.

Zhang K, Fang H, Chen Z, Taylor JSA, Wooley KL (2008). Shape effects of nanoparticles conjugated with cell-penetrating peptides (HIV tat PTD) on CHO cell uptake'. *Bioconjugate Chem.* 19(9), 1880–1887.

Zhang Y, Wei S, Liu F, Du Y, Liu S, Ji Y, Yokoi T, Tatsumi T, Xiao FS (2009). Superhydrophobic nanoporous polymers as efficient adsorbents for organic compounds. *Nano Today.* 4(2), 135–142.

Zhou Y, Dai Z (2018). New strategies in the design of nanomedicines to oppose uptake by the mononuclear phagocyte system and enhance cancer therapeutic efficacy. *Chem. Asian J.* 13(22), 3333–3340.

Zielinska A, Carreiró F, Oliveira AM, Neves A, Pires B, Venkatesh DN, Durazzo A, Lucarini M, Eder P, Silva AM, Santini A, Soutu EB (2020). Polymeric nanoparticles: Production, characterization, toxicology and ecotoxicology. *Molecules.* 25(16), 3731.

2 Synthesis of Materials by Synthetic Approach — Materials Synthesis Using Chemical Approaches

Firdos Alam Khan

2.1 INTRODUCTION

The discovery of different types of spectroscopic techniques has enhanced innovation of the nanomaterials and biomaterials recently. The US-based computer company namely IBM developed the scanning tunneling microscopy (STM) in the year 1982; the discovery of STM has helped to get the image of a single atom on flat surfaces (Binnig and Rohrer, 1982). Then atomic force microscopy (AFM) was designed in the year 1988, and AFM has become the most critical scanning probe microscope technique (Binnig et al., 1986) for molecular imaging. The computer configuration has been improved over the years, which makes it possible to design hard discs with a high storage capacity. The better storage discs have inspired the capacity of electrostatic and magnetic forces to be better applied and used for various applications. This has caused the development of electrostatic and magnetic-force microscopy (Butt et al., 2005). Nanotechnology is quickly progressing and becoming part of virtually every materials science field. Different types of materials and nanomaterials are being produced in laboratories where their structures, shapes, and sizes are examined by using advanced machines and tools.

The application of nanotechnology in the vast fields of materials science offers many advantages of producing various nanomaterials with different shapes and sizes, along with better commercial utilities (Marques et al., 2021). There are many applications of nanomaterials, especially in developing cosmetics, environmental remediation, scratch-free paints, surface coatings, electronics products, sports equipment, and biosensors (Sharifi et al., 2012). In this chapter, we have discussed the elementary concepts and methods of producing different types of nanomaterials. This chapter provides a fundamental understanding for researchers of the different methods of production of the various nanomaterials (Figure 2.1).

DOI: 10.1201/9781003317715-2

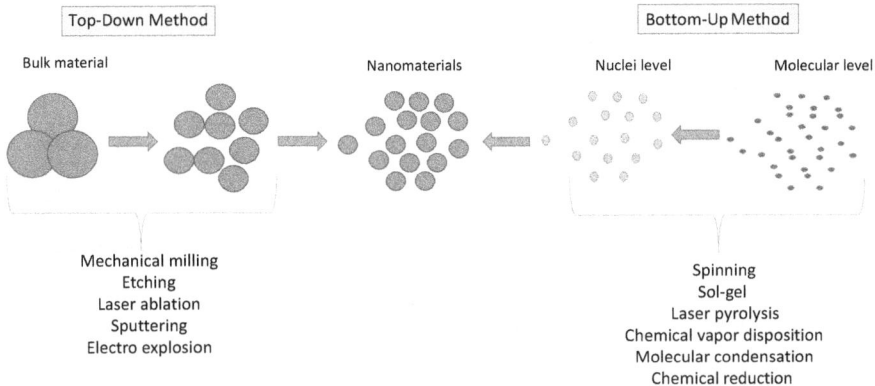

FIGURE 2.1 Method of synthesizing nanomaterials by top-down methods and bottom-up methods.

2.2 PRODUCTION OF NANOMATERIALS BY BOTTOM-UP APPROACHES

Nanomaterials can be produced by different bottom-up approaches, as described individually later.

2.2.1 CHEMICAL VAPOR DEPOSITION (CVD)

This is a chemical vaporization method (CVD), where chemicals are deposited on the surface to produce carbon-based nanomaterials, where a squeaky or thin film is produced through the chemical reactions of vapor phase precursors (Jones and Hitchman, 2008; Baig et al., 2021). A precursor is basically a well-thought-out material for the CVD application, and the precursor has better volatility, high chemical purity, good stability, low cost, and long shelf life. Furthermore, the decomposition of precursors does not generate any kind of residual impurities during chemical reactions (Jones and Hitchman, 2008; Baig et al., 2021). During the preparation of carbon nanotubes by using the CVD method, a substrate is normally placed in an oven and at a high temperature. Then a carbon-containing material, like hydrocarbon gas, is slowly released into the chemical reaction as a precursor, and at a high temperature, the gas releases carbon atoms that recombine to produce carbon nanotubes on the substrate (Shah and Tali, 2016). It has been reported that the nature of the catalyst plays a critical role in shaping the structure and morphology of different types of nanomaterials. In the preparation of graphene nanomaterials, nickel and cobalt catalysts provide multilayer graphene, whereas a copper catalyst provides mono-layer graphene nanomaterials (Ago, 2015). Generally, CVD is an excellent method for producing high-quality materials or nanomaterials (Machac et al., 2020), and this method is also famous for the production of two-dimensional nanomaterials (Wu et al., 2016) (Figure 2.2).

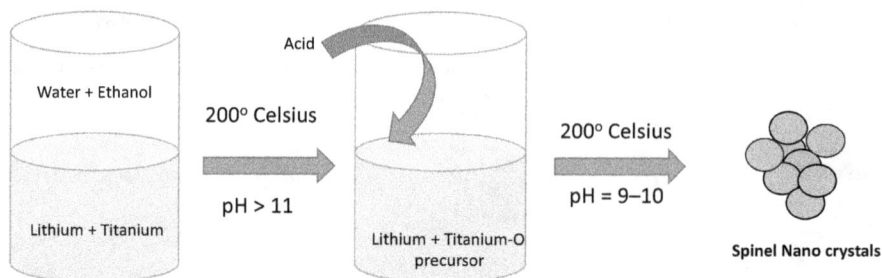

FIGURE 2.2   Synthesis of nanocrystals.

2.2.2   SOLVOTHERMAL AND HYDROTHERMAL PROCEDURE

This method of production of nanomaterials requires a hydrothermal process, which has been extensively applied in the production of nanomaterials or nanostructured materials (Wu et al., 2011; Cao et al., 2016). In this method, nanostructured materials undergo a series of steps of heterogeneous reactions in an aqueous medium, with high pressure and temperature, in a completely sealed vessel (Li et al., 2015a). This method is similar to the hydrothermal method, and the only difference is that it is performed in a non-aqueous solution. Both hydrothermal and solvothermal methods are generally performed in sealed systems (Chen and Holt-Hindle, 2010). The microwave-assisted hydrothermal method has attracted the researchers for production of nanomaterials, which has benefits of both hydrothermal and microwave methods (Meng et al., 2016). In addition, both hydrothermal and solvothermal methods are useful for the production of different types of nanowires, nanorods, nanosheets, and nanospheres (Dong et al., 2020; Jiang et al., 2018; Chai et al., 2018) (Figure 2.3).

2.2.3   SOL-GEL METHOD FOR NANOMATERIAL PRODUCTION

This sol-gel method basically involves a wet chemical technique, which has been mostly used in the production of nanomaterials. The application of this method helps researchers produce various types of very high-quality metal oxide–based nanomaterials. During the production of the metal oxide nanoparticles, the liquid precursor is converted into a sol structure, and this sol structure is finally converted into a gel-like structure (Danks et al., 2016). Metal alkoxides are conventional precursors for the preparation of nanomaterials by using the sol-gel method. The preparation of nanoparticles using the sol-gel method can be finished in numerous steps. Step 1: the hydrolysis of the metal oxide takes place in water or alcohol to form a sol-like structure. Step 2: the condensation of the materials will occur where the sol structure will become viscous to form porous-like structures and during the condensation period, which is also called as poly-condensation process, where hydroxo-(M–OH–M)/oxo-(M–O–M) bridges will form, which finally produced metal–hydroxo-/metal–oxo-polymer in the solution (Tseng et al., 2010). Step 4: during the aging process, poly-condensation of the sol structure continues, with significant changes in the structure, properties, and porosity of the sol. During the aging process,

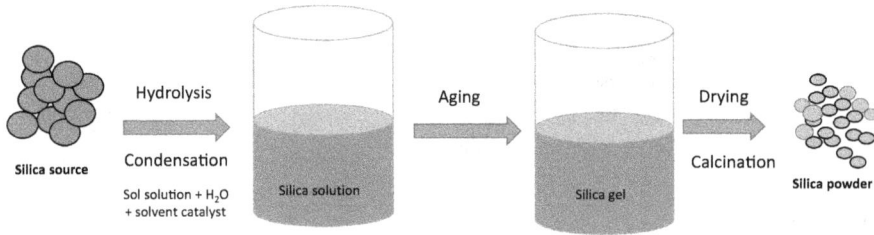

FIGURE 2.3 Synthesis of nanocrystals by solvothermal method.

it has been found that the porosity of material decreases, and the distance between the particles increases. Step 5: after the aging of materials, the materials are dried where water and organic solvents are removed from the gel. Step 6: during this step, calcination is performed to obtain nanoparticles (Parashar et al., 2020), where materials are converted to powder formation using the sol-gel method (Znaidi, 2010). There are several factors that affect the final nanomaterials by the sol-gel method, which are the type of nature of precursor, rate of hydrolysis, time duration of aging, and pH values (De Coelho Escobar and dos Santos, 2014). Most important, this method is economical and has many advantages, such as that the final product is always homogeneous in nature, the temperature requirement is low and the processing temperature is low, and it's very simple and easy to produce both composites and complex nanomaterials (Parashar et al., 2020).

2.2.4 SOFT AND HARD TEMPLATING PROCEDURE

This soft and hard template procedure has been extensively used to prepare nanoporous materials, and this is a simple conventional method for the preparation of nanomaterials. There are many advantages of using the soft template method, such as straightforward implementation, relatively mild experimental conditions, and the development of materials with a variety of sizes and shapes (Liu et al., 2013a). The nanoporous materials can be produced by using adequately soft materials, such as block co-polymers, flexible organic molecules, and anionic, cationic, and nonionic surfactants. It has been found that protuberant interactions between the soft templates and the precursors happen through different bonding, such as hydrogen bonding, van der Waals forces, and electrostatic forces respectively (Poolakkandy and Menamparambath, 2020). In addition, soft templates can also be used in the preparation of three-dimensional mesoporous nanostructures. One of the best examples is the involvement of mesoporous solids, such as lamellar, cubic, and hexagonal mesoporous silica, in the production of alkyl-tri-methyl-ammonium surfactant (Kresge et al., 1992; Beck et al., 1992). Usually, two processes, called cooperative self-assembly and liquid-crystal templating, are adopted for the synthesis of well-arranged mesoporous materials via a soft templating method (Li and Zhao, 2013). There are several factors that affect the mesoporous material structures derived from three-dimensionally arranged micelles, such as the concentrations of surfactant and precursor, the ratio of surfactant to precursor, surfactant structure, and environmental

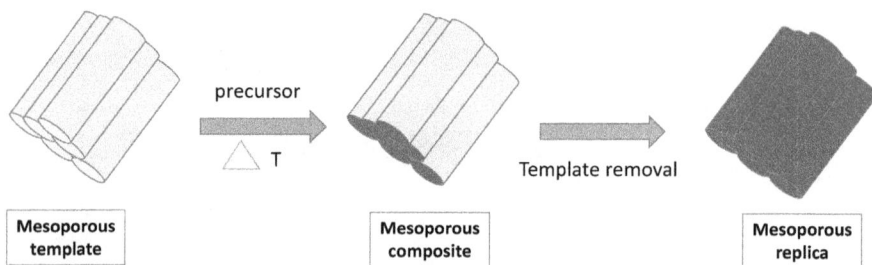

FIGURE 2.4   Synthesis of mesoporous composite by nanocasting.

conditions under which chemical reactions take place (Liu et al., 2013b). It is possible to modify the size of pores by using surfactant carbon chain length or introducing auxiliary pore-expanding agent's nanoporous materials. A range of nanostructured materials, such as mesoporous polymeric carbonaceous nanospheres (Beck et al., 1992), single crystal nanorods (Lv et al., 2004), porous alumina (Martins et al., 2010), and mesoporous N-doped graphene (Tang et al., 2019), can be prepared by using the soft template method (Figure 2.4).

2.2.5   NANOCASTING

This method is generally used to prepare well-designed nanomaterials, where hard casting templates are used, and the casting template is filled with precursors or molecules to prepare nanostructures for different applications (Poolakkandy and Menamparambath, 2020). The choice of the hard template is important for preparing well-organized mesoporous nanomaterials. While making the hard template, it's important that the template maintains a mesoporous structure during the precursor conversion step, and they should be effortlessly removable without disturbing the shaped nanomaterials. There are different types of materials that have been used to construct the template, such as carbon nanotubes, particles, colloidal crystals, carbon black, silica, and wood shells (Szczęśniak et al., 2020). There are three different methods to produce nanomaterials using templates, and in the first step, a suitable unique template is selected, and a targeted precursor is filled into the template mesopores to convert them into an inorganic solid structure. In the last step, the template is removed to accomplish the mesoporous copy (Yamauchi and Kuroda, 2008). By using mesoporous templates, exclusive nanomaterials, such as nanowires, nanorods, metal oxides nanomaterials, and other nanomaterials, can be produced (Figure 2.4) (Hurst et al., 2006).

2.2.6   REVERSE MICELLE PROCEDURE

The nanomaterials can be produced by the reverse micelle method with the desired shapes and sizes. The process of making nanomaterials includes the involvement of an oil-in-water emulsion in the normal micelles, where hydrophobic tails are pointed toward a core that has trapped oil droplets within it. Though reverse micelles are

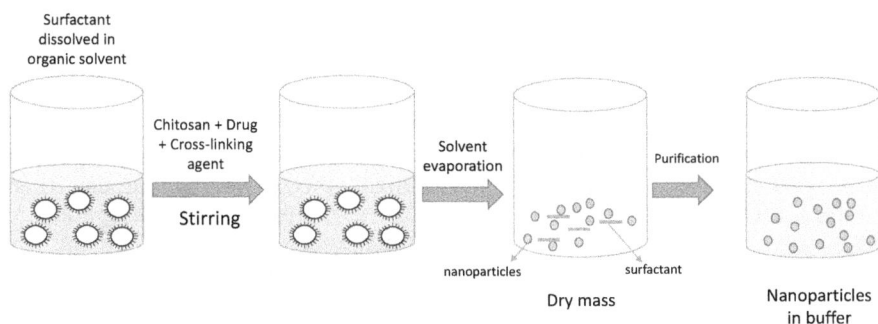

FIGURE 2.5 Synthesis of nanoparticles by reverse micelle method.

formed in the case of a water-in-oil emulsion, in which the hydrophilic heads are directed toward a core that comprises water (Malik et al., 2012). The core of the reverse micelles acts as a nanoreactor for the production of nanoparticles, and it acts as the water pool for synthesizing nanomaterials. The size of these nanoreactors can be controlled by changing the water-to-surfactant ratio, eventually affecting the size of the nanoparticles synthesized through this method. In case the water concentration is decreased, this consequences in smaller water droplets, resulting in the development of smaller nanoparticles (Soleimani et al., 2019). Therefore, the reverse micelle method delivers a simplistic way of manufacturing uniform nanoparticles with precisely controlled size. The nanoparticles that are produced by the reverse micelle method are astonishingly fine and mono-dispersed in nature (Nguyen, 2013), which proves the synthesis of magnetic lipase immobilized nanoparticles through the reverse micelle method (Figure 2.5) (Yi et al., 2017).

2.2.7 CHEMICAL CO-PRECIPITATION METHOD

This method involves using chemical co-precipitation to mix two or more different materials that finally forms precipitation in an aqueous solvent, especially base (Andhare et al., 2020). The classic method to prepare magnetic nanoparticles involves the chemical co-precipitation method, and in this method, the Fe^{2+} and Fe^{3+} salts are mixed in the NaOH base solution (Anbarasu et al., 2015). Interestingly, the morphology, size, and composition of the materials can be altered by altering the pH, temperature, ligands, precursor salt, and chemical ratios (Gnanaprakash et al., 2007). Nanoparticles can be stabilized by an addition of an appropriate surfactant, such as oleic acid, ligand aptamer, poly-ethylene glycol acrylate, and NaOH (Bloemen et al., 2012). Moreover, complex metals can be synthesized by using this realizable method. The preparation of iron chromite is obtained by the mixture of iron III salt and chromate. The salts from metal ions are formed and then precipitated by using an ammonium base in the aqueous solution. Thereafter, precipitated materials can be decomposed at a high temperature to yield iron III chromite (Tang et al., 2020). It has been reported that the characteristics of chemical materials prepared by using the co-precipitation method are generally an insoluble form and contain smaller-sized particles. The insolubility appearance of the materials usually comes from the high supersaturation of the materials (Othman et al., 2009), and the size of materials may change from smaller to larger. Moreover, during the nucleation step, large-sized nanoparticles are formed. The factors that affect the prepared particles are (1) aggregation and (2) Oswald ripening (Hu et al., 2014). There are many advantages of the co-precipitation methods, like this method is very simple and direct, and the control size of the particles is based on their compositions. In addition, the surface of the particles can be changed/modified with various functionalities. The chemical compositions normally require a low temperature to synthesize particles to avoid the involvement of organic solvents, and this method generates a number of impurities during the precipitation steps. This method is also time-consuming and not consistent in reproducibility and scalability (Maleki et al., 2018).

2.2.8 BALL MILLING OR MECHANICAL METHOD

The ball milling or mechanical method produces nanomaterials, as in this method, materials are ground or milled in a closed container. The production of the materials needed small pebbles, which are normally made of glass or ceramics or stainless steel, to create shear force during grinding. The bulk materials are placed inside the closed vessel for the preparation of fine materials, and during the grinding process, the bulk materials are converted to fine and small nanomaterials (Delogu et al., 2017). This method can be used to prepare metallic hydrides and nitrides, and the prepared nitrides hold indispensable properties that offer a range of applications. For example, the hardness and stability of the nitrides are used to cut tools and tool coating in micro-electronic applications. This is usually synthesized by using the reactive ball milling method (Sun et al., 2009), and the bulk metallic powder is generally placed in a closed vessel under the purging of the nitrogen gas atmosphere that is subjected to high-energy ball milling. During this process, the metallic powders are disintegrated to form tiny nanoparticles, and oxygen-free active surfaces are produced on the nanomaterials (Pentimalli et al., 2017). Moreover, nanotubes are ground to prepare very tiny powder by crashing two or more pebbles in a closed vessel that generates a very high pressure to produce fine nanotubes (Bi et al., 2021). In addition, the quality of the nanotubes is increased by conjugating functional materials and molecules on the surface of the nanotube in the vessel (Ma et al., 2009).

There are a few factors that affect the dispersion of nanotubes, which are the size of the pebbles, speed of rotation, time of milling, and amount of nanotube added during the chemical reaction (Gou et al., 2012). Because of this, nanotubes of less than 100 nm in size can be prepared by the grinding process. This method can be applied where carbon nanotubes are transformed into fine carbon nanomaterials, and few damages occur on the surface of the nanomaterials during the preparation stage (Hecht et al., 2011). This method is also used in the production of the mechanical alloying method, which is basically a top-down approach. The decrease of particle size is usually done in the grinding step by the collision of pebbles that generates a frictional force that results in the increase of pressure, temperature, and internal energy, respectively (Piras et al., 2019). The grinding or milling speed can be amplified through surface functionalization of the alkyl or aryl group on the surface of the single-walled carbon, which gives high solubility in organic solvents (Karousis et al., 2010; Li et al., 2015b). In addition, metastable materials can be produced using the high-energy ball milling method by maintaining thermal equilibrium. This method somewhat varies from the conventional ball milling methods because the conventional methods cannot yield adequate energy to mill the materials. For example, nickel-niobium alloy can be prepared by using high-energy ball milling (Koch et al., 1983). There are many advantages of this method; for example, it makes a fine powder, and this method is suitable for milling toxic materials, and it's possible to mill abrasive materials. There is also some contamination received from the wear and tear in ball collision, and the method also generates too much noise, and also this method is very time-consuming (Delogu et al., 2017).

2.2.9 PHYSICAL VAPOR DEPOSITION METHOD

This method of producing nanomaterials where the surface coating is done by vapor deposition to prepare ultra-thin material film is called the physical vapor deposition (PVD) method. This method is applied to produce ultra-thin films and surface coating, and this method is used to produce metal vapor that can be deposited on the conductive layer as ultra-thin films and alloy coatings. It is carried in a vacuum vessel with a clean atmosphere, where vacuum deposition occurs in the chamber and the metals are deposited in the localized area of materials (Fox-Rabinovich et al., 2020). This method is designed to deposit metal on the surface and reactive gas, such as oxygen, nitrogen, or methane, passed in the vacuum vessel. With the use of plasma, the high-energetic beam is bombarded on the metal surfaces, ensuring hard and dense coatings. This method is used to synthesize nanoparticles and also to produce nanoformulations (El-Eskandarany et al., 2020). It has been reported that thin-film formation is characterized by the metal ions in the vapor phase obtained from the condensed phase film (Venables and Spiller, 1983). This PVD method comprises evaporation and a sputtering process to produce thin ultra-films. The PVD method comprises a sputtering process that is leftover in the vapor phase under supersaturation (Abegunde et al., 2019). There are many advantages of the PVD techniques, such as having better-quality properties as compared with the substrate material, being able to use inorganic and few organic materials, and being an eco-friendly method to produce as compared to the electroplating technique (Knotek et al., 1993; Tillotson et al., 2001). There are a few shortcomings of this technique, such as difficulty in coating with complex nanostructures, and this PDV method is an expensive method with low output (Mattox, 1999; Yi et al., 2017).

2.2.10 LITHOGRAPHY

This method of lithography is used in printing, where a stamp-covered stamp has both hydrophobic and hydrophilic regions, where the hydrophobic area takes up the ink, while the hydrophilic area will not (Kim et al., 2016; Sun et al., 2021). Normally, during the process, lithography duplicates the pattern that looks like the substrate patterning (Lee et al., 2012). While doing this process, two different types of masks are used, positive and negative, which are normally used to pattern the surface.

A positive photoresist material is in a soluble form when exposed to light, whereas a negative photoresist is in an insoluble form and makes the photoresist unbending (Jang et al., 2007). There are various types of lithography that are used to pattern the surfaces, such as photo-lithography, UV lithography, soft lithography, and scanning probe lithograph (Pimpin and Srituravanich, 2012; Prawer et al., 2000; Rahman and Padavettan, 2012). Photo-lithography is basically a light-based technique, where an image develops on a light projection into the photoresist coated on the substrate, like a silicon wafer (Paik et al., 2020; Hakim and Shanks, 2009; Rane et al., 2018). This method is a widely used technique, especially in the nanoelectronics industries to pattern semiconductors. In UV lithography, a specific type of wavelength is normally used, where submicron-level pattering is possible in the photoresist condition (Del Barrio and Sánchez-Somolinos, 2019; Mochalov et al., 2020; Muüller et al., 2020). Under UV-light exposure, there is a change in the solubility of the solution called developer. After the exposure to the UV light, photo-crosslinking occurs on the photoresist, and the unreacted pattern is etched away (Vollenbroek and Spiertz, 1988; Kara and Öztürk, 2019). There are a few shortcomings of this method, as during the production, free radicals are generated, which may cause damage to cellular DNA (Sha et al., 2001; Koponen et al., 2016). Another technique is e-beam lithography, where scanning electron beams are applied to pattern the surface without a mask and attain a correctness of less than 1 nanometer (Altissimo, 2010; Kickelbick, 2007; Kim et al., 2021). There are two methods for scanning an electron beam, the raster scanning method and the vector scanning method; in the case of the raster scanning method, the image is divided into pixel form, and the image is printed either in a left-to-right fashion or top-to-bottom fashion. In the case of the raster scanning, the beam scans the entire surface of the image (Ferrera, 2000) (Figure 2.6).

There is an elastomeric stamp to deposit ink on a substrate, which is called soft lithography, and this method of preparing nanomaterials has many advantages over other patterning methods, such as being economical, being simpler, and having a high throughout. This method has a precision of making nanomaterials with a wide

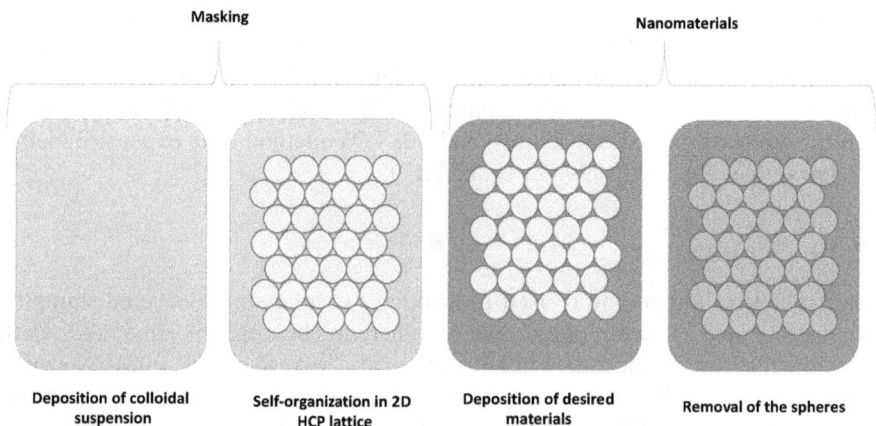

Masking   Nanomaterials

| Deposition of colloidal suspension | Self-organization in 2D HCP lattice | Deposition of desired materials | Removal of the spheres |

FIGURE 2.6 Synthesis of nanoparticles by lithography.

range, from nanometer (nm) to micrometer (mm) resolution, to pattern the substrate (Whitesides et al., 2001; Kwiatkowski and Lukehart, 2002). There are many shortcomings of this method, such as that it requires another lithography method to construct the stamp master. There is another benefit, such as that the same pattern can be used for making many duplicates (Sahin et al., 2018). It is possible to modify the image surface with the help of an atomic resolution, where the probe is used similar to atomic force microscopy and scanning tunneling microscopy (Quate, 1997; Lee and Hwang, 2008). In this technique, it is used to fabricate graphene nanoribbons by catalyzing graphene oxide in the presence of hydrogen using platinum-coated atomic force microscopy (Zhang et al., 2012; Sun et al., 2009). One of the advantages of scanning probe lithography is having the ability to produce topographies with patterns on non-planar surfaces (Kuhnel et al., 2018; Li et al., 2013b; Liu et al., 2013b). Moreover, this method is simple in solution environments and direct cross-examination of protein-binding proceedings. Integrated circuits with nanopatterning have been synthesized using micro and nanolithography (Lyles, 2013). Lithography is done by deposition to achieve a high-resolution tomography, and there are two types, such as masked lithography and mask-less lithography (Zhao et al., 2020).

REFERENCES

Abegunde O.O., Akinlabi E.T., Oladijo O.P., Akinlabi S., Ude A.U. Overview of thin film deposition techniques. *AIMS Mater. Sci.* 2019;6:174–199. Doi: 10.3934/matersci.2019.2.174.

Ago H. *Frontiers of Graphene and Carbon Nanotubes.* Springer, Japan, Tokyo, 2015; pp. 3–20.

Altissimo M. E-beam lithography for micro-/nanofabrication. *Biomicrofluidics.* 2010;4:026503. Doi: 10.1063/1.3437589.

Anbarasu M., Anandan M., Chinnasamy E., Gopinath V., Balamurugan K. Synthesis and characterization of polyethylene glycol (PEG) coated Fe_3O_4 nanoparticles by chemical co-precipitation method for biomedical applications. *Spectrochim. Acta Part A Mol. Biomol. Spectrosc.* 2015;135:536–539. Doi: 10.1016/j.saa.2014.07.059.

Andhare D., Jadhav S., Khedkar M., Somvanshi S.B., More S., Jadhav K. Structural and chemical properties of $ZnFe_2O_4$ nanoparticles synthesised by chemical co-precipitation technique. In *Proceedings of the Journal of Physics: Conference Series, International Web Conference on Advanced Material Science and Nanotechnology (NANOMAT—2020); Nandgaon Khandeshwar, India. 20–21 June 2020.* IOP Publishing, Bristol, UK, 2020; p. 012014.

Baig N., Kammakamak I., Falath W. Nanomaterials: A review of synthesis methods, properties, recent progress, and challenges. (*Review Article*) *Mater. Adv.* 2021;2:1821–1871. Doi: 10.1039/D0MA00807A.

Beck J.S., Vartuli J.C., Roth W.J., Leonowicz M.E., Kresge C.T., Schmitt K.D., Chu C.T.W., Olson D.H., Sheppard E.W., McCullen S.B., Higgins J.B., Schlenker J.L. A new family of mesoporous molecular sieves prepared with liquid crystal templates. *J. Am. Chem. Soc.* 1992;114:10834–10843. Doi: 10.1021/ja00053a020.

Bi S., Xiao B., Ji Z., Liu B., Liu Z., Ma Z. Dispersion and damage of carbon nanotubes in carbon nanotube/7055Al composites during high-energy ball milling process. *Acta Metall. Sin. (Engl. Lett.).* 2021;34:196–204. Doi: 10.1007/s40195-020-01138-5.

Binnig G., Quate C.F., Gerber C. Atomic force microscope. *Phys. Rev. Lett.* 1986;56:930–933.

Binnig G., Rohrer H. Scanning tunneling microscope. *US Pat.* US4343993A, 1982.

Bloemen M., Brullot W., Luong T.T., Geukens N., Gils A., Verbiest T. Improved functionalization of oleic acid-coated iron oxide nanoparticles for biomedical applications. *J. Nanoparticle Res.* 2012;14:1–10. Doi: 10.1007/s11051-012-1100-5.

Butt H.J., Cappella B., Kappl M. Force measurements with the atomic force microscope. *Surf. Sci. Rep.* 2005;59:1–152.

Cao S., Zhao C., Han T., Peng L. Hydrothermal synthesis, characterization and gas sensing properties of the WO3 nanofibers. *Mater. Lett.* 2016;169:17–20 CrossRef CAS.

Chai B., Xu M., Yan J., Ren Z. Remarkably enhanced photocatalytic hydrogen evolution over MoS2 nanosheets loaded on uniform CdS nanospheres. *Appl. Surf. Sci.* 2018;430:523–530.

Chen A., Holt-Hindle P. Platinum-based nanostructured materials: Synthesis, properties, and applications. *Chem. Rev.* 2010;110:3767–3804.

Danks A.E., Hall S.R., Schnepp Z. The evolution of 'sol–gel' chemistry as a technique for materials synthesis. *Mater. Horiz.* 2016;3:91–112 RSC.

De Coelho Escobar C., dos Santos J.H.Z. Effect of the sol-gel route on the textural characteristics of silica imprinted with Rhodamine B. *J. Sep. Sci.* 2014;37:868–875.

Del Barrio J., Sánchez-Somolinos C. Light to shape the future: From photolithography to 4D printing. *Adv. Opt. Mater.* 2019;7:1900598. Doi: 10.1002/adom.201900598.

Delogu F., Gorrasi G., Sorrentino A. Fabrication of polymer nanocomposites via ball milling: Present status and future perspectives. *Prog. Mater. Sci.* 2017;86:75–126. Doi: 10.1016/j.pmatsci.2017.01.003.

Dong Y., Du X., Liang P., Man X. One-pot solvothermal method to fabricate 1D-VS4 nanowires as anode materials for lithium ion batteries. *Inorg. Chem. Commun.* 2020;115:107883.

El-Eskandarany M.S., Al-Salem S.M., Ali N. Top-down reactive approach for the synthesis of disordered ZrN nanocrystalline bulk material from solid waste. *Nanomaterials.* 2020;10:1826. Doi: 10.3390/nano10091826.

Ferrera J.F.U. *Ph.D. Thesis.* Massachusetts Institute of Technology, Cambridge, MA, 2000. Nanometer-Scale Placement in Electron-Beam Lithography.

Fox-Rabinovich G., Gershman I., Veldhuis S. Thin-film PVD coating metamaterials exhibiting similarities to natural processes under extreme tribological conditions. *Nanomaterials.* 2020;10:1720. Doi: 10.3390/nano10091720.

Gnanaprakash G., Mahadevan S., Jayakumar T., Kalyanasundaram P., Philip J., Raj B. Effect of initial pH and temperature of iron salt solutions on formation of magnetite nanoparticles. *Mater. Chem. Phys.* 2007;103:168–175. Doi: 10.1016/j.matchemphys.2007.02.011.

Gou J., Zhuge J., Liang F. *Manufacturing Techniques for Polymer Matrix Composites (PMCs).* Elsevier, Amsterdam, The Netherlands, 2012; pp. 95–119. Processing of Polymer Nanocomposites.

Hakim S.H., Shanks B.H. A comparative study of macroporous metal oxides synthesized via a unified approach. *Chem. Mater.* 2009;21:2027–2038. Doi: 10.1021/cm801691g.

Hecht D.S., Hu L., Irvin G. Emerging transparent electrodes based on thin films of carbon nanotubes, graphene, and metallic nanostructures. *Adv. Mater.* 2011;23:1482–1513. Doi: 10.1002/adma.201003188.

Hu Y., Li Q., Lee B., Jun Y.-S. Aluminum affects heterogeneous Fe (III)(Hydr) oxide nucleation, growth, and Ostwald ripening. *Environ. Sci. Technol.* 2014;48:299–306. Doi: 10.1021/es403777w.

Hurst H.J., Payne E.K., Qin L., Mirkin C.A. Multisegmented one-dimensional nanorods prepared by hard-template synthetic methods. *Angew. Chem., Int. Ed.* 2006;45:2672–2692.

Jang J.H., Ullal C.K., Maldovan M., Gorishnyy T., Kooi S., Koh C., Thomas E.L. 3D micro- and nanostructures via interference lithography. *Adv. Funct. Mater.* 2007;17:3027–3041. Doi: 10.1002/adfm.200700140.

Jiang Y., Peng Z., Zhang S., Li F., Liu Z., Zhang J., Liu Y., Wang K. A facile approach for the synthesis of Zn2SnO4/BiOBr hybrid nanocomposites with improved visible-light photocatalytic performance. *Ceram. Int.* 2018;44:6115–6126.

Jones A.C., Hitchman M.L. *Chemical Vapour Deposition*, ed. A.C. Jones, M.L. Hitchman. Royal Society of Chemistry, Cambridge, 2008; pp. 1–36.

Kara F., Öztürk B. Comparison and optimization of PVD and CVD method on surface roughness and flank wear in hard-machining of DIN 1.2738 mold steel. *Sens. Rev.* 2019;29:24–33. Doi: 10.1108/SR-12-2017-0266.

Karousis N., Tagmatarchis N., Tasis D. Current progress on the chemical modification of carbon nanotubes. *Chem. Rev.* 2010;110:5366–5397. Doi: 10.1021/cr100018g.

Kickelbick G. Introduction to hybrid materials. *Hybrid Mater.* 2007;1:2.

Kim H.-Y., Kim D.-S., Hwang N.-M. Comparison of diamond nanoparticles captured on the floating and grounded membranes in the hot filament chemical vapor deposition process. *RSC Adv.* 2021;11:5651–5657. Doi: 10.1039/D0RA09649K.

Kim S., Sojoudi H., Zhao H., Mariappan D., McKinley G.H., Gleason K.K., Hart A.J. Ultrathin high-resolution flexographic printing using nanoporous stamps. *Sci. Adv.* 2016;2:e1601660. Doi: 10.1126/sciadv.1601660.

Knotek O., Löffler F., Krämer G. Process and advantage of multicomponent and multilayer PVD coatings. *Surf. Coat. Technol.* 1993;59:14–20. Doi: 10.1016/0257-8972(93)90048-S.

Koch C., Cavin O., McKamey C., Scarbrough J. Preparation of "amorphous" Ni60Nb40 by mechanical alloying. *Appl. Phys. Lett.* 1983;43:1017–1019. Doi: 10.1063/1.94213.

Koponen S.E., Gordon P.G., Barry S.T. Principles of precursor design for vapour deposition methods. *Polyhedron.* 2016;108:59–66. Doi: 10.1016/j.poly.2015.08.024.

Kresge C.T., Leonowicz M.E., Roth W.J., Vartuli J.C., Beck J.S. Ordered mesoporous molecular sieves synthesized by a liquid-crystal template mechanism. *Nature.* 1992;359:710–712.

Kühnel M., Fröhlich T., Füßl R., Hoffmann M., Manske E., Rangelow I.W., Reger J., Schäffel C., Sinzinger S., Zöllner J.-P. Towards alternative 3D nanofabrication in macroscopic working volumes. *Meas. Sci. Technol.* 2018;29:114002. Doi: 10.1088/1361-6501/aadb57.

Kwiatkowski K.C., Lukehart C.M. *Nanostructured Materials and Nanotechnology.* Elsevier, Amsterdam, The Netherlands, 2002; pp. 57–91. Nanocomposites Prepared by Sol-Gel Methods: Synthesis and Characterization.

Lee J.-I., Hwang N.-M. Generation of negative-charge carriers in the gas phase and their contribution to the growth of carbon nanotubes during hot-filament chemical vapor deposition. *Carbon.* 2008;46:1588–1592. Doi: 10.1016/j.carbon.2008.07.006.

Lee K.-H., Kim S.-M., Jeong H., Jung G.-Y. Spontaneous nanoscale polymer solution patterning using solvent evaporation driven double-dewetting edge lithography. *Soft Matter.* 2012;8:465–471. Doi: 10.1039/C1SM06431B.

Li J., Sun X., Liu S., Li X., Li J.-G., Huo D. A homogeneous co-precipitation method to synthesize highly sinterability YAG powders for transparent ceramics. *Ceram. Int.* 2015a;41:3283–3287. Doi: 10.1016/j.ceramint.2014.10.076.

Li J., Wu Q., Wu J. *Handbook of Nanoparticles.* Springer International Publishing, Cham, 2015b; pp. 1–28.

Li W., Zhao D. Ordered mesoporous molecular sieves synthesized by a liquid-crystal template mechanism. *Chem. Commun.* 2013;49:943–946 RSC.

Liu L., Yang T., Wang D.-W., Lu G.Q., Zhao D., Qiao S.Z. Preparation and characterization of hollow MgO/SiO2 nanocomposites and using as reusable. Catalyst for synthesis of 1H-isochromene. *Nat. Commun.* 2013a;4:2798.

Liu Y., Goebl J., Yin Y. Templated synthesis of nanostructured materials. *Chem. Soc. Rev.* 2013b;42:2610–2653 RSC.

Lv R., Cao C., Zhai H., Wang D., Liu S., Zhu H. One-dimensional nanostructures: Principles and applications. *Solid State Commun.* 2004;130:241–245.

Lyles V.D. *Ph.D. Thesis.* Louisiana State University and Agricultural and Mechanical College, Baton Rouge, LA, 2013. Surface studies of Organic Thin Films Using Scanning Probe Microscopy and Nanofabrication.

Ma P.C., Wang S.Q., Kim J.-K., Tang B.Z. In-situ amino functionalization of carbon nanotubes using ball milling. *J. Nanosci. Nanotechnol.* 2009;9:749–753. Doi: 10.1166/jnn.2009.C017.

Machac P., Cichon S., Lapcak L., Fekete L. Graphene prepared by chemical vapour deposition process. *Graphene Technol.* 2020;5:9–17. CrossRef.

Maleki H., Haselpour M., Fathi R. The effect of calcination conditions on structural and magnetic behavior of bismuth ferrite synthesized by co-precipitation method. *J. Mater. Sci. Mater. Electron.* 2018;29:4320–4326. Doi: 10.1007/s10854-017-8379-z.

Malik M.A., Wani M.Y., Hashim M.A. Microemulsion method: A novel route to synthesize organic and inorganic nanomaterials. *Arabian J. Chem.* 2012;5:397–417.

Marques A.C., Vale M., Vicente D., Schreck M., Tervoort E., Niederberger M. Porous silica microspheres with immobilized titania nanoparticles for in-flow solar-driven purification of wastewater. *Global Chall.* 2021:2000116.

Martins L., Alves Rosa M.A., Pulcinelli S.H., Santilli C.V. Characterization of the as-synthesized mesoporous TiO2 materials. *Microporous Mesoporous Mater.* 2010;132:268–275.

Mattox D.M. Physical vapor deposition (PVD) processes. *Met. Finish.* 1999;97:417–430. Doi: 10.1016/S0026-0576(99)80043-9.

Meng L.-Y., Wang B., Ma M.-G., Lin K.-L. Fast microwave-assisted hydrothermal synthesis of TiNb 2 O 7 nanoparticles. *Mater. Today Chem.* 2016;1–2:63–83.

Mochalov L., Logunov A., Kitnis A., Vorotyntsev V. Plasma-chemistry of arsenic selenide films: Relationship between film properties and plasma power. *Plasma Chem. Plasma Process.* 2020;40:407–421. Doi: 10.1007/s11090-019-10035-4.

Muüller R., Gelme O., Scholz J.-P., Huber F., Mundszinger M., Li Y., Madel M., Minkow A., Kaiser U., Herr U. Epitaxial ZnO layer growth on Si (111) substrates with an intermediate AlN nucleation layer by methane-based chemical vapor deposition. *Cryst. Growth Des.* 2020;20:6170–6185. Doi: 10.1021/acs.cgd.0c00907.

Nguyen T-D. From formation mechanisms to synthetic methods toward shape-controlled oxidenanoparticles. *Nanoscale.* 2013;5:9455. RSC.

Othman M., Helwani Z., Fernando W. Synthetic hydrotalcites from different routes and their application as catalysts and gas adsorbents: A review. *Appl. Organomet. Chem.* 2009;23:335–346. Doi: 10.1002/aoc.1517. [CrossRef] [Google Scholar].

Paik S., Kim G., Chang S., Lee S., Jin D., Jeong K.-Y., Lee I.S., Lee J., Moon H., Lee J. Near-field sub-diffraction photolithography with an elastomeric photomask. *Nat. Commun.* 2020;11:1–13. Doi: 10.1038/s41467-020-14439-1.

Parashar M., Shukla V.K., Singh R. Metal oxides nanoparticles via sol–gel method: A review on synthesis, characterization and applications. *J. Mater. Sci.: Mater. Electron.* 2020;31:3729–3749.

Pentimalli M., Imperi E., Zaccagnini A., Padella F. Nanostructured metal hydride–polymer composite as fixed bed for sorption technologies. Advantages of an innovative combined approach by high-energy ball milling and extrusion techniques. *Renew. Energy.* 2017;110:69–78. Doi: 10.1016/j.renene.2016.07.074.

Pimpin A., Srituravanich W. Review on micro-and nanolithography techniques and their applications. *Eng. J.* 2012;16:37–56. Doi: 10.4186/ej.2012.16.1.37.

Piras C.C., Fernández-Prieto S., De Borggraeve W.M. Ball milling: A green technology for the preparation and functionalisation of nanocellulose derivatives. *Nanoscale Adv.* 2019;1:937–947. Doi: 10.1039/C8NA00238J.

Poolakkandy R.R., Menamparambath M.M. Soft-template-assisted synthesis: A promising approach for the fabrication of transition metal oxides. *Nanoscale Adv.* 2020;2:5015–5045 RSC.

Prawer S., Nugent K., Jamieson D., Orwa J., Bursill L.A., Peng J. The Raman spectrum of nanocrystalline diamond. *Chem. Phys. Lett.* 2000;332:93–97. Doi: 10.1016/S0009-2614(00)01236-7.

Quate C.F. Scanning probes as a lithography tool for nanostructures. *Surf. Sci.* 1997;386:259–264. Doi: 10.1016/S0039-6028(97)00305-1.

Rahman I.A., Padavettan V. Synthesis of silica nanoparticles by sol-gel: Size-dependent properties, surface modification, and applications in silica-polymer nanocomposites—A review. *J. Nanomater.* 2012;2012:8. Doi: 10.1155/2012/132424.

Rane A.V., Kanny K., Abitha V., Thomas S. *Synthesis of Inorganic Nanomaterials.* Elsevier, Amsterdam, The Netherlands, 2018; pp. 121–139. Methods for Synthesis of Nanoparticles and Fabrication of Nanocomposites.

Sahin O., Ashokkumar M., Ajayan P.M. *Fundamental Biomaterials: Metals.* Elsevier, Amsterdam, The Netherlands, 2018; pp. 67–78. Micro-and Nanopatterning of Biomaterial Surfaces.

Sha D., Hsieh L., Chen K. Wafer rework strategies at the photolithography stage. *Int. J. Ind. Eng. Theory Appl. Pract.* 2001;8:122–130.

Shah K.A., Tali B.A. Synthesis of carbon nanotubes by catalytic chemical vapour deposition: A review on carbon sources, catalysts and substrates. *Mater. Sci. Semicond. Process.* 2016;41:67–82. CrossRef CAS.

Sharifi S., Behzadi S., Laurent S., Laird Forrest M., Stroeve P., Mahmoudi M. Toxicity of nanomaterials. *Chem. Soc. Rev.* 2012;41:2323–2343 RSC.

Soleimani Zohr Shiri M., Henderson W., Mucalo M.R. A review of the lesser-studied microemulsion-based synthesis methodologies used for preparing nanoparticle systems of the noble metals, Os, Re, Ir and Rh. *Materials.* 2019;12:1896. CrossRef PubMed.

Sun J., Wang M., Zhao Y., Li X., Liang B. Synthesis of titanium nitride powders by reactive ball milling of titanium and urea. *J. Alloy. Compd.* 2009;482:L29–L31. Doi: 10.1016/j.jallcom.2009.04.043.

Sun L., Yuan G., Gao L., Yang J., Chhowalla M., Gharahcheshmeh M.H., Gleason K.K., Choi Y.S., Hong B.H., Liu Z. Chemical vapour deposition. *Nat. Rev. Methods Primers.* 2021;1:1–20. Doi: 10.1038/s43586-020-00005-y.

Szczęśniak B., Choma J., Jaroniec, M. Major advances in the development of ordered mesoporous materials. *Chem. Commun.* 2020;56:7836–7848.

Tang T., Zhang T., Li W., Huang X., Wang X., Qiu H., Hou Y. Mesoporous N-doped graphene prepared by a soft-template method with high performance in Li–S batteries. *Nanoscale.* 2019;11:7440–7446.

Tang Y., Zhao J., Zhou J., Zeng Y., Zhang W., Shi B. Highly efficient removal of Cr (III)-poly (acrylic acid) complex by coprecipitation with polyvalent metal ions: Performance, mechanism, and validation. *Water Res.* 2020;178:115807. Doi: 10.1016/j.watres.2020.115807.

Tillotson T., Gash A., Simpson R., Hrubesh L., Satcher J., Jr., Poco J. Nanostructured energetic materials using sol-gel methodologies. *J. Non Cryst. Solids.* 2001;285:338–345. Doi: 10.1016/S0022-3093(01)00477-X.

Tseng TK., Lin Y.S., Chen Y.J., Chu H. A review of photocatalysts prepared by sol–gel method for VOCs removal. *Int. J. Mol. Sci.* 2010;11:2336.

Venables J., Spiller G. Nucleation and growth of thin films. *Surf. Mobilities Solid Mater.* 1983;86:341–404.

Vollenbroek F.A., Spiertz E.J. *Electronic Applications.* Springer, Berlin, Heidelberg, Germany, 1988; pp. 85–111. Photoresist Systems for Microlithography.

Whitesides G.M., Ostuni E., Takayama S., Jiang X., Ingber D.E. Soft lithography in biology and biochemistry. *Annu. Rev. Biomed. Eng.* 2001;3:335–373. Doi: 10.1146/annurev.bioeng.3.1.335.

Wu Q., Wongwiriyapan W., Park J.-H., Park S., Jung S.J., Jeong T., Lee S., Lee Y.H., Song Y.J. In situ chemical vapor deposition of graphene and hexagonal boron nitride heterostructures. *Curr. Appl. Phys.* 2016;16:1175–1191.

Wu X., (Max) Lu G.Q., Wang L. Shell-in-shell TiO_2 hollow spheres synthesized by one-pot hydrothermal method for dye-sensitized solar cell application. *Energy Environ. Sci.* 2011;4:3565.

Yamauchi Y., Kuroda K. Rational design of mesoporous metals and related nanomaterials by a soft-template approach. *Chem. Asian J.* 2008;3:664–676.

Yi S., Dai F., Zhao C., Si, Y. A reverse micelle strategy for fabricating magnetic lipase-immobilized nanoparticles with robust enzymatic activity. *Sci. Rep.* 2017;7:9806.

Zhang K., Fu Q., Pan N., Yu X., Liu J., Luo Y., Wang X., Yang J., Hou J. Direct writing of electronic devices on graphene oxide by catalytic scanning probe lithography. *Nat. Commun.* 2012;3:1–6. Doi: 10.1038/ncomms2200.

Zhao C., Liu Q., Cheung K.M., Liu W., Yang Q., Xu X., Man T., Weiss P.S., Zhou C., Andrews A.M. Narrower nanoribbon biosensors fabricated by chemical lift-off lithography show higher sensitivity. *ACS Nano.* 2020;15:904–915. Doi: 10.1021/acsnano.0c07503.

Znaidi L. Sol–gel-deposited ZnO thin films: A review. *Mater. Sci. Eng. B.* 2010;174:18–30. CrossRef CAS.

3 Synthesis of Materials by Using Green Technology or Biological Approaches

Firdos Alam Khan

3.1 INTRODUCTION

There have been emerging trends in the global market for various applications of nanomaterials, and it has been reported by economic analysts that the growth of nanomaterials will increase in the coming years. There are various types of nanomaterials that have been produced with different applications, but the production of nanoparticles (NPs) showed the most promising results (Inshakova and Inshakov, 2017; Barhoum et al., 2022). There are different types of NPs that are synthesized for a variety of applications, such as in the production for aerospace, automotive industries, food packaging, sporting goods, textiles, cosmetics, electronics, and information technology products. Bearing in mind the current progress in research, there has been use of NPs for biomedical applications (Yadid et al., 2019; Ahmeda et al., 2020; Materón et al., 2021) and agricultural (Hofmann et al., 2020; Šebesta et al., 2021) products. NPs are showing enormous prospects in the global market, and global demand for NPs is increasing also in developing countries (Salamanca-Buentello et al., 2005). In spite of many beneficial applications of NPs in biomedical applications, there are a few potentially harmful effects associated with nanomaterials that pose serious prospects in clinical and animal applications (Tang et al., 2015). Notwithstanding the sign that NPs might be harmful, there is still wide-scale production of various nanomaterials for various applications, especially in industrial-scale production. There are different types of nanomaterial production, but in the conventional synthesis method, physical and chemical methods, are used, where a large amount of energy is needed, and this method also generates chemical pollution (Jamkhande et al., 2019). The application of the biological or green synthesis method appears to be a better option than synthetic, where NPs are produced with less level of pollution and a more economical method. The green synthesis method is eco-friendly and cost-effective, with low energy consumption in comparison with the conventional methods (Jamkhande et al., 2019; Parveen et al., 2016). In the green synthesis of NPs, mostly living organisms are used, which are plants and microorganisms that are generally accessible and economical. Furthermore, the application of biomass waste has also

DOI: 10.1201/9781003317715-3

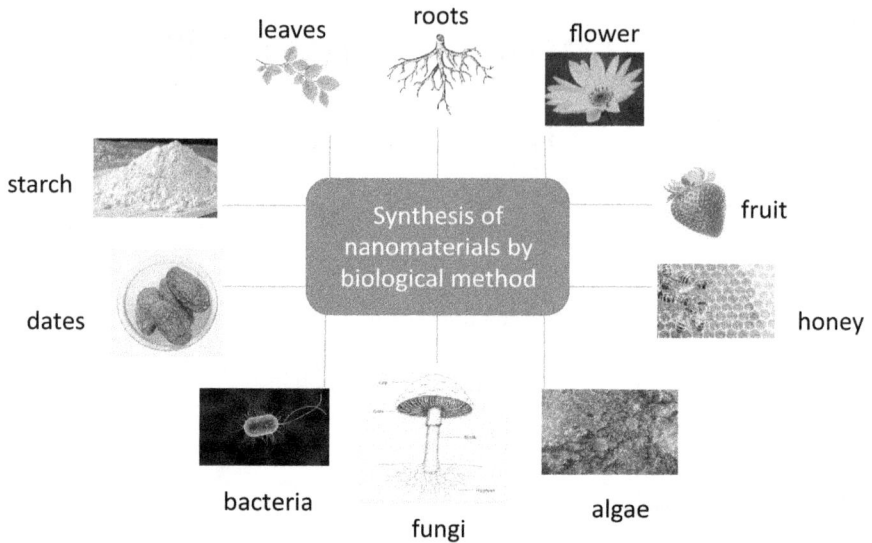

FIGURE 3.1   Application of different natural products in the synthesis of nanomaterials.

been used in NP synthesis by using green synthesis (Figure 3.1). There is also the use of bio-based compounds to coat the surface of NPs during the green synthesis process (Javed et al., 2020). Consequently, this additional layer of coating helps to enhance the biological properties of NPs compared to those that are produced by using chemical reactions. Furthermore, the involvement of bio-based compounds averts the contamination of NPs with toxic by-products, as these by-products can be hazardous compounds that ascribe to the NPs during the physical and chemical synthesis (Samuel et al., 2022). Nevertheless, one of the reasons that green synthesis has remained in the research stage is that there are various parameters, such as the composition of biological reducing agents, the concentration of initial precursor salts, speed of agitation, reaction time, pH, and temperature. These parameters generally induce inconsistency during production. Hence, the optimization of biological methods is a complex process that needs to be validated and automated for industrial-level production of NPs. In addition, the application of living organisms in NP production makes it difficult to replicate the process, as the living organisms may generate a different growth profile under varied culture conditions.

3.2   SIGNIFICANCE OF GREEN SYNTHESIS

There are three ways in which living organisms can be used to produce NPs: (1) intracellular synthesis, (2) extracellular synthesis, and (3) the use of specific biochemicals for the production of NPs. The endogenous synthesis process is primarily the application of different types of organisms to extract metals from the growing culture medium and hyper-accumulate them. Different types of microorganisms and plants are used in biomining applications to remove commercially viable metals from the soil or land, where conventional methods of mining would not have been very effective and economical (Tognacchini et al., 2020; Yan et al., 2020). Research studies have suggested that due to the bio-accumulation mechanism, plants can easily retain metals in the form of nanoparticles (Abdallah et al., 2020). The synthesis happens inside the cell cytosol, and also due to its high reductive ability, several types of cellular enzymes and biomolecules generally take part in the synthesis process. It has been reported that the application of living cells of the *Chlamydomonas reinhardtii* microalga has been used to obtain silver-gold NPs. It was shown that the addition of silver and gold salts to the algal culture resulted in cell sedimentation because of the internalization of the metallic ions in the cytoplasm of plant cells. Therefore, the reduction process in this situation happens intra-cellularly, and the synthesized NPs are then released into the extra-cellular matrix of the plant cell. Finally, for the stability of silver-gold NPs, it is very important that the extracellular matrix, which is rich in polysaccharides, covers the NP surface (Dahoumane et al., 2014).

Furthermore, phyto-mined metals are usually extracted by the biomass combustion method, followed by the sintering or smelting process. Nevertheless, these methods are unsuitable because of the extreme temperature and pressure used in these cases, and these extreme temperatures and pressure may cause a negative effect to maintain the nano size of the metallic NPs (Sheoran et al., 2013; Akinbile et al., 2021). Owing to maintaining the structure and properties of NPs, there are other methods developed that are mild in action. For example, it has been shown that a difference was introduced based on the filtration and centrifugation steps. During this process, plant materials were ground and mixed with SDS (1%), and the resulting mixture was filtrated. Thereafter, extracts were centrifuged, and the pellet was obtained, which was later subjected to a lyophilization process. Lastly, ultra-centrifugation in sucrose density gradients was performed to separate NPs from the plant materials (Abdallah et al., 2020). Moreover, a method of enzymatic digestion was proposed to able to get concentrated gold NPs intracellularly, which were accumulated into *Brassica juncea*. Hence, 1-β-endoglucanase from *Trichoderma viridae* was used to solubilize the plant biomass for attaining NPs at a suitable concentration that is appropriate for the catalytic reaction. Nonetheless, it was reported that only 55% to 60% of the biomass can be converted into a soluble form. The size of the NPs was maintained even though NPs were not purified by enzymatic treatment (Marshall et al., 2007). Additionally, the separation of NPs from cells is not constantly essential when an endogenous synthesis is accomplished for catalytic purposes (Zhu et al., 2016; Stephen et al., 2019).

The synthesis of NPs by the intracellular method has some limitations, which make it inappropriate for industrial-level application. The morphology of the NPs is difficult to control, and there are also complications concerning the effectiveness of extraction, isolation, and purification of NPs (Pantidos, 2014). These issues can be resolved by using an in vitro approach, where the synthesis of NPs by using green synthesis is broadly based on the presence of internal biomolecules in the plant cells to act as reducing agents and capping agents. Additionally, the method of in vitro basically involves plant extracts containing the total biocomposition of the organism that was used. Moreover, this method of NPs synthesis was also performed by using a single biomolecule, like quercetin (Tasca and Antiochia, 2020), resveratrol (Thipe et al., 2019), or curcumin (Khan et al., 2019).

It has been reported that living plants release certain biomolecules into the environment in response to metal stress, and the exogenous synthesis of NPs utilizes the secondary metabolites released by plants to chelate metallic ions. These biomolecules are secreted by the plants to decrease the toxicity produced by the metallic ions, and these biomolecules then converted them into less toxic nanoparticles. For example, it was reported that gold NPs were produced when parts of germinated seeds and roots of seedlings of *Vigna unguiculata* were submerged in different concentrations of chloroauric acid. Additionally, during plant seed germination and the early development of plant seedlings, there are reports of phenolic compounds that might explain the existence of the NPs (Shabnam et al., 2014). Likewise, silver NPs have been produced when peanut (*Arachis hypogaea*) seedlings' roots were treated with silver nitrate (Raju et al., 2014). Interestingly, these are methods of NP synthesis for industrial-level production (Basavegowda and Lee, 2014; Valdez-Salas et al., 2020).

3.3 ORGANISMS USED IN BIOLOGICALLY SYNTHESIZED NANOMATERIALS

3.3.1 BACTERIA

To be able to produce metallic and metal oxide NPs, different bacterial species have been used. There are several studies that have been performed where different bacterial strains of *Aeromonas, Bacillus, Desulfovibrio, Enterobacter, Escherichia, Klebsiella, Lactobacillus, Pseudomonas, Rhodobacter, Rhodopseudomonas, Shewanella, Ureibacillus,* or *Weissella* have been used to produce NPs (Li et al., 2011). There are other types of bacterial strains that are isolated, which are *Alcaligenes, Alteromonas, Ochrobactrum,* and *Stenotrophomonas* (Gahlawat and Choudhury, 2019). Furthermore, different species of *Bacillus,* such as *B. subtilis, B. pumilus, B. persicus,* and *B. licheniformis,* have been used widely to harvest silver or gold NPs (Elbeshehy et al., 2015; Jain and Chauhan, 2017). In addition, *B. amyloliquefaciens* has been used for the synthesis of cadmium sulfide NPs (Singh et al., 2011) (Figure 3.2). There are still no well-studied phenomena to know how many different types of metallic ions can be produced by a bacterial cell. There are a few bacterial strains that are involved in the production of only one or a few types of NP, while other strains can mediate the formation of many more types of NPs. For example, *Pseudomonas aeruginosa* can synthesize seven types of NPs by extracellular method, and they are

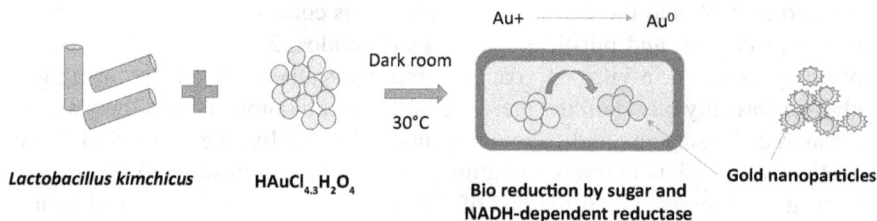

FIGURE 3.2 Green synthesis of gold nanoparticles using bacteria.

silver, palladium, iron, nickel, platinum, rhodium, and ruthenium, respectively. This *Pseudomonas aeruginosa* can also produce a large volume of cobalt and lithium particles by using intracellular methods (Srivastava and Sivashanmugam, 2020).

It has been found that most of the bacterial strains that are involved in the synthesis of NPs are terrestrial organisms. There is a report on the use of reference strains and other types of bacteria to enhance the ability to bioleach metals and bioaccumulate metals. Nevertheless, recently, there has been a report of the application of marine bacterial cultures in the synthesis of silver, gold, copper, and cadmium sulfide NPs (Gahlawat and Choudhury, 2019). Additionally, the extracellular polymeric substances (EPS) extracted from a marine strain of *P. aeruginosa* were effectively used to produce cadmium sulfide NPs. Interestingly, the sulfhydryl functional groups of the EPS play a major role in the mechanism of NP formation, as they signify binding locations for metallic ions (Raj et al., 2015). Interestingly, genetic manipulation is an easy and simple method in bacterial cells compared to animal and human cells. Bacterial genetic materials have already been applied in creating transgenic cells to be able to generate NPs. Consequently, the *mms6* gene, which contributes to the formation of magnetosome in *Magnetospirillum magneticum* bacteria, was inserted in human mesenchymal stem cells, and the intracellular formation of iron NPs with magnetic properties was revealed. NPs with sizes between 10 and 500 nm were accumulated in vacuoles of the cells (Elfick et al., 2017).

3.3.2 MICRO-FUNGI AND ACTINOMYCETES

Recently, there has been growing interest in the application of many fungal strains in their ability to reduce metallic ions. It has been reported that many different fungal species, such as *Aspergillus, Cladosporium, Colletotrichum, Fusarium, Penicillium, Phoma, Trichoderma*, and *Trichothecium* (Narayanan and Sakthivel, 2010), are used in NP synthesis. There are also reports of using ascomycetes of the *Brevibacterium, Corynebacterium, Kocuria*, and *Neurospora* genera (Li et al., 2011) in NP synthesis. Additionally, the cluster of fungi that yield NPs is accomplished by some actinomycetes (mycelial bacteria), as they share some features with prokaryotes. Interestingly, NPs synthesized by actinomycete-mediated approaches are considered to be stable, with good poly-disperse distribution and high bactericidal activity. Nevertheless, the potential application of actinomycetes that are involved in NP production has not been explored at a high capability. Many microorganisms have been used widely in the biosynthesis of silver and gold NPs, whereas a few of them have been applied in the synthesis of zinc and some bimetallic NPs. The most studied actinomycetes are *Nocardia, Nocardiopsis, Rhodococcus, Streptomyces*, and *Thermoactinomyces* in the NPs synthesis (Golinska et al., 2014).

3.3.3 YEASTS

The application of yeasts in NP synthesis has been extensively used, especially in the production of cadmium sulfide or lead sulfide NPs. Nonetheless, yeasts have also been used in the synthesis of gold, titanium dioxide, antimony trioxide (Sb_2O_3), or other NPs (Hulkoti and Taranath, 2014). Silver NPs have been produced by using different *Candida* strains, such as *C. albicans*, *C. glabrata*, *C. lusitaniae*, and *C. utilis* (Gahlawat and Choudhury, 2019). There is an application of yeast-mediated synthesis of different types of NPs, and they are *Pichia jadinii*, *Saccharomyces cerevisiae*, *Schizosaccharomyces pombe*, or *Yarrowia lipolytica* (Narayanan and Sakthivel, 2010). Other yeasts, such as the *Cryptococcus*, *Magnusiomyces*, *Phaffia*, *Rhodosporidium*, and *Rhodotorula* genera, have been applied in NP synthesis (Gahlawat and Choudhury, 2019).

3.3.4 MICRO-ALGAE AND CYANOBACTERIA

Micro-algae have been applied in many biomedical applications, especially in the removal of nutrients, organic carbon, and heavy metals from wastewater. In addition, these micro-algae have potential applications in the manufacturing of biofuels (Khan et al., 2018; Jacob et al., 2021). There are many advantages of micro-algal cultures, especially in the green synthesis of NPs, and some of the benefits are that these micro-algae have a high tolerance to metallic ions (Danouche et al., 2020) and also have a high growth rate and efficiency in producing different biomolecules (Mehariya et al., 2021). The application of micro-algal has led to greater consideration in nano-biotechnological research and development. Among different micro-algae, the use of *Chlorella vulgaris* seems to be the most studied micro-alga for its ability to reduce metal ions, and this has been involved in the green synthesis of many types of NPs (Gahlawat and Choudhury, 2019; Arsiya et al., 2017). There are other *Chlorella* species, such as *C. pyrenoidosa* and *C. kessleri*, which have also been proved to be effective as nanofactories in the synthesis of silver and copper NPs (Patel et al., 2015; Kusumaningrum et al., 2018; Salas-Herrera et al., 2019).

In addition, there is also the use of different types of micro-algae, such as *Botryococcus* sp., *Chlamydomonas* sp., *Coelastrum* sp., *Scenedesmus* sp., *Neochloris oleoabundans*, *Galdieria* sp., *Dunaliella tertiolecta*, or *Tetraselmis suecica*, in the metallic NP synthesis (Jacob et al., 2021; Patel et al., 2015). The diatoms signify a group of uni-cellular algae distinguishable by micro- and nano-patterned siliceous cell walls, and these structures are formed by the deposition of silica, bio-generated from ortho-silicic acid, which is taken up from the environment (Kröger and Poulsen, 2008). There are different species of diatoms that are extensively used in gold NP synthesis, such as *Stephanopyxis turris* (Pytlik et al., 2017), *Amphora copulate* (Roychoudhury et al., 2016), *Navicula atomus* (Schröfel et al., 2011), and *Diadesmis gallica* (Fischer et al., 2016). In addition, *Navicula* sp. (Chetia et al., 2017), *Chaetoceros* sp., *Skeletonema* sp., and *Thalassiosira* sp. (Mishra et al., 2020) have been used for the production of silver nanomaterials. As diatoms acquire unique features of a 3D structure, they are also used as scaffolds for the anchoring of metallic NPs, biosilica-based nanocomposites for drug delivery (Briceno et al., 2021), biosensing (Chen et al., 2022), and catalysis (Fischer et al., 2016) purposes. Cyanobacteria represent a large taxonomic group containing photosynthetic organisms, and these microorganisms are found to be most suitable for the biological synthesis of nanoparticles. There are many nanotechnological potentials that are still not well explored, as current studies are focused on cyanobacteria-mediated NP synthesis. The ability to reduce metallic ions was found in different cyanobacterial species, such as *Anabaena*,

Cylindrospermopsis, Limnothrix, Lyngbya, Synechococcus, Synechocystis, and *Arthrospira* genera, respectively (Patel et al., 2015; Zayadi and Bakar, 2020).

3.3.5 Plants

There are several plants that are known to accumulate heavy metals from contaminated water or environments. It has been reported that some plants have phyto-mining potential, and it was found that plants can store metals in the nanoparticles inside plant cells. It has been reported that different plants, such as *Sesbania drummondii, Ipomoea lacunosa, Festuca rubra*, and *Arabidopsis thaliana*, are applied in NP synthesis. *Medicago sativa* is the most studied plant species for the production of NPs, which is followed by *Brassica juncea*, and these species have been applied in the synthesis of silver, gold, copper, and platinum NPs (Mohammadinejad et al., 2019). Additionally, there are many plant species with phyto-mining potentials that have not been used in nanoparticles production, such as *Acanthopanax sciadophylloides, Maytenus founieri*, and *Clethra barbinervis* (Mohammadinejad et al., 2019; Iravani, 2011).

The NPs are synthesized by using plant extracts, and plants that belong to the angiosperm taxonomic group are most widely used in nanoparticle production. The diversity of plant extracts that have been applied so far in NP synthesis is remarkably high. For example, extracts from more than 30 different plant species have been used only for the synthesis of titanium dioxide NPs (Miu and Dinischiotu, 2021; Miu and Dinischiotu, 2022). It appears that plants having medicinal properties show a higher preference, as these plants contain different biomolecules that possess biomedical potentials that can be used for NP production through the capping method. It has been reported in many studies that certain medicinal plants can produce various types of NPs, especially silver or zinc oxide nanoparticles. The biological application of these green-synthesized NPs has also been examined, and it has been found that these NPs showed antibacterial activity in many studies, whereas a few studies have reported anticancer, antileishmania, antioxidant, or anticoagulant potentials. There are a few examples of medicinal plants that are used as nanofactories, such as *Prunella vulgaris, Suaeda maritima, Bauhinia acuminata, Taraxacum laevigatum*, and *Carum copticum* (Agarwal and Gayathri, 2017).

In addition to the medicinal plants, there are a few plants that are used as food that have the capability to produce NPs (Figure 3.3); for example, there are different types of fruit trees, such as the apple tree *(Malus domestica)*, orange tree *(Citrus sinensis)*, walnut tree *(Juglans regia)*, and peach tree *(Prunus persic)*, that have been applied in the synthesis of silver, titanium dioxide, zinc oxide, and iron oxide NPs, respectively (Mirza et al., 2018; Mobeen and Sundaram, 2019; Darvishi et al., 2019; Mariadoss et al., 2019). Iron oxide NPs can be produced from the plant beet, *Beta vulgaris*; pumpkin; and *Cucurbita moschata* extracts (De Lima Barizão et al., 2020). There are certain spice plants, like the rosemary, *Rosmarinus officinalis*, and ginger, *Zingiber officinale*, that have been used to synthesize iron-containing NPs and copper-containing bimetallic NPs (Farshchi et al., 2018; Ismail et al., 2018). There are several angiosperms, like *Eichhornia crassipes* and *Linaria maroccana*, with no precise significance to human beings that have been shown to be effective as intermediaries for NP production (Prabhakar et al., 2017; Garmanchuk et al., 2019).

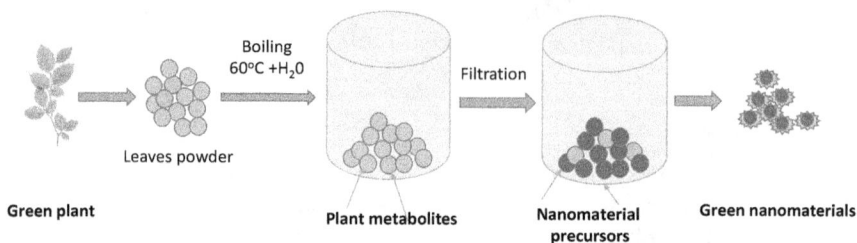

FIGURE 3.3 Procedure of synthesis of green nanomaterials using plant leaves.

Furthermore, other parts of the plant, such as gymnosperms, pteridophytes (also known as ferns), bryophytes (mosses), and macroalgae that have been reported to possess the ability to mediate the production of NPs. These plant parts can be used to produce silver NPs, gold NPs, platinum NPs, and palladium NPs. There have been growing trends in the utilization of these plant organisms for NP production; the use of gymnosperms showed the most promising candidates for the green synthesis of NPs, and also, *Cycas circinalis, Ginkgo biloba, Pinus, Thuja orientalis*, and *Torreya nucifera* have shown potential application in NP production. With regard to pteridophytic plants, there are at least different genera, such as *Adiantum, Pteris*, and *Nephrolepis*, that have shown great potential in NP production. In addition, there are a few methods that have been recently developed to produce silver NPs by using extracts from the plant *Anthoceros* species, *Riccia* species, or *Fissidens minutus*. It has been reported that, compared to the mosses and ferns, the macro-algae are better exemplified in nanotechnological research. The production of green synthesis of NPs can be achieved by using *capillacea, Jania rubens, Ulva fasciata, Colpomenia sinuosa, Pterocladia Ulva intestinalis*, and different species of *Sargassum* (Das et al., 2017).

3.4 FACTORS INFLUENCING GREEN NANOMATERIALS

There are several factors influencing the production of NPs, as it has been reported that increasing the concentration of the reducing agent normally increases the production of NPs. Therefore, highly concentrated biological extracts can help to produce larger-sized NPs, as it has been shown that increasing the concentration of fungal filtrate of *Trichoderma viride* from 10% to 100 % increased the size of gold NPs by almost six times (Kumari et al., 2016). Similarly, it has been found that silver NPs, with different concentrations of *Plantago major* extracts, showed larger nanoparticles sizes (Sukweenadhi et al., 2021). It has been suggested that the increased size of NPs could be due to a secondary reduction process that occurs on the metal nuclei; because of the surplus of reducing phytochemicals observed, surpassing a concentration of 20% of *Azadirachta indica* plant extract causes the agglomeration of copper NPs; thus, larger structures are formed. Nevertheless, a little reductant concentration does not provide sufficient biomolecules to start the conversion of ions (Nagar and Devra, 2018). Though a low level of biomolecules might be adequate to activate the reduction step for the aggregation and precipitation of nanoparticles and precipitation, they can be quickly exhausted by the metallic ions in the capping process (Yuan et al., 2017). In contrast, a disproportionate amount of biochemicals can impair the nucleation step (Satpathy et al., 2019).

It has been reported that the reducing power of biologically derived extracts is linked to their composition as well as the amount of biochemicals. Therefore, the solvent used for obtaining the extract can influence the production of NPs. It has been recently shown that the average size of silver NPs can reach 20 nm by using the ethanol-based extract of *Acacia cyanophylla*. In contrast, with the aqueous-based extract, NPs can be produced with an average size of around 87 nm (Jalab et al., 2021). The difference between ethanol and aqueous extract may be due to polarity, as ethanol is less polar than water, and the biomolecules are anticipated to be more concentrated and also diverse in the ethanol-based extracts compared with the aqueous-based ones. The diversity and higher content of biomolecules in the ethanol-based extracts derived from different plants were also established experimentally (Cieniak et al., 2015; Atu et al., 2022). The production of palladium NPs using a methanol-based extract of *Eryngium caeruleum* have taken 60 minutes, whereas it took 100 minutes in the ethanol-based extract–mediated synthesis (Saleh et al., 2021).

The biomolecules that are used in the production of NPs may differ based on the organism used for their extraction. Nonetheless, this is not binding for the biomolecule precursors, which are basically salts containing the ion of interest. It has been reported that a decrease in the average size of NPs is proportional to the increase in the concentration of precursors (Rao and Tang, 2017). Once the precursor amount is high, additional nuclei are formed, and the capping agents operate rapidly to stabilize them. Nevertheless, when the concentration of the precursor is too high, the level of phytochemicals becomes insufficient to stabilize a large number of nuclei. Consequently, the larger NPs are shaped due to the accumulation of nuclei. It is shown that increasing the concentration of copper chloride by 7.5 mM can decrease the NP size to almost 45 nm (Nagar and Devra, 2018). Similarly, the increase of silver nitrate amount in the reaction mixture leads to the formation of larger silver NPs, as shown by spectroscopic analyses (Rao and Tang, 2017; Kumar et al., 2016). Comparable results were achieved for gold NP synthesis as well, where the application of chloroauric acid mixed with *T. viride* fungal extract showed that the growth of nanoparticles is promoted by a high precursor concentration. It was reported that when a reaction was done at 30°C, with a concentration of 250 mg/L chloroauric acid, the average size of the gold NPs was 34 nm, whereas at 500 mg/L chloroauric acid, the NPs were 85.2 nm in size. Interestingly, at 50°C and with the same concentrations, the size of gold nanoparticles increased by about 150%, showing that the metal salt concentration works together with other reaction parameters to mediate the size of NPs (Kumari et al., 2016).

Consequently, the characteristics of NPs produced through the green synthesis method appear to be better when using proper precursors. Nevertheless, the information regarding the effect of different precursor salts on green NP features is inadequate. It was reported that ZnO nanospheres with a diameter of about 107 nm have been achieved when zinc acetate and *Anacardium occidentale* leaf extract were mixed. The use of zinc chloride has led to the synthesis of ZnO nanorods that were 167 nm in length and 68 nm in width. Nevertheless, both samples faced aggregation (Droepenu et al., 2021). The ZnO NPs synthesized from zinc sulfate had a nanorod morphology and an average size of 30 nm when *Justicia adhatoda* leaf extract was used. Inversely, the NPs achieved by the same method, but starting from zinc nitrate or zinc acetate, were cubic and 15–20 nm in size. Furthermore, their inclination to form agglomerates was detected. Amusingly, the use of different precursors can have an influence also on the biological activity of NPs. The antimicrobial activity of ZnO NPs achieved from zinc nitrate was more noticeable against bacterial strains, whereas the ones produced using zinc sulfate were well-organized against dissimilar strains of *Aspergillus* (Pachaiappan et al., 2021). The effect of different precursors on ZnO NP morphology was also established by using *Laurus nobilis* leaf extract as a reducing agent (Fakhari et al., 2019). It was discovered that the effect of different precursors on the shape of iron (III) oxide particles using synthetic reagents as cubic and octahedral nanoparticles were formed from ferrous sulfate, solubilized in ethylene glycol, and capped with potassium hydroxide. In contrast, spherical nanoparticles happened when ferric chloride was used instead (Fatima et al., 2018).

REFERENCES

Abdallah B.B., Zhang X., Andreu I., Gates B.D., El Mokni R., Rubino S., Landoulsi A., Chatti A. Differentiation of nanoparticles isolated from distinct plant species naturally growing in a heavy metal polluted site. *J. Hazard. Mater.* 2020;386:121644. Doi: 10.1016/j.jhazmat.2019.121644.

Agarwal H., Gayathri M. Biological synthesis of nanoparticles from medicinal plants and its uses in inhibiting biofilm formation. *Asian, J. Pharm. Clin. Res.* 2017;10:64–68. Doi: 10.22159/ajpcr.2017.v10i5.17469.

Ahmeda A., Zangeneh A., Zangeneh M.M. Green synthesis and chemical characterization of gold nanoparticle synthesized using *Camellia sinensis* leaf aqueous extract for the treatment of acute myeloid leukemia in comparison to daunorubicin in a leukemic mouse model. *App. Organomet. Chem.* 2020;34:e5290. Doi: 10.1002/aoc.5290.

Akinbile B.J., Makhubela B.C.E., Ambushe A.A. Phytomining of valuable metals: Status and prospective-a review. *Int. J. Environ. Anal. Chem.* 2021;2021:1–21. Doi: 10.1080/03067319.2021.1917557.

Arsiya F., Sayadi M.H., Sobhani S. Green synthesis of palladium nanoparticles using *Chlorella vulgaris*. *Mater. Lett.* 2017;186:113–115. Doi: 10.1016/j.matlet.2016.09.101.

Atu S., Pertiw K.R., Qolbia M., Saf S. Phytochemical analysis both of water and ethanol extract from some herbs combinations, nanoemulsion formulation, and antioxidant effects. *Open Access Maced. J. Med. Sci.* 2022;10:95–100. Doi: 10.3889/oamjms.2022.7886.

Barhoum A., García-Betancourt M.L., Jeevanandam J., Hussien E.A., Mekkawy S.A., Mostafa M., Omran M.M., Abdalla M.S., Bechelany M. Review on natural, incidental, bioinspired, and engineered nanomaterials: History, definitions, classifications, synthesis, properties, market, toxicities, risks, and regulations. *Nanomaterials.* 2022;12:177. Doi: 10.3390/nano12020177.

Basavegowda N., Lee Y.R. Synthesis of gold and silver nanoparticles using leaf extract of *Perilla frutescens*—A biogenic approach. *J. Nanosci. Nanotechnol.* 2014;14:4377–4382. Doi: 10.1166/jnn.2014.8646.

Briceno S., Chavez-Chico E.A., Gonzalez G. Diatoms decorated with gold nanoparticles by *In-situ* and *Ex-situ* methods for in vitro gentamicin release. *Mater. Sci. Eng. C.* 2021;123:112018. Doi: 10.1016/j.msec.2021.112018.

Chen T., Wu F., Li Y., Rozan H.E., Chen X., Feng C. Gold nanoparticle-functionalized diatom biosilica as label-free biosensor for biomolecule detection. *Front. Bioeng. Biotechnol.* 2022;10:894636. Doi: 10.3389/fbioe.2022.894636.

Chetia L., Kalita D., Ahmed G.A. Synthesis of Ag nanoparticles using diatom cells for ammonia sensing. *Sens. Bio-Sens. Res.* 2017;16:55–61. Doi: 10.1016/j.sbsr.2017.11.004.

Cieniak C., Walshe-Roussel B., Liu R., Muhammad A., Saleem A., Haddad P.S., Cuerrier A., Foster B.C., Arnason J.T. Phytochemical comparison of the water and ethanol leaf extracts of the Cree medicinal plant, *Sarracenia purpurea* L. (Sarraceniaceae) *J. Pharm. Pharm. Sci.* 2015;18:484–493. Doi: 10.18433/J35W27.

Dahoumane S.A., Wijesekera K., Filipe C.D.M., Brennan J.D. Stoichiometrically controlled production of bimetallic gold-silver alloy colloids using micro-alga cultures. *J. Colloid Interface Sci.* 2014;416:67–72. Doi: 10.1016/j.jcis.2013.10.048.

Danouche M., El Ghachtouli N., El Baouchi A., El Arroussi H. Heavy metals phycoremediation using tolerant green microalgae: Enzymatic and non-enzymatic antioxidant systems for the management of oxidative stress. *J. Environ. Chem. Eng.* 2020;8:104460. Doi: 10.1016/j.jece.2020.104460.

Darvishi E., Kahrizi D., Arkan E. Comparison of different properties of zinc oxide nanoparticles synthesized by the green (using *Juglans regia* L. leaf extract) and chemical methods. *J. Mol. Liq.* 2019;286:110831. Doi: 10.1016/j.molliq.2019.04.108.

Das R.K., Pachapur V.L., Lonappan L., Naghdi M., Pulicharla R., Maiti S., Cledon M., Dalila L.M.A., Sarma S.J., Brar S.K. Biological synthesis of metallic nanoparticles: Plants, animals and microbial aspects. *Nanotechnol. Environ. Eng.* 2017;2:18. Doi: 10.1007/s41204-017-0029-4.

De Lima Barizão A.C., Silva M.F., Andrade M., Brito F.C., Gomes R.G., Bergamasco R. Green synthesis of iron oxide nanoparticles for tartrazine and bordeaux red dye removal. *J. Environ. Chem. Eng.* 2020;8:103618. Doi: 10.1016/j.jece.2019.103618.

Droepenu E.K., Asare E.A., Wee B.S., Wahi R.B., Ayertey F., Kyene M.O. Biosynthesis, characterization, and antibacterial activity of ZnO nanoaggregates using aqueous extract from *Anacardium occidentale* leaf: Comparative study of different precursors. *Beni-Suef Univ. J. Basic Appl. Sci.* 2021;10:1. Doi: 10.1186/s43088-020-00091-7.

Elbeshehy E.K., Elazzazy A.M., Aggelis G. Silver nanoparticles synthesis mediated by new isolates of Bacillus spp., nanoparticle characterization and their activity against Bean Yellow Mosaic Virus and human pathogens. *Front Microbiol.* 2015 May 13;6:453. doi: 10.3389/fmicb.2015.00453. PMID: 26029190; PMCID: PMC4429621

Elfick A., Rischitor G., Mouras R., Azfer A., Lungaro L., Uhlarz M., Herrmannsdorfer T., Lucocq J., Gamal W., Bagnaninchi P. et al. Biosynthesis of magnetic nanoparticles by human mesenchymal stem cells following transfection with the magnetotactic bacterial gene *mms6*. *Sci. Rep.* 2017;7:39755. Doi: 10.1038/srep39755.

Fakhari S., Jamzad M., Fard H.K. Green synthesis of zinc oxide nanoparticles: A comparison. *Green Chem. Lett. Rev.* 2019;12:19–24. Doi: 10.1080/17518253.2018.1547925.

Farshchi H.K., Azizi M., Jaafari M.R., Nemati S.H., Fotovat A. Green synthesis of iron nanoparticles by Rosemary extract and cytotoxicity effect evaluation on cancer cell lines. *Biocatal. Agric. Biotechnol.* 2018;16:54–62. Doi: 10.1016/j.bcab.2018.07.017.

Fatima H., Lee D.W., Yun H.J., Kim K.S. Shape-controlled synthesis of magnetic Fe_3O_4 nanoparticles with different iron precursors and capping agents. *RSC Adv.* 2018;8:22917. Doi: 10.1039/C8RA02909A.

Fischer C., Adam M., Mueller A.C., Sperling E., Wustmann M., van Pee K.H., Kaskel S., Brunner E. Gold nanoparticle-decorated diatom biosilica: A favorable catalyst for the oxidation of D-glucose. *ACS Omega.* 2016;1:1253–1261. Doi: 10.1021/acsomega.6b00406.

Gahlawat G., Choudhury A.R. A review on the biosynthesis of metal and metal salt nanoparticles by microbes. *RSC Adv.* 2019;9:12944–12967. Doi: 10.1039/C8RA10483B.

Garmanchuk L.V., Borovaya M.N., Nehelia A.O., Inomistova M., Khranovska N.M., Tolstanova G.M., Blume Y.B., Yemets A.I. CdS quantum dots obtained by "green" synthesis: Comparative analysis of toxicity and effects on the proliferative and adhesive activity of human cells. *Cytol. Genet.* 2019;53:132–142. Doi: 10.3103/S0095452719020026.

Golinska P., Wypij M., Ingle A.P., Gupta I., Dahm H., Rai M. Biogenic synthesis of metal nanoparticles from actinomycetes: Biomedical applications and cytotoxicity. *Appl. Microbiol. Biotechnol.* 2014;98:8083–8097. Doi: 10.1007/s00253-014-5953-7.

Hofmann T., Lowry G.V., Ghoshal S., Tufenkji N., Brambilla D., Dutcher J.R., Gilbertson L.M., Giraldo J.P., Kinsella J.M., Landry M.P. et al. Technology readiness and overcoming barriers to sustainably implement nanotechnology-enabled plant agriculture. *Nat. Food.* 2020;1:416–425. Doi: 10.1038/s43016-020-0110-1.

Hulkoti N.I., Taranath T.C. Biosynthesis of nanoparticles using microbes—a review. *Colloids Surf. B Biointerfaces.* 2014;121:474–483. Doi: 10.1016/j.colsurfb.2014.05.027.

Inshakova E., Inshakov O. *MATEC Web of Conferences.* Volume 129. EDP Sciences, Les Ulis, France, 2017; p. 02013. World Market for Nanomaterials: Structure and Trends.

Iravani S. Green synthesis of metal nanoparticles using plants. *Green Chem.* 2011;13:2638–2650. Doi: 10.1039/c1gc15386b.

Ismail M., Khan M.I., Khan S.B., Khan M.A., Akhtar K., Asiri A.M. Green synthesis of plant supported Cu–Ag and Cu–Ni bimetallic nanoparticles in the reduction of nitrophenols and organic dyes for water treatment. *J. Mol. Liq.* 2018;260:78–91. Doi: 10.1016/j.molliq.2018.03.058.

Jacob J.M., Ravindran R., Narayanan M., Samuel S.M., Pugazhendhi A., Kumar G. Microalgae: A prospective low cost green alternative for nanoparticle synthesis. *Curr. Opin. Environ. Sci. Health.* 2021;20:100163. Doi: 10.1016/j.coesh.2019.12.005.

Jain U., Chauhan N. Glycated hemoglobin detection with electrochemical sensing amplified by gold nanoparticles embedded N-doped graphene nanosheet. *Biosens Bioelectron.* 2017 Mar 15;89(Pt 1):578–584. doi: 10.1016/j.bios.2016.02.033. Epub 2016 Feb 12. PMID: 26897102.

Jalab J., Abdelwahed W., Kitaz A., Al-Kayali R. Green synthesis of silver nanoparticles using aqueous extract of *Acacia cyanophylla* and its antibacterial activity. *Heliyon.* 2021;7:e08033. Doi: 10.1016/j.heliyon.2021.e08033.

Jamkhande P.G., Ghule N.W., Bamer A.H., Kalaskar M.G. Metal nanoparticles synthesis: An overview on methods of preparation, advantages and disadvantages, and applications. *J. Drug Deliv. Sci. Technol.* 2019;53:101174. Doi: 10.1016/j.jddst.2019.101174.

Javed R., Zia M., Naz S., Aisida S.O., Ain N., Ao Q. Role of capping agents in the application of nanoparticles in biomedicine and environmental remediation: Recent trends and future prospects. *J. Nanobiotechnol.* 2020;18:172. Doi: 10.1186/s12951-020-00704-4.

Khan M.I., Shin J.H., Kim J.D. The promising future of microalgae: Current status, challenges, and optimization of a sustainable and renewable industry for biofuels, feed, and other products. *Microb. Cell Fact.* 2018;17:36. Doi: 10.1186/s12934-018-0879-x.

Khan M.J., Shameli K., Sazili A.Q., Selamat J., Kumari S. Rapid green synthesis and characterization of silver nanoparticles arbitrated by curcumin in an alkaline medium. *Molecules.* 2019;24:719. Doi: 10.3390/molecules24040719.

Kröger N., Poulsen N. Diatoms—From cell wall biogenesis to nanotechnology. *Annu. Rev. Genet.* 2008;42:83–107. Doi: 10.1146/annurev.genet.41.110306.130109.

Kumar V., Singh D.K., Mohan S., Hasan S.H. Photo-induced biosynthesis of silver nanoparticles using aqueous extract of *Erigeron bonariensis* and its catalytic activity against Acridine Orange. *J. Photochem. Photobiol. B Biol.* 2016;155:39–50. Doi: 10.1016/j.jphotobiol.2015.12.011.

Kumari M., Mishra A., Pandey S., Singh S.P., Chaudhry V., Mudiam M.K.R., Shukla S., Kakkar P., Nautiyal C.S. Physico-chemical condition optimization during biosynthesis lead to development of improved and catalytically efficient gold nano particles. *Sci. Rep.* 2016;6:27575. Doi: 10.1038/srep27575.

Kusumaningrum H.P., Zainuri M., Marhaendrajaya I., Subagio A. Nanosilver microalgae biosynthesis: Cell appearance based on SEM and EDX methods. *J. Phys. Conf. Ser.* 2018;1025:012084. Doi: 10.1088/1742-6596/1025/1/012084.

Li X., Xu H., Chen Z.S., Chen G. Biosynthesis of nanoparticles by microorganisms and their applications. *J. Nanomater.* 2011;2011:270974. Doi: 10.1155/2011/270974.

Mariadoss A.V.A., Vinayagam R., Vijayakumar S., Balupillai A., Jebaraj F., Kumar S., Ghidan A.Y., Al-Antary T.M., David E. Green synthesis, characterization and antibacterial activity of silver nanoparticles by *Malus domestica* and its cytotoxic effect on (MCF-7) cell line. *Microb. Pathog.* 2019;135:103609. Doi: 10.1016/j.micpath.2019.103609.

Marshall A.T., Haverkamp R.G., Davies C.E., Parsons J.G., Gardea-Torresdey J.L., van Agterveld D. Accumulation of gold nanoparticles in *Brassic juncea. Int. J. Phytoremediation.* 2007;9:197–206. Doi: 10.1080/15226510701376026.

Materón E.M., Miyazaki C.M., Carr O., Joshi N., Picciani P.H.S., Dalmaschio C.J., Davis F., Shimizu F.M. Magnetic nanoparticles in biomedical applications: A review. *Appl. Surf. Sci. Adv.* 2021;6:100163. Doi: 10.1016/j.apsadv.2021.100163.

Mehariya S., Goswami R.K., Karthikeysan O.P., Verma P. Microalgae for high-value products: A way towards green nutraceutical and pharmaceutical compounds. *Chemosphere.* 2021;280:130553. Doi: 10.1016/j.chemosphere.2021.130553.

Mirza A.U., Kareem A., Nami S.A.A., Khan M.S., Rehman S., Bhat S.A., Mohammad A., Nishat N. Biogenic synthesis of iron oxide nanoparticles using *Agrewia optiva* and *Prunus persica* phyto species: Characterization, antibacterial and antioxidant activity. *J. Photochem. Photobiol. B Biol.* 2018;185:262–274. Doi: 10.1016/j.jphotobiol.2018.06.009.

Mishra B., Saxena A., Tiwari A. Biosynthesis of silver nanoparticles from marine diatoms *Chaetoceros* sp., *Skeletonema* sp., *Thalassiosira* sp., and their antibacterial study. *Biotechnol. Rep.* 2020;28:e00571. Doi: 10.1016/j.btre.2020.e00571.

Miu B.A., Dinischiotu A. Green synthesized titanium dioxide nanoparticles and their future applications in biomedicine, agriculture and industry. *Rev. Biol. Biomed. Sci.* 2021;4:1–21. Doi: 10.31178/rbbs.2021.4.1.1.

Miu B.A., Dinischiotu A. New green approaches in nanoparticles synthesis: An overview. *Molecules.* 2022 Oct. 1;27(19):6472. Doi: 10.3390/molecules27196472. PMID: 36235008; PMCID: PMC9573382.

Mobeen Amanulla A., Sundaram R. Green synthesis of TiO_2 nanoparticles using orange peel extract for antibacterial, cytotoxicity and humidity sensor applications. *Mater. Today Proc.* 2019;8:323–331. Doi: 10.1016/j.matpr.2019.02.118.

Mohammadinejad R., Shavandi A., Raie D.S., Sangeetha J., Soleimani M., Hajibehzad S.S., Thangadurai D., Hospet R., Popoola J.O., Arzani A. et al. Plant molecular farming: Production of metallic nanoparticles and therapeutic proteins using green factories. *Green Chem.* 2019;21:1845–1865. Doi: 10.1039/C9GC00335E.

Nagar N., Devra V. Green synthesis and characterization of copper nanoparticles using *Azadirachta indica* leaves. *Mater. Chem. Phys.* 2018;213:44–51. Doi: 10.1016/j.matchemphys.2018.04.007.

Narayanan K.B., Sakthivel N. Biological synthesis of metal nanoparticles by microbes. *Adv. Colloid Interface. Sci.* 2010;156:1–13. Doi: 10.1016/j.cis.2010.02.001.

Pachaiappan R., Rajendran S., Ramalingam G., Vo D.V.N., Priya P.M., Soto-Moscoso M. Green synthesis of zinc oxide nanoparticles by *Justicia adhatoda* leaves and their antimicrobial activity. *Chem. Eng. Technol.* 2021;44:551–558. Doi: 10.1002/ceat.202000470.

Pantidos N. Biological synthesis of metallic nanoparticles by bacteria, fungi and plants. *J. Nanomed. Nanotechnol.* 2014;5:233. Doi: 10.4172/2157-7439.1000233.

Parveen K., Banse V., Ledwani L. Green synthesis of nanoparticles: Their advantages and disadvantages. *AIP Conf. Proc.* 2016;1724:020048. Doi: 10.1063/1.4945168.

Patel V., Berthold D., Puranik P., Gantar M. Screening of cyanobacteria and microalgae for their ability to synthesize silver nanoparticles with antibacterial activity. *Biotechnol. Rep.* 2015;5:112–119. Doi: 10.1016/j.btre.2014.12.001.

Prabhakar R., Samadder S.R., Jyotsana. Aquatic and terrestrial weed mediated synthesis of iron nanoparticles for possible application in wastewater remediation. *J. Clean. Prod.* 2017;168:1201–1210. Doi: 10.1016/j.jclepro.2017.09.063.

Pytlik N., Kaden J., Finger M., Naumann J., Wanke S., Machill S., Brunner E. Biological synthesis of gold nanoparticles by the diatom Stephanopyxis turris and in vivo SERS analyses. *Algal Res.* 2017;28:9–15. Doi: 10.1016/j.algal.2017.10.004.

Raj R., Dalei K., Chakraborty J., Das S. Extracellular polymeric substances of a marine bacterium mediated synthesis of CdS nanoparticles for removal of cadmium from aqueous solution. *J. Colloid Interface Sci.* 2016;462:166–175. Doi: 10.1016/j.jcis.2015.10.004.

Raju D., Paneliya N., Mehta U.J. Extracellular synthesis of silver nanoparticles using living peanut seedling. *Appl. Nanosci.* 2014;4:875–879. Doi: 10.1007/s13204-013-0269-y.

Rao B., Tang R.C. Green synthesis of silver nanoparticles with antibacterial activities using aqueous *Eriobotrya japonica* leaf extract. *Adv. Nat. Sci. Nanosci. Nanotechnol.* 2017;8:015014. Doi: 10.1088/2043-6254/aa5983.

Roychoudhury P., Nandi C., Pal R. Diatom-based biosynthesis of gold-silica nanocomposite and their DNA binding affinity. *J. Appl. Phycol.* 2016;28:2857–2863. Doi: 10.1007/s10811-016-0809-4.

Salamanca-Buentello F., Persad D.L., Court E.B., Martin D.K., Daar A.S., Singer P.A. Nanotechnology and the developing world. *PloS Med.* 2005;2:e97. Doi: 10.1371/journal.pmed.0020097.

Salas-Herrera G., González-Morales S., Benavides-Mendoza A., Castañeda-Facio A.O., Fernández-Luqueño F., Robledo-Olivo A. Impact of microalgae culture conditions over the capacity of copper nanoparticle biosynthesis. *J. Appl. Phycol.* 2019;31:2437–2447. Doi: 10.1007/s10811-019-1747-8.

Saleh E.A.M., Khan A.U., Tahir K., Almehmadi S.J., Al-Abdulkarim H.A., Alqarni S., Muhammad N., Dawsari A.M.A., Nazir S., Ullah A. Phytoassisted synthesis and characterization of palladium nanoparticles (Pd NPs); with enhanced antibacterial, antioxidant and hemolytic activities. *Photodiagnosis Photodyn. Ther.* 2021;36:102542. Doi: 10.1016/j.pdpdt.2021.102542.

Samuel M.S., Ravikumar M., John J.A., Selvarajan E., Patel H., Chander P.S., Soundarya J., Vuppala S., Balaji R., Chandrasekar N. A review on green synthesis of nanoparticles and their diverse biomedical and environmental applications. *Catalysts.* 2022;12:459. Doi: 10.3390/catal12050459.

Satpathy S., Patra A., Ahirwar B., Hussain M.D. Process optimization for green synthesis of gold nanoparticles mediated by extract of *Hygrophila spinosa* T. Anders and their biological applications. *Phys. E Low-Dimens. Syst. Nanostruct.* 2019;121:113830. Doi: 10.1016/j.physe.2019.113830.

Schröfel A., Kratošová G., Bohunická M., Dobročka E., Vávra I. Biosynthesis of gold nanoparticles using diatoms—Silica-gold and EPS-gold bionanocomposite formation. *J. Nanopart. Res.* 2011;13:3207–3216. Doi: 10.1007/s11051-011-0221-6.

Šebesta M., Kolenčík M., Sunil B.R., Illa R., Mosnáček J., Ingle A.P., Urík M. Field application of ZnO and TiO$_2$ nanoparticles on agricultural plants. *Agronomy.* 2021;11:2281. Doi: 10.3390/agronomy11112281.

Shabnam N., Pardha-Saradhi P., Sharmila P. Phenolics impart Au^{3+}-stress tolerance to cowpea by generating nanoparticles. *PloS One.* 2014;9:e85242. Doi: 10.1371/journal.pone.0085242.

Sheoran V., Sheoran A.S., Poonia P. Phytomining of gold: A review. *J. Geochem. Explor.* 2013;128:42–50. Doi: 10.1016/j.gexplo.2013.01.008.

Singh B.R., Dwivedi S., Al-Khedhairy A.A., Musarrat J. Synthesis of stable cadmium sulfide nanoparticles using surfactin produced by *Bacillus amyloliquifaciens* strain KSU-109. *Colloids Surf. B Biointerfaces.* 2011;85:207–213. Doi: 10.1016/j.colsurfb.2011.02.030.

Srivastava P., Sivashanmugam K. Combinatorial drug therapy for controlling *Pseudomonas aeruginosa* and its association with chronic condition of diabetic foot ulcer. *Int. J. Low. Extrem. Wounds.* 2020 Mar;19(1):7–20. doi: 10.1177/1534734619873785. Epub 2019 Sep 19. PMID: 31535600.

Srivastava S.K., Constanti M. Room temperature biogenic synthesis of multiple nanoparticles (Ag, Pd, Fe, Rh, Ni, Ru, Pt, Co, and Li) by *Pseudomonas aeruginosa* SM1. *J. Nanopart. Res.* 2012;14:831. Doi: 10.1007/s11051-012-0831-7.

Stephen A.J., Rees N.V., Mikheenko I., Macaskie L.E. Platinum and palladium bio-synthesized nanoparticles as sustainable fuel cell catalysts. *Front. Energy Res.* 2019;7:66. Doi: 10.3389/fenrg.2019.00066.

Sukweenadhi J., Setiawan K.I., Avanti C., Kartini K., Rupa E.J., Yang D.C. Scale-up of green synthesis and characterization of silver nanoparticles using ethanol extract of *Plantago major* L. leaf and its antibacterial potential. *S. Afr. J. Chem. Eng.* 2021;38:1–8. Doi: 10.1016/j.sajce.2021.06.008.

Tang S., Wang M., Germ K.E., Du H.M., Sun W.J., Gao W.M., Mayer G.D. Health implications of engineered nanoparticles in infants and children. *World J. Pediatr.* 2015;11:197–206. Doi: 10.1007/s12519-015-0028-0.

Tasca F., Antiochia R. Biocide activity of green quercetin-mediated synthesized silver nanoparticles. *Nanomaterials.* 2020;10:909. Doi: 10.3390/nano10050909.

Thipe V.C., Panjtan Amiri K., Bloebaum P., Raphael Karikachery A., Khoobchandani M., Katti K.K., Jurisson S.S., Katti K.V. Development of resveratrol-conjugated gold nanoparticles: Interrelationship of increased resveratrol corona on anti-tumor efficacy against breast, pancreatic and prostate cancers. *Int. J. Nanomed.* 2019;14:4413–4428. Doi: 10.2147/IJN.S204443.

Tognacchini A., Rosenkranz T., van der Ent A., Machinet G.E., Echevarria G., Puschenreiter M. Nickel phytomining from industrial wastes: Growing nickel hyperaccumulator plants on galvanic sludges. *J. Environ. Manage.* 2020;254:109798. Doi: 10.1016/j.jenvman.2019.109798.

Valdez-Salas B., Beltran-Partida E., Mendez-Trujillo V., González-Mendoza D. Silver nanoparticles from *Hpytus suaveolens* and their effect on biochemical and physiological parameter in mesquite plants. *Biocatal. Agric. Biotechnol.* 2020;28:101733. Doi: 10.1016/j.bcab.2020.101733.

Yadid M., Feiner R., Dvir T. Gold nanoparticle-integrated scaffolds for tissue engineering and regenerative medicine. *Nano Lett.* 2019;19:2198–2206. Doi: 10.1021/acs.nanolett.9b00472.

Yan C., Wang F., Liu H., Liu H., Pu S., Lin F., Geng H., Ma S., Zhang Y., Tian Z. et al. Deciphering the toxic effects of metals in gold mining area: Microbial community tolerance mechanism and change of antibiotic resistance genes. *Environ. Res.* 2020;189:109869. Doi: 10.1016/j.envres.2020.109869.

Yuan C.G., Huo C., Yu S., Gui B. Biosynthesis of gold nanoparticles using *Capsicum annuum* var. *grossum* pulp extract and its catalytic activity. *Phys. E Low-Dimens. Syst. Nanostruct.* 2017;85:19–26. Doi: 10.1016/j.physe.2016.08.010.

Zayadi R.A., Bakar F.A. Comparative study on stability, antioxidant and catalytic activities of bio-stabilized colloidal gold nanoparticles using microalgae and cyanobacteria. *J. Environ. Chem. Eng.* 2020;8:103843. Doi: 10.1016/j.jece.2020.103843.

Zhu J., Wood J., Deplanche K., Mikheenko I., Macaskie L.E. Selective hydrogenation using palladium bioinorganic catalyst. *Appl. Catal. B Environ.* 2016;199:108–122. Doi: 10.1016/j.apcatb.2016.05.060.

4 Chemical Characterizations of Materials—Tools, Machines, Processes, Methods

Firdos Alam Khan

4.1 INTRODUCTION

Materials with a three-dimensional structure and ranges from 1 to 100 nm are considered nanomaterials, per the International Organization for Standardization (ISO) guidelines (Dolez, 2015). The field of nanotechnology has been there since 2600 BC, as it has many applications in the production of colors for fabrics, window panels, nanowires, and batteries. The word "nanotechnology" was first coined by Richard Feynman in 1959. However, nanotechnology was recognized globally in 1974 by Norio Taniguchi for its application in the development of semiconductor processes (Dolez, 2015). Soon after the discovery of the nanotechnology field, there has been continuous growth in the production of nanomaterials, and the global market for nanomaterials reached $64.2 billion by the year 2019 (Dolez, 2015). There are different parameters to examine nanomaterials so that they can be easily classified. The various parameters can be applied to their source, dimensions, material origin, and possible toxicity level (Ligler and White, 2013; Jayawardena et al., 2021; Scida et al., 2011). As for their origin, the categories that apply to their origin are anthropogenic or natural. The anthropogenic category is divided, in accordance with their intentional or unintentional formation, into incidental and engineered nanomaterials (Dolez, 2015). Those that have natural origin are called ultra-fine particles, and they originated from erupting volcanos, breaking sea waves, sandstorms, forest fires, or soils. Another origin of natural nanomaterials is living organisms, such as ferritin or the nanocrystalline constituent of bones. These materials are associated with magneto-reception and are considered to have a ferromagnetic crystalline structure (Jayawardena et al., 2021; Scida et al., 2011; Valentini and Palleschi, 2008).

It has been suggested that human activity is accountable for the manufacture of unplanned products that include nanomaterials. The various examples of the application of nanomaterials are in the development of incinerators, metal fume, internal combustion engines, polymer fume, food transformation processes, and electric

DOI: 10.1201/9781003317715-4

motors (Dolez, 2015; Valentini and Palleschi, 2008). The production of nanomaterials involves high temperatures, rapid cooling, and the presence of vaporizable materials, which leads to the emission of incidental nanomaterials (Dolez, 2015). There is a difference between natural nanomaterials and incidental nanomaterials or manufactured nanomaterials, in the case of manufactured nanomaterials, the shape, size, dimension, and composition can be altered or modified, whereas the shape, size, dimension, and composition of natural nanomaterials cannot be altered or modified. The manufactured nanomaterials can be derived from multiple origins, such as metal oxides, metals carbon, polymers, and semiconductors (Scida et al., 2011). Nanomaterials can be designed in different shapes and sizes based on their desired applications. In addition, the surface of manufactured nanomaterials can be treated or coated or conjugated and functionalized with drugs or biomolecules. Moreover, nanomaterials can be produced in different shapes, such as wires, tubes, rods, rings, spheres, fibers, needles, plates, and shells (Lorente et al., 2012; Albanese et al., 2012; Guo et al., 2014).

The metal nanoparticles can be produced in a size ranging from 1 to 100 nm for different biomedical applications. Metallic nanoparticles can be used alone or in combination with other nanomaterials or polymers to improve targeting, improve signal amplification, increase sensitivity, improve detection, and also quantify different biomolecules (Guo et al., 2014; Fritea et al., 2021). The carbon-based nanomaterials have added advantage over other nanomaterials, as they have better mechanical strength, high conductivity, better chemical versatility, and better optical properties. Examples of carbon-based nanomaterials are carbon nanotubes and graphene, which are normally applied in chemical reactions (Crevillen et al., 2019).

The external appearance and size of the nanomaterials play an important role in various biomedical applications. The dimension of nanomaterials is generally used to categorize them with other nanomaterials. In case the exterior dimension of the nanomaterial is less than 100 nm, then it is considered a zero-dimensional nanoparticle (0D). Quantum dots (QDs) generally fall into this category, as they are 10 nm in diameter (Vladitsi et al., 2022; Dolez, 2015). In addition to QDs, spheres, dendrimers (which are highly symmetrical), branching macro-molecules, and hollow spheres are listed under 0D nanomaterials. Moreover, carbon fullerenes, sodium tungsten, cubes palladium, zinc oxide rings, vanadium oxide star-shaped crystal formations, molybdenum disulfides, silicon carbide, or magnesium oxide are those 0D nanomaterials that do not have dimensions. Independently, nanomaterials can be used as a cell marker, as an emulsifier, or as a strengthening filler within a solid matrix (Dolez, 2015).

The one-dimensional (1D) nanomaterials have two exterior dimensions, whereas the third usually occurs at the micro-scale, and nanofibers, nanotubes, nanowires, and nanorods are considered as 1D nanomaterials. The inorganic materials that are used to prepare nanofibers and aluminum oxide, titanium dioxide, carbon, titanium dioxide, nylon, and polyurethane are good examples of 1D nanomaterials (Jayawardena et al., 2021; Scida et al., 2011).

Nanotubes possess unique features and appear as a cylindrical shape, with pentagons, hexagons, or heptagons shapes. Among different nanomaterials, carbon-based nanotubes are considered the most favorable materials for making nanotubes, while boron nitride has also been used to produce nanotubes. Nanotubes can also be prepared from sulfides of molybdenum, tungsten, copper, nickel chloride, cadmium chloride, and cadmium iodine, respectively. Nanowires possess the highest ratio of any other material, where 1D nanomaterials are used with a ratio of 1000:1, especially in electronics product development. Moreover, thin films, nanocoatings, and nanoplates are 2D nanomaterials, with only one exterior dimension present at the nanoscale. These thin films are used for coating ceramic or metallic tiles or surfaces (Crevillen et al., 2019; Kurakula et al., 2014). They are frequently applied in electrical engineering, such as to make electronic components, where insulating or conducting surfaces is essential. The surface optical reflectivity or features of the nanomaterials can be modified. Lastly, 3D nanomaterials, which are also called nanocomposites and nanostructured nanomaterials, possess internal nanoscale features but no outward dimension at the nanoscale. These nanocomposites are multiphase solid materials comprising at least one nanoscale exterior dimension (Zhu et al., 2010; Summers, 2010; do Nascimento et al., 2010). Nanofillers that spread in a bulk matrix are commonly referred to as nanocomposites. Nanofillers are accessible in 0D, 1D, and 2D nanomaterials. Polymers, ceramics, and metals can all be used as matrices. The final product can be a nanofiber or a nanofilm with a 1D, 2D, or 3D structure.

4.2   CHEMICAL CHARACTERIZATION OF NANOMATERIALS

With the rising demand for nanomaterials, several techniques have been introduced and applied to produce nanomaterials in large quantities. Recently, advancements in analytical tools, techniques, and apparatus have helped researchers in providing methods for the physical-chemical characterization of nanomaterials (Brar and Verma, 2011). The progress of analytical methodologies for the examination of nanomaterials allowing the European Commission Recommendation is critical (Rauscher et al., 2019).

4.3   ELECTRON MICROSCOPY

Electron microscopy has been widely used to understand the structure, morphology, and surface of nanomaterials. It has been reported that electron microscopy is considered one of the potent techniques for nanomaterial analysis because of its ability to picture the nanomaterials and, consequently, get evidence on the size, shape, and structure of the nanomaterials. There are two different types of electron microscopy, scanning electron microscopes (SEM) and transmission electron microscopy (TEM) that have been used in nanomaterial analysis. SEM, coupled with a field emission electron gun, may match with a spatial resolution of TEM of less than 1.0 nm (Brar and Verma, 2011). On the contrary, the prime advantage of microscopy exists in the potential of connecting it with other spectroscopic instruments that give information about the structure and the origin of nanomaterials (Brar and Verma, 2011). The chemical composition and structural morphology of selenium nanomaterials were examined under TEM equipped with EDX microscopy (Correia and Loeschner, 2018). The sample was prepared using mesh copper grinds with holey carbon coatings, and a few milliliters of the sample were allowed to dry for the microscopic analysis (Correia and Loeschner, 2018). These TEM-EDX data were used for the single-particle analysis while connected with inductively coupled plasma-mass spectrometry (ICP-MS), which was used to precisely measure the size of the unidentified nanoparticles.

4.4 OPTICAL MICROSCOPY

Optical microscopy is another technique to examine the structural features of nanomaterials. The application of enhanced dark-field hyper-spectral imaging (EDF-HSI) has shown promising results in nanomaterial analysis. It has been reported that when nanomaterials were examined under EDF-HSI, along with optical spectroscopy, it showed a better and brighter image of the nanomaterials, and their near-infrared spectra can also be examined. Moreover, the nanoparticle illumination intensity has been increased to 150 times because of high-intensity dark-field surroundings. The atmospheric pressure is critical for achieving the best EDF-HSI image. Another advantage of this method is that it can be used in both liquid and solid forms of nanomaterials, with slight and easy preparation (Tiede et al., 2009).

The capabilities of EDF-HIS were compared with other analytical tools, such as energy-dispersed X-ray spectroscopy, SEM, and Raman spectroscopy. In one study, ceria and alumina nanomaterials were treated to epidermal cells derived from porcine skin tissue, and the results showed that EDFM-HIS showed better nanomaterial imaging, which help to better under tissue and nanomaterial interaction. They also provide initial confirmation of EDFM-HSI mapping as a novel and somewhat raised technique for recognizing ENMs in biological samples as well as a foundation for future protocol development using EDFM-HSI for ENM semiquantitative method (Peña et al., 2016).

4.5 LIGHT SCATTERING

The nanomaterials that are present in the liquid and dispersion forms can be examined by multi-angle light scattering (MALS) and dynamic light scattering (DLS) methods. During the analysis, the average amounts of the dispersed incident light gathered at multiple angles are used to calculate size metrics, such as the axis of rotation by using MALS. Nevertheless, the DLS method uses a time-dependent difference in scattering intensity to estimate the phase transition of the nanomaterials. It has been reported that fluctuation is persuaded by both beneficial and harmful interferences and is comparable to an identical hydrodynamic diameter (Brar and Verma, 2011). Furthermore, hyphenation is regularly applied with size-separation devices, including hydrodynamic chromatography (HDC) or the field-flow fractionation (FFF) method. An analytical method for detecting nanoplastics in the tissues of fish that uses FFF in conjunction with a MALS detector has been recently developed, and the maximum detection limit of this method was 52 µg/gram fish. Another type of nanoplastic prepared in the solution used with the AF4-MALS technique is polyethylene (PE); then it was found that the background dispersion was too big for the detection of polyethylene nanomaterials (Correia and Loeschner, 2018). In another study, the DLS detector was used in combination with a sedimentation FFF in order to detect SiO_2 nanomaterials in the lung tissue after enzyme digestions. The results of this study showed that SdFF and tissue digestion methods can show unidentified metal oxide nanoparticles and differentiate nanoparticles with 100 nm in diameter (Deering et al., 2008).

4.6 X-RAY TOMOGRAPHY

To be able to get an enhanced image of the nanomaterials, X-ray-based techniques have been developed, and they are X-ray fluorescence (XRF) and transmission X-ray microscopy (TXRM). The application of XRF can create two-dimensional images that are precise representations of the TXRM technique and can generate three-dimensional images by measuring the elemental distribution of the monitored analytes. Moreover, the spatial resolution of a synchrotron-generated XRF beam normally falls in the range of 1 to 10 m; however, some XRF beams have a spatial resolution of up to 100 m. It has been found that beamlines for sub-micrometer analysis are available and can provide a spatial resolution of up to 100 nm (Servin et al., 2018). For example, CeO_2 nanomaterial deposition was done on rat lung tissue (Deering et al., 2008), earthworms (Servin et al., 2018), and zebrafish. The uptake of TiO_2 and multi-walled nanotubes was examined (Da Silva et al., 2018) with the help of the XRF technique (Da Silva et al., 2018), as this technique delivered significant evidence for the absorption of Au nanosheets by the skin. It has been found that these imaging techniques cannot differentiate the analyte's physical conditions, as a high signal concentration of the analyte does not suggest its presence in a particulate form. Nevertheless, tomography is useful for mapping nanomaterial distribution within living organisms in order to comprehend the molecular mechanisms that contribute to their creation (Mahmoud et al., 2018; Lombi et al., 2011).

4.7 SPECTROSCOPY

The spectroscopy technique is also widely used to analyze nanomaterials. Inductively coupled plasma (ICP) spectroscopy is an analytical technique used to detect and measure elements to analyze chemical reactions. The application of ICP, coupled with mass spectroscopy (MS), is the most regularly used technique for nanomaterial analysis. These methods are used to analyze biological matrices (McRae et al., 2009). The asymmetric flow field-flow fractionation (AF4) hyphenated to inductively coupled plasma mass spectrometry (AF4-ICP-MS) has been used for the determination of Au nanoparticles (Schmidt et al., 2011). Gamma-mercapto-propyl-trimethoxysilane (gamma-MPTS) was used to prepare modified silica-coated magnetic nanoparticles in cultured cells and were analyzed by the ETV-ICP-MS (Henss et al., 2018). In addition, silver nanoparticles were examined in animal and human tissues by using this technique (Peters et al., 2014; Vidmar et al., 2018).

The field-flow fractionation coupled with the ICP-MS (AF4-ICP-MS) method is used to analyze the metal particles and metalloproteins in different biofluids (Loeschner et al., 2015). In another study, rat liver and kidney tissues were analyzed by using sp-ICP-MS for the determination of cadmium and selenium (Arslan et al., 2011). Based on the various research publications, it has been found that sp-ICP-MS is the most often used technique for metallic nanoparticles. This technique has been used for the determination of mercury and selenium nanoparticles in whale liver and brain tissues (Gajdosechova et al., 2016). In another study, silver nanoparticles and gold nanoparticles were examined in beef, *Daphnia manga*, and *Lumbriculus variegatus*, and selenium nanoparticles in yeast (Gray et al., 2013); platinum nanoparticles in human urine and blood serum (Fernández-Trujilloa et al., 2021); silver nanoparticles in human tissue (Abdolahpur Monikh et al., 2019); silver and gold nanoparticles in human tissues (Bocca et al., 2020); gold nanoparticles and silver nanoparticles in human blood samples (Witzler et al., 2018); and silver nanoparticles in chicken meat (Ramos et al., 2017) by using these methods. In addition, inductively coupled plasma-optical emission spectrometry (ICP-OES) was used for determining aluminum III in hair, water samples, and human urine, reaching a level of development (LOD) of 60 picogram/mL (Xu et al., 2013).

REFERENCES

Abdolahpur Monikh F., Chupani L., Zuskova E., Peters R., Vancova M., Vijver M.G., Porcal P., Peijnenburg W.J.G.M. Method for Extraction and Quantification of Metal-Based Nanoparticles in Biological Media: Number-Based Biodistribution and Bioconcentration. *Environ. Sci. Technol.* 2019;53:946–953. doi: 10.1021/acs.est.8b03715. [PubMed] [CrossRef] [Google Scholar].

Albanese A., Tang P.S., Chan W.C.W. The Effect of Nanoparticle Size, Shape, and Surface Chemistry on Biological Systems. *Annu. Rev. Biomed. Eng.* 2012;14:1–16. doi: 10.1146/annurev-bioeng-071811-150124. [PubMed] [CrossRef] [Google Scholar].

Arslan Z., Ates M., McDuffy W., Agachan M.S., Farah I.O., Yu W.W., Bednar A.J. Probing Metabolic Stability of CdSe Nanoparticles: Alkaline Extraction of Free Cadmium from Liver and Kidney Samples of Rats Exposed to CdSe Nanoparticles. *J. Hazard. Mater.* 2011:S0304389411005498. doi: 10.1016/j.jhazmat.2011.05.003. [PMC free article] [PubMed] [CrossRef] [Google Scholar].

Bocca B., Battistini B., Petrucci F. Silver and Gold Nanoparticles Characterization by SP-ICP-MS and AF4-FFF-MALS-UV-ICP-MS in Human Samples Used for Biomonitoring. *Talanta.* 2020;220:121404. doi: 10.1016/j.talanta.2020.121404. [PubMed] [CrossRef] [Google Scholar].

Brar S.K., Verma M. Measurement of Nanoparticles by Light-Scattering Techniques. *TrAC Trends Anal. Chem.* 2011;30:4–17. doi: 10.1016/j.trac.2010.08.008. [CrossRef] [Google Scholar].

Correia M., Loeschner K. Detection of Nanoplastics in Food by Asymmetric Flow Field-Flow Fractionation Coupled to Multi-Angle Light Scattering: Possibilities, Challenges and Analytical Limitations. *Anal Bioanal. Chem.* 2018;410:5603–5615. doi: 10.1007/s00216-018-0919-8. [PubMed] [CrossRef] [Google Scholar].

Crevillen A.G., Escarpa A., García C.D. *Carbon-Based Nanomaterials in Analytical Chemistry*. The Royal Society of Chemistry, London, 2019; pp. 1–36. Carbon-Based Nanomaterials in Analytical Chemistry; Chapter 1 [Google Scholar].

Da Silva G.H., Clemente Z., Khan L.U., Coa F., Neto L.L.R., Carvalho H.W.P., Castro V.L., Martinez D.S.T., Monteiro R.T.R. Toxicity Assessment of TiO_2-MWCNT Nanohybrid Material with Enhanced Photocatalytic Activity on Danio Rerio (Zebrafish) Embryos. *Ecotoxicol. Environ. Saf.* 2018;165:136–143. doi: 10.1016/j.ecoenv.2018.08.093. [PubMed] [CrossRef] [Google Scholar].

Deering C.E., Tadjiki S., Assemi S., Miller J.D., Yost G.S., Veranth J.M. A Novel Method to Detect Unlabeled Inorganic Nanoparticles and Submicron Particles in Tissue by Sedimentation Field-Flow Fractionation. *Part. Fibre Toxicol.* 2008;5:18. doi: 10.1186/1743-8977-5-18. [PMC free article] [PubMed] [CrossRef] [Google Scholar].

do Nascimento G.M., de Oliveira R.C., Pradie N.A., Lins P.R.G., Worfel P.R., Martinez G.R., Di Mascio P., Dresselhaus M.S., Corio P. Single-Wall Carbon Nanotubes Modified with Organic Dyes: Synthesis, Characterization and Potential Cytotoxic Effects. *J. Photochem. Photobiol. A Chem.* 2010;211:99–107. doi: 10.1016/j.jphotochem.2010.01.019. [CrossRef] [Google Scholar].

Dolez P.I. *Nanoengineering.* Elsevier, Amsterdam, The Netherlands, 2015; pp. 3–40. Nanomaterials Definitions, Classifications, and Applications. [Google Scholar].

Fernández-Trujilloa S., Jiménez-Morenoa M., Ríos A., del Carmen Rodríguez Martín-Doimeadios R. A Simple Analytical Methodology for Platinum Nanoparticles Control in Complex Clinical Matrices via SP-ICP-MS. *Talanta.* 2021;231:122370. doi: 10.1016/j.talanta.2021.122370. [PubMed] [CrossRef] [Google Scholar].

Fritea L., Banica F., Costea T., Moldovan L., Dobjanschi L., Muresan M., Cavalu S. Metal Nanoparticles and Carbon-Based Nanomaterials for Improved Performances of Electrochemical (Bio)Sensors with Biomedical Applications. *Materials.* 2021;14:6319. doi: 10.3390/ma14216319. [PMC free article] [PubMed] [CrossRef] [Google Scholar].

Gajdosechova Z., Lawan M.M., Urgast D.S., Raab A., Scheckel K.G., Lombi E., Kopittke P.M., Loeschner K., Larsen E.H., Woods G. et al. In Vivo Formation of Natural HgSe Nanoparticles in the Liver and Brain of Pilot Whales. *Sci. Rep.* 2016;6:34361. doi: 10.1038/srep34361. [PMC free article] [PubMed] [CrossRef] [Google Scholar].

Gray E.P., Coleman J.G., Bednar A.J., Kennedy A.J., Ranville J.F., Higgins C.P. Extraction and Analysis of Silver and Gold Nanoparticles from Biological Tissues Using Single Particle Inductively Coupled Plasma Mass Spectrometry. *Environ. Sci. Technol.* 2013;47:14315–14323. doi: 10.1021/es403558c. [PubMed] [CrossRef] [Google Scholar].

Guo Q., Ghadiri R., Weigel T., Aumann A., Gurevich E., Esen C., Medenbach O., Cheng W., Chichkov B., Ostendorf A. Comparison of in Situ and Ex Situ Methods for Synthesis of Two-Photon Polymerization Polymer Nanocomposites. *Polymers.* 2014;6:2037–2050. doi: 10.3390/polym6072037. [CrossRef] [Google Scholar].

Henss A., Otto S.-K., Schaepe K., Pauksch L., Lips K.S., Rohnke M. High Resolution Imaging and 3D Analysis of Ag Nanoparticles in Cells with ToF-SIMS and Delayed Extraction. *Biointerphases.* 2018;13:03B410. doi: 10.1116/1.5015957. [PubMed] [CrossRef] [Google Scholar].

Jayawardena H.S.N., Liyanage S.H., Rathnayake K., Patel U., Yan M. Analytical Methods for Characterization of Nanomaterial Surfaces. *Anal. Chem.* 2021;93:1889–1911. doi: 10.1021/acs.analchem.0c05208. [PMC free article] [PubMed] [CrossRef] [Google Scholar].

Kurakula M., Sobahi T., El-Helw A., Abdelaal M. Development and Validation of a RP-HPLC Method for Assay of Atorvastatin and Its Application in Dissolution Studies on Thermosensitive Hydrogel-Based Nanocrystals. *Trop. J. Pharm. Res.* 2014;13:1681. doi: 10.4314/tjpr.v13i10.16. [CrossRef] [Google Scholar].

Ligler F.S., White H.S. Nanomaterials in Analytical Chemistry. *Anal. Chem.* 2013;85:11161–11162. doi: 10.1021/ac403331m. [PubMed] [CrossRef] [Google Scholar].

Loeschner K., Harrington C.F., Kearney J.-L., Langton D.J., Larsen E.H. Feasibility of Asymmetric Flow Field-Flow Fractionation Coupled to ICP-MS for the Characterization of Wear Metal Particles and Metalloproteins in Biofluids from Hip Replacement Patients. *Anal. Bioanal. Chem.* 2015;407:4541–4554. doi: 10.1007/s00216-015-8631-4. [PubMed] [CrossRef] [Google Scholar].

Lombi E., Scheckel K.G., Kempson I.M. In Situ Analysis of Metal(Loid)s in Plants: State of the Art and Artefacts. *Environ. Exp. Bot.* 2011;72:3–17. doi: 10.1016/j.envexpbot.2010.04.005. [CrossRef] [Google Scholar].

Lorente A.I.L., Simonet B.M., Valcarel M. Determination of Nanoparticles in Biological Matrices. *Front Biosci.* 2012;E4:1024–1042. doi: 10.2741/e438. [PubMed] [CrossRef] [Google Scholar].

Mahmoud N.N., Harfouche M., Alkilany A.M., Al-Bakri A.G., El-Qirem R.A., Shraim S.A., Khalil E.A. Synchrotron-Based X-Ray Fluorescence Study of Gold Nanorods and Skin Elements Distribution into Excised Human Skin Layers. *Colloids Surf. B Biointerfaces.* 2018;165:118–126. doi: 10.1016/j.colsurfb.2018.02.021. [PubMed] [CrossRef] [Google Scholar].

McRae R., Bagchi P., Sumalekshmy S., Fahrni C.J. In Situ Imaging of Metals in Cells and Tissues. *Chem. Rev.* 2009;109:4780–4827. doi: 10.1021/cr900223a. [PMC free article] [PubMed] [CrossRef] [Google Scholar].

Peters R.J.B., Rivera Z.H., van Bemmel G., Marvin H.J.P., Weigel S., Bouwmeester H. Development and Validation of Single Particle ICP-MS for Sizing and Quantitative Determination of Nano-Silver in Chicken Meat. *Anal Bioanal. Chem.* 2014;406:3875–3885. doi: 10.1007/s00216-013-7571-0. [PubMed] [CrossRef] [Google Scholar].

Peña M.D.P.S., Gottipati A., Tahiliani S., Neu-Baker N.M., Frame M.D., Friedman A.J., Brenner S.A. Hyperspectral Imaging of Nanoparticles in Biological Samples: Simultaneous Visualization and Elemental Identification. *Microsc Res Tech.* 2016 May;79(5):349–358. doi: 10.1002/jemt.22637. Epub 2016 Feb 11. PMID: 26864497.

Ramos K., Ramos L., Gómez-Gómez M.M. Simultaneous Characterisation of Silver Nanoparticles and Determination of Dissolved Silver in Chicken Meat Subjected to in Vitro Human Gastrointestinal Digestion Using Single Particle Inductively Coupled Plasma Mass Spectrometry. *Food Chem.* 2017;221:822–828. doi: 10.1016/j.foodchem.2016.11.091. [PubMed] [CrossRef] [Google Scholar].

Rauscher H., Mech A., Gibson N., Gilliland D., Held A., Kestens V., Koeber R., Linsinger T.P.J., Stefaniak E.A., European Commission et al. *Identification of Nanomaterials through Measurements: Points to Consider in the Assessment of Particulate Materials According to the European Commission's Recommendation on a Definition of Nanomaterial.* Publications Office of the European Union, Luxembourg, 2019. [Google Scholar].

Schmidt B., Loeschner K., Hadrup N., Mortensen A., Sloth J.J., Bender Koch C., Larsen E.H. Quantitative Characterization of Gold Nanoparticles by Field-Flow Fractionation Coupled Online with Light Scattering Detection and Inductively Coupled Plasma Mass Spectrometry. *Anal. Chem.* 2011;83:2461–2468. doi: 10.1021/ac102545e. [PubMed] [CrossRef] [Google Scholar].

Scida K., Stege P.W., Haby G., Messina G.A., García C.D. Recent Applications of Carbon-based Nanomaterials in Analytical Chemistry: Critical Review. *Anal. Chim. Acta.* 2011;691: 6–17. doi: 10.1016/j.aca.2011.02.025. [PMC free article] [PubMed] [CrossRef] [Google Scholar].

Servin A.D., Castillo-Michel H., Hernandez-Viezcas J.A., De Nolf W., De La Torre-Roche R., Pagano L., Pignatello J., Uchimiya M., Gardea-Torresdey J., White J.C. Bioaccumulation of CeO_2 Nanoparticles by Earthworms in Biochar-Amended Soil: A Synchrotron Microspectroscopy Study. *J. Agric. Food Chem.* 2018;66:6609–6618. doi: 10.1021/acs.jafc.7b04612. [PubMed] [CrossRef] [Google Scholar].

Summers H. Can Cells Reduce Nanoparticle Toxicity? *Nano Today.* 2010;5:83–84. doi: 10.1016/j.nantod.2010.01.003. [CrossRef] [Google Scholar].

Tiede K., Hassellöv M., Breitbarth E., Chaudhry Q., Boxall A.B. Considerations for Environmental Fate and Ecotoxicity Testing to Support Environmental Risk Assessments for Engineered Nanoparticles. *J. Chromatogr. A.* 2009 Jan 16;1216(3):503–509. doi: 10.1016/j.chroma.2008.09.008. Epub 2008 Sep 7. PMID: 18805541.

Valentini F., Palleschi G. Nanomaterials and Analytical Chemistry. *Anal. Lett.* 2008;41:479–520. doi: 10.1080/00032710801912805. [CrossRef] [Google Scholar].

Vidmar J., Buerki-Thurnherr T., Loeschner K. Comparison of the Suitability of Alkaline or Enzymatic Sample Pre-Treatment for Characterization of Silver Nanoparticles in Human Tissue by Single Particle ICP-MS. *J. Anal. At. Spectrom.* 2018;33:752–761. doi: 10.1039/C7JA00402H. [CrossRef] [Google Scholar].

Vladitsi M., Nikolaou C., Kalogiouri N.P., Samanidou V.F. Analytical Methods for Nanoma-
    terial Determination in Biological Matrices. *Methods Protoc.* 2022 July 15;5(4):61. doi:
    10.3390/mps5040061. PMID: 35893587; PMCID: PMC9326673.
Witzler M., Küllmer F., Günther K. Validating a Single-Particle ICP-MS Method to Measure
    Nanoparticles in Human Whole Blood for Nanotoxicology. *Anal. Lett.* 2018;51:587–
    599. doi: 10.1080/00032719.2017.1327538. [CrossRef] [Google Scholar].
Xu H., Wu Y., Wang J., Shang X., Jiang X. Simultaneous Preconcentration of Cadmium and
    Lead in Water Samples with Silica Gel and Determination by Flame Atomic Absorption
    Spectrometry. *J. Environ. Sci.* 2013;25:S45–S49. doi: 10.1016/S1001-0742(14)60624-0.
    [PubMed] [CrossRef] [Google Scholar].
Zhu X., Chang Y., Chen Y. Toxicity and Bioaccumulation of TiO_2 Nanoparticle Aggregates
    in Daphnia Magna. *Chemosphere.* 2010;78:209–215. doi: 10.1016/j.chemosphere.
    2009.11.013. [PubMed] [CrossRef] [Google Scholar].

5 Structural Characterization of Materials—Tools, Machines, Processes, Methods, and Examples of Characterization

Sultan Akhtar

5.1 INTRODUCTION

Structural characterization is the structural and morphological analyses of materials in order to understand their properties. Several techniques have been developed to study the structural and morphological information of the materials (Akhtar and Ali, 2020). The materials are composed of tiny particles, referred to as nanoparticles, and they required special instrumentations and tools for their characterization and analysis (Kumar and Dixit, 2017). In this regard, X-rays diffraction (XRD) and Fourier transform infrared spectroscopy (FTIR), scanning electron microscopy (SEM), energy dispersive X-rays spectroscopy (EDX), and transmission electron microscopy (TEM) are the main and important techniques for the characterization of such materials. In this chapter, we will describe these instruments by covering the following topics: tools, machines, processes, methods, and examples of characterization. A detailed description of each characterization of each technique will be provided with examples. The pictorial preparation of the main parts of the instruments, along with a schematic diagram will be displayed. The important parts of these characterization techniques are the sample preparation and the operation. A detailed description of sample preparation for each instrument is provided. After reading, the reader will understand most of the steps of the sample preparation and their importance for the successful characterization of nanomaterials.

5.2 X-RAY DIFFRACTION (XRD)

The properties of the materials depend on the morphology and crystalline structure of the materials. X-ray diffraction (XRD) is a technique that utilizes X-rays to study the crystalline structure, no-crystalline, and chemical composition of the materials. In the XRD technique, the samples are scanned by varying the scan angle and

DOI: 10.1201/9781003317715-5

recording the diffracted beam in the form of a spectrum. Typically, the wavelengths (λ) of the X-rays used in the XRD method are in the range of nanometers. When the X-rays interact with the atoms of the samples, the X-rays are diffracted depending on the arrangement of the atoms and the angle at which they strike the sample. The working principle of this technique is based on the interference phenomenon (Berne and Pecora, 2000; Misture and Snyder, 2001; Richard, 2009).

The intensity of the diffracted beam varies by the path difference of the two waves and phase or angle. For instance, if the two diffracted waves are meeting in such a way that they are in the phase, meaning that they have the same crusts and troughs, then the resultant intensity will be the sum of the two intensities. The phenomenon is referred to as constructive interference, and the resultant intensity will be enhanced. Contrarily, if the two waves are superimposed in such a way that they are out of phase, then the resultant intensity will be the difference between the two intensities (Figure 5.1). Thus, the XRD data is an *x-y* plot between the intensity and scattering angle, 2θ (degrees). The XRD pattern is often analyzed by a famous mathematical formulation known as Bragg's equation. From Bragg's equation, we can extract the following information about the samples, such as the nature of the material, atomic arrangement, crystallite size, and chemical composition. The electronic database known as Joint Committee on Powder Diffraction Standards (JCPDS) has the XRD pattern of more than 60,000 crystallographic phases. The PDF file (example: JCPDS No. 19–0628) consists of the three strongest characteristic lines of the existing phase. The XRD technique is used for specimens of powders, thin films, and solids.

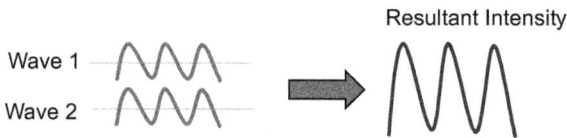

5.2.1 BASIC PARTS OF THE XRD MACHINE

The main unit of an XRD instrument is shown in Figure 5.2A and Figure 5.2B. It consists of the following main components: an X-ray tube, collimator, sample

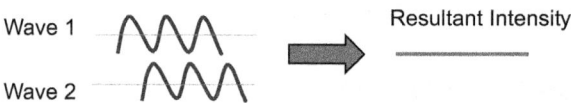

FIGURE 5.1 Schematic illustration of the basic principle of the XRD technique: (A) in constructive interference, the intensity of the resultant wave is increased (= sum of the two waves); while (B) there is a decrease in the case of destructive interference (= difference of the intensity of the two waves).

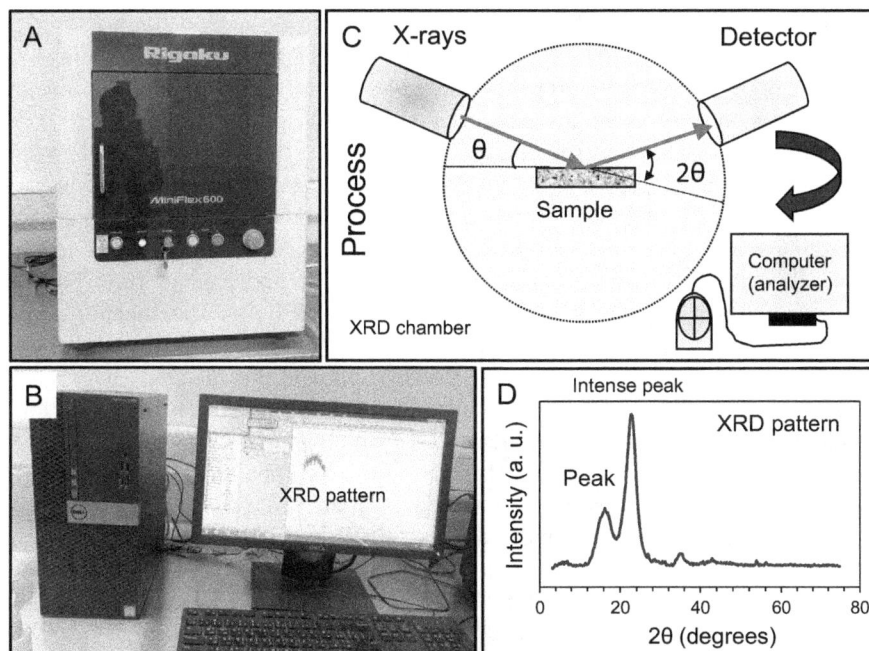

FIGURE 5.2 (A, B, C) Digital photos of the XRD instrument, along with a schematic representation of working with the XRD technique; (D) an XRD pattern showing the intense peak and other low-intensity peaks appearing under different 2-theta angles.

stage, detector, and computer. A short description of each part is provided as follows:

1. X-ray tube: This is where energetic electrons are collided with atoms of a target (usually copper) and produce X-rays.
2. Collimator: The function of a collimator is to produce a parallel beam of X-rays for the XRD method.
3. Sample stage: The place where the samples are mounted for XRD experiments.
4. Detector: A detector is used to detect the XRD signal to make the XRD pattern.
5. Computer: The collected data during the scan is drawn on the computer in the form of an XRD pattern.

5.2.2 WORKING PRINCIPLE OF THE XRD INSTRUMENT

In XRD, a parallel beam of X-rays is produced and directed toward a sample. The fast-moving beam of X-rays is then interacted with atoms of the sample and diffracted in different directions, depending on the arrangement of the atoms. It is a fact that all samples are composed of atoms in the form of a periodic manner (crystalline) or present in a random arrangement (amorphous) (Figure 5.2C) (Misture and Snyder, 2001).

Angles made by incident X-rays with the surface of the specimen are θ; then the angle of the diffracted beam will be 2θ. The diffracted angle, 2θ, is dependent on the arrangement of the atoms, the type of atoms, and so on. The diffracted beam is then detected by a detector and transferred to a computer to produce a digital XRD pattern (see Figure 5.2D). For a specific specimen, assume that atoms are arranged in a periodic atomic layer, known as lattice planes. The gap between two atomic layers is called interplane spacing and is denoted by d. By Bragg's law, the constrictive interference happened when the path difference is an integral multiple of wavelengths. We can describe this situation as follows: $AB = d\ sin\theta$ and $BC = d\ sin\theta$. The path difference of the two waves will be $(AB + BC) = 2d\ sin\theta$. By the statement of Bragg's laws, the constructive interface will occur when $2d\ sin\theta = n\ \lambda$ is satisfied. Where n is an integer, λ is the wavelength of the X-ray beam, and θ is the angle between the incoming beam and the normal to the sample planes. In general, the scattering angle 2θ is lower for wider interparticle distance d, which applies that the planes with a wider d appeared at small angles at the start of the XRD pattern. In the XRD technique, the angle of incoming waves is varied to produce all possible reflections for a given sample. By measuring θ and d of every single crystallographic phase, we can find out the crystallographic information and then compare it with standard available data in the digital library in the Powder Diffraction File (PDF) database (Slimani et al., 2023).

5.3 FOURIER TRANSFORM INFRARED (FTIR) SPECTROSCOPY

Fourier transform infrared (FTIR) is a technique to investigate the molecular bonding of organic/inorganic materials. IR is a region of electromagnetic radiation that lies between the red edge of the visible spectrum (wavelength of 700 nm to 1 mm). This means that wavelengths of the IR waves are longer than visible light and shorter than radio waves. During the FTIR experiment, a specimen is exposed to IR radiations in order to produce a spectrum of the specimen. During this scanning, a portion of the radiation is transmitted, while the rest of the radiation is absorbed by the specimen depending on bonding. FTIR is a molecular fingerprint of the specimen, which is a result of transmittance and absorbance at a molecular level. A wide range of information could be extracted from the FTIR spectrum, which includes identifying the material properties, quality of the specimen, and number/ratio of the individual ingredients in a mixture (Amenabar et al., 2013; Talari et al., 2017).

5.3.1 BASIC PARTS OF THE FTIR INSTRUMENT

The main unit of the FTIR instrument is shown in Figure 5.3A, along with a schematic representation of the workings of the FTIR technique. The FTIR machine is composed of the following main components: source, interferometer, sample stage, detector, and computer. A short description of each part is given as follows:

- Source: The FTIR source is used to produce IR energy in the form of a beam.

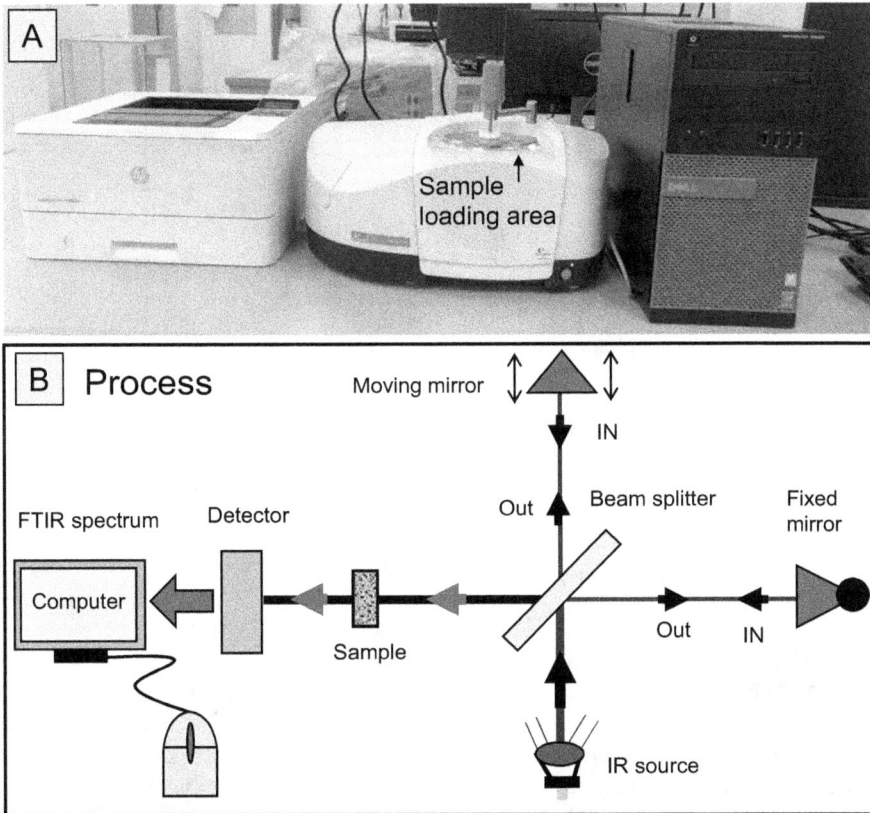

FIGURE 5.3 (A) A photo of the main unit of the FTIR instrument, along with (B) a schematic illustration of working with the FTIR technique.

- Interferometer: A distinct signal containing all IR frequencies is produced by the interferometer. The interferogram signal is produced by the interference of two beams that hold the information of each IR frequency. Collecting the interferogram signals means the simultaneous measurement of all IR frequencies.
- Sample chamber: This is the region of the instrument where samples are mounted in order to start the FTIR experiments. The IR beam reaches the sample chamber to produce interferogram signals for the FTIR spectrum. Only certain IR frequencies are absorbed/transmitted depending on the nature of the chemical bonding present in the specimen.
- The detector: This is used to collect the IR signals, which are transferred into a computer for further purposes.
- The computer: The signal sent by the detector is plotted in the form of an FTIR spectrum and analyzed for sample identification. The interferogram is decoded into the individual frequencies in a computer using a Fourier transform, a mathematical formulation.

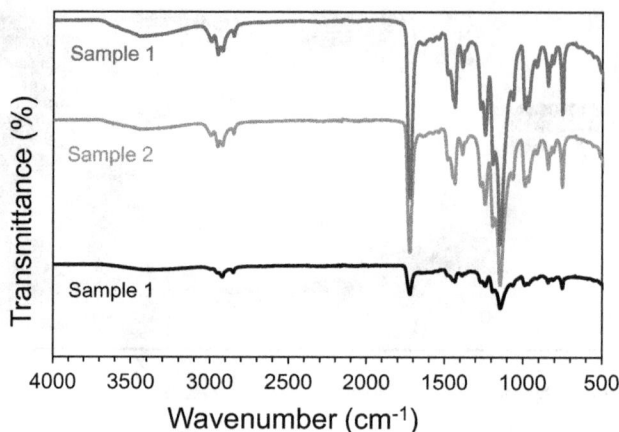

FIGURE 5.4 FTIR spectra of three samples to compare the intensity of the same bands in different samples.

5.3.2 WORKINGS OF THE FTIR INSTRUMENT

For FTIR scans, IR waves are produced by an IR light source in the form of a beam. The IR beam is then moved through the interferometer for spectral encoding. The interferogram is created after spectral encoding. The workings of an interferometer and the creation of the FTIR plot is described as follows (see Figure 5.3B). In an interferometer, a partially reflecting mirror, known as a beam splitter of the interferometer, splits the incident of one IR beam into two beams. These two beams are then reflected from two separate mirrors; one of the mirrors is fixed, and the other is moveable. After reflecting from the respective mirrors, both beams meet each other at the beam splitter.

Now, the IR beam passes into the specimen chamber. The signal from the interferometer is the result of interference of these two beams, referred to as interferogram. The interferogram occupies the information of each IR frequency that is falling on the specimen from the source. The beam is either passed through or bounces off the specimen surface, depending on the analysis requirement. A desired range of IR frequencies representing a distinctive property of the specimen is absorbed. The interferogram signal is detected by a special-purpose detector and decoded in the computer to transform into meaningful data using a mathematical tool known as Fourier transformation. After the signal transformation, the FTIR signal in the form of a spectrum is available for manipulation and expositions (see Figure 5.4) (Fouda et al., 2022; Zupančič et al., 2022; Haris and Severcan, 1999).

5.4 SCANNING ELECTRON MICROSCOPY (SEM)

All electron microscopes use electrons instead of light, as in the case of optical microscopes forming the images of the specimens. The images formed in the electron microscope often show a better image quality in terms of resolution and clarity as compared to optical microscopy (OM) due to the small wavelengths of electrons.

Simply, electron microscopes can be categorized into two types: (1) scanning electron microscopes (SEM) and transmission electron microscopes (TEM). In this section, SEM will be discussed in detail (e.g., along with the tools, machines, process, working principle (method), example of characterization, and sample preparation). And a detailed discussion of the second type of electron microscope, TEM, is in the next section. SEM is a very important machine for extracting useful information from specimens with a wide area in terms of surface topography, surface morphology, surface features, structures, and chemical composition. A pictorial representation of the SEM working and the main signals produced in the SEM are provided in Figure 5.5. The basic unit of the SEM instrument and the coating machine are also shown in this figure (see Figure 5.1). An SEM machine consists of the following main parts: an electron gun, an electron column electromagnetic lens system, a chamber (a small house for samples), detectors to detect the signals, and vacuum pumps to produce the vacuum (not shown in this figure).

In an SEM machine, an electron gun is used to produce the electrons, which are normally situated on the top of the machine. These electrons are then moved downward toward the sample by applying a high voltage; typically, 20–30 kV is used to accelerate the electrons in the SEM. The electrons produced by the gun are referred to as primary electrons, which are then focused on a narrow beam using electromagnetic lenses. The electric coils are used to scan the specimen and to produce the SEM

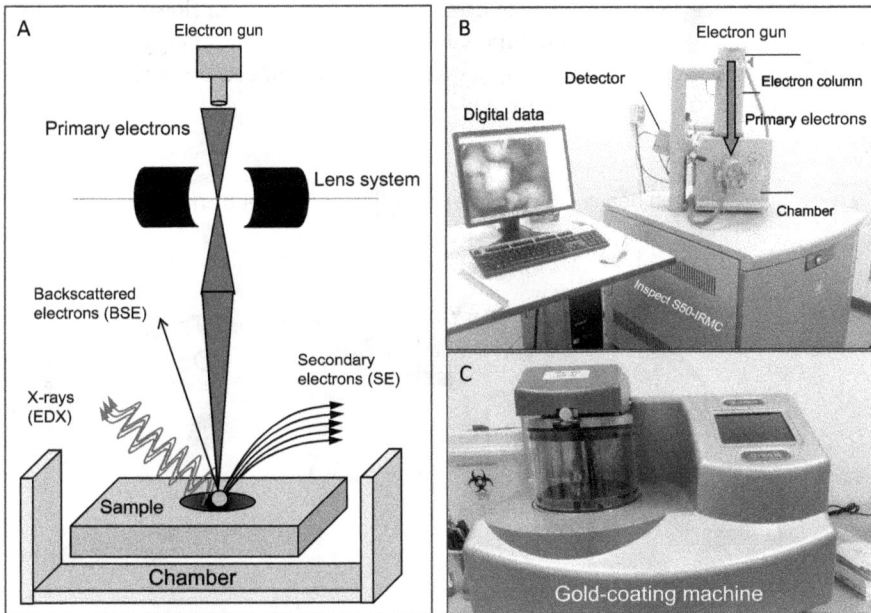

FIGURE 5.5 (A) Schematic illustration of the SEM instrument and basic signals of the SEM after striking the electron beam with specimens (SE, BSE, EDX, etc.); (B) digital photo of the SEM instrument, along with its important parts; and (C) gold sputter coating machine is also shown.

data from the area of interest. Upon striking the electron beam to the sample surface, different kinds of signals are produced; the signals produced on the top of the sample surface are secondary electrons (SE), backscattered electrons (BSE), X-rays, and so on. The working principle of the SEM and how these signals are produced after interaction with samples are described in Figure 5.6. In fact, in each sample, either from materials science or life science, the fine detail is exhibited in the layer of atoms, the smallest unit of the material. The electrons of the SEM strike the sample surface (atoms) and eject the innermost electrons of the atoms and produce the vacancy. The electron from the upper shell jumps to occupy that empty position and releases the extra energy in the form of X-rays. These X-rays are utilized in the technique known as EDX for elemental analysis. The ejected electrons from the atoms are known as secondary electrons (SE) and are used for the formation of SE images, providing topographical and morphological information.

SE and BSE signals are utilized to produce images of the samples, respectively, for surface morphology and topography, and chemical composition. X-rays are collected in order to produce EDX spectra and EDX mapping images of the specimen with chemical composition and distribution of composed elements with micrometer precision. EDX is commonly used in materials science and sometimes also performed in life science to obtain a chemical structural analysis of the cells/tissues, and the technique stands for energy dispersive X-rays spectroscopy. In the EDX spectrum, we obtained the data of the element of the samples in the form of peaks spread based on their energy, which is the fingerprint of each individual element of the samples. For example, the C peak will appear first in any EDX spectrum (low energy side) as compared to gold due to its low atomic number and, hence, low energy. Furthermore, if the intensity of the EDX peak is higher for a specific element, this suggests a higher content of this element in the compound.

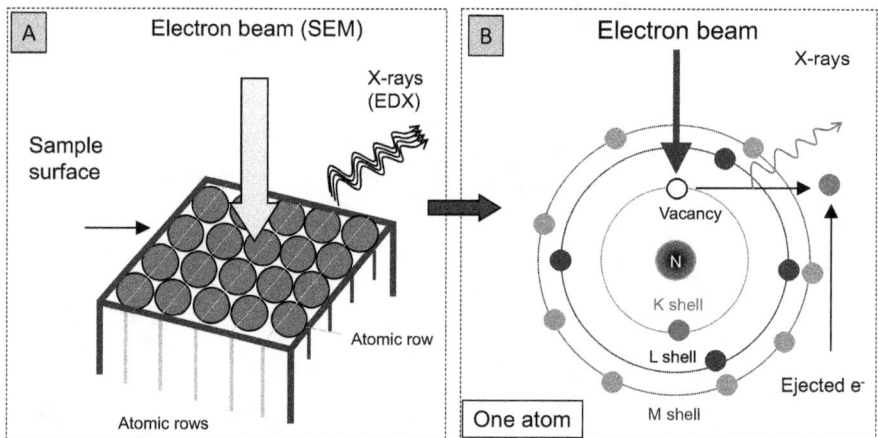

FIGURE 5.6 Working principle of SEM: sample-electron interaction: (A) schematic description of the sample-electron interaction showing the detailed structure of the sample (atoms); and (B) the arrangement of electrons in an atom and the production of SEM signals (SE and EDX).

5.4.1 Sample Preparation of Materials and Life Science Specimens (SEM)

Powder samples: For SEM examination, either it is SE, BSE, or EDX analysis, samples are prepared by dropping a small quantity of the powder onto the metallic stub (SEM stub) using a double-sided carbon tape. Extra powder is blown away, and the prepared stubs holding the samples are transferred into the SEM chamber for examination.

Liquid samples (nanoparticles in dispersion): In the case of samples in the liquid media (for example, any kind of nanoparticles), a drop of dispersion is deposited onto an SEM stub having a double-sided carbon tape. Sample stubs are dried well in the fume hood at room temperature and transferred into the SEM chamber for examination.

Biological samples: The biological samples are collected from the animals (e.g., mice or rabbits) and chemically prepared for SEM analysis. Different preparation steps are adopted in order to complete the preparation of samples for the successful investigation of biological samples. A detailed description of the biological sample preparation is illustrated step-by-step in Figure 5.7. These steps consisted of (1) samples collection, (2) immersion in glutaraldehyde (first fixative), (3) immersion in sodium cacodylate (buffer), (4) placement into osmium tetroxide (OsO_4) (second fixative), (5) dehydration into graded ethanol (30%, 50%, 70%, 90%) and absolute ethanol (100%), (6) drying process using critical drying machine, (7) gold coating of the prepared sample, and (8) finally, transferring into the SEM for examination.

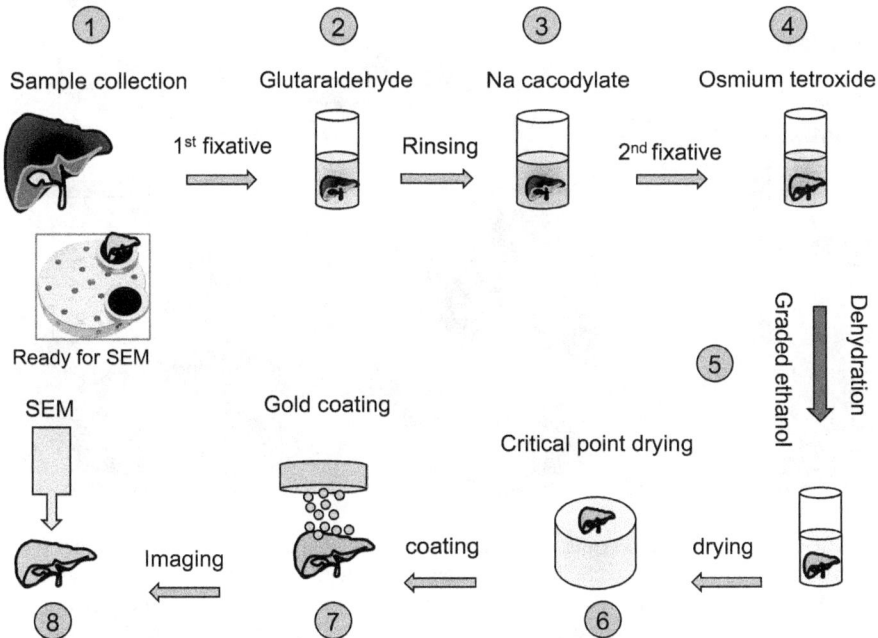

FIGURE 5.7 A detailed, step-by-step description of the biological sample preparation: (1) sample collection, immersion in (2) glutaraldehyde, (3) Na cacodylate, (4) osmium tetroxide (OsO_4), (5) dehydration, (6) drying, (7) gold coating, and (8) transferring into SEM.

It is noted that if the SEM analyses required the investigation of the internal structure, then the samples must be fractured or cut into small pieces (~ 2 mm) inside the glutaraldehyde for cross-sectional preparation. For all biological samples and for non-conductive samples (paper, polymers, plastics, ceramics, etc.), the samples are coated with gold using a gold coating machine prior to the SEM examination to improve the image quality by making them electrically conductive.

Examples of SEM instrument: As an example, the biological specimens, liver, and femur bone collected from the adult mice were prepared. The details of the animal given are as follows: The experiment was performed on adult male mice (C57BL6; aged 4 months); the weight is ~ 28g; they are housed in groups of five in a room, with a controlled temperature of 22 to 24°C and relative humidity (40% to 70%). The mice were fed a rodent maintenance diet (ARASCO, Saudi Arabia), provided with water ad libitum, adapted for 7–10 days, and monitored during the period of the study periodically.

Figure 5.8 shows the SEM analysis of the prepared fractured bone and liver specimens. The specimens were prepared by adopting the protocol, as described earlier in Figure 5.3. The cross-sections were prepared by fracturing the specimen inside

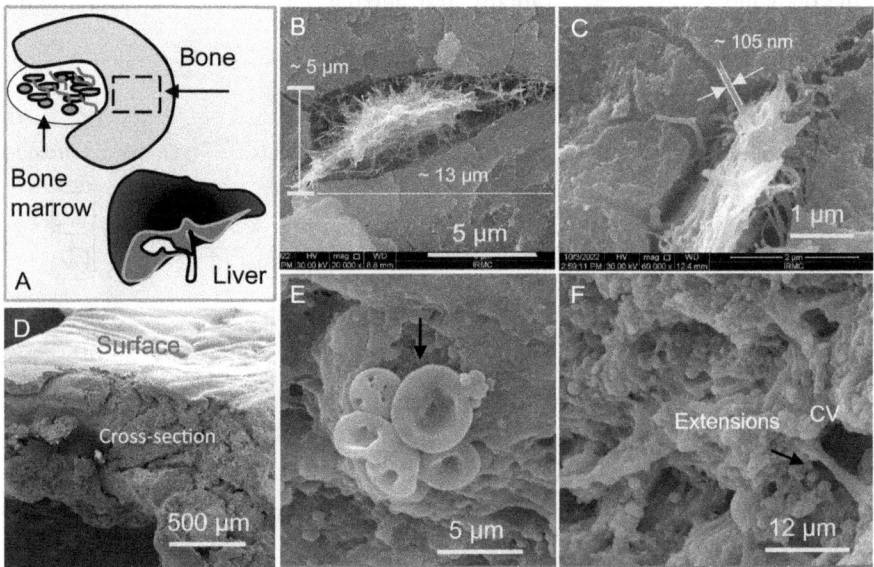

FIGURE 5.8 Biological sample preparation for SEM analysis: (A) schematic diagrams of the cross-sectional view of the femur bone showing the hard bone and bone marrow and liver; (B) SEM micrographs of the cross-sectional view of the femur bone showing the hard bone and bone marrow in the middle; (C) osteocyte cells are visible, along with the dendric network and canals; (D–F) SEM micrographs of the liver, with the surface view and cross-sectional views showing characteristic features of the tissue. EDX spectrum taken from the cross-section of the hard Ca/P enrich the characteristics of the bone. Gold (Au) peak appeared because of the gold coating. (SEM working voltage: 20 kV.)

the glutaraldehyde during immersion in the first chemical fixation and continuing to follow the remaining steps of the preparation: Figure 5.8A is the schematic representation of the bone cross-section and liver. SEM examination revealed the successful preparation, as both the specimens showed their fine internal structures. The cross-section of the mice femur showed the hard bone (extremes) and the bone marrow in the middle (Figure 5.8B). The thickness of the bone is estimated at ~ 2 mm in diameter. The characteristic cells of the bone, osteocytes, are revealed by SEM when a part of the hard bone was zoomed at a high magnification (Figure 5.8C). The size of the osteocytes and the dendric network is measured. The dendric processes are passing through the canals (path; ~ 105 nm) to establish the interconnection network and communication with other cells. Figures 5.8D–5.8F show the SEM micrographs of the liver, surface view and cross-sectional views, revealing the characteristic features of the tissue. The EDX spectrum (Figure 5.8G) of the hard bone is displaying the calcium/phosphorous (Ca/P) enriched characteristics of the bone, along with natural light elements (C, N, and O). Gold (Au) peak appeared due to the gold coating, as it was applied due to the nature of the samples.

5.5   TRANSMISSION ELECTRON MICROSCOPY (TEM)

Though the SEM is a user-friendly machine and provides sample information on a large area of interest with sub-micrometer precision; however, the resolution and quality of SEM images are limited due to technology-based principles. Transmission electron microscopy (TEM) is a useful technique of characterization to obtain high-quality electronic data with a sub-nanometer resolution of the nanomaterials. Both SEM and TEM instruments are important: SEM is used to scan the large area of the sample in order to find out and select the area of interest or sample features that we want to study and then perform TEM to get the data of the sample on a small area but with a high precision and high resolution for detailed structure and morphology. Both techniques, SEM and TEM, are varied in their working principle. In SEM, the sample surface is scanned and generates the electronic signals on top of the sample to make the electronic images or X-ray spectrum. However, in TEM, an energetic beam of electrons is interacted with a thin sample (usually, a sample thickness of ~ 100 nm) and is transmitted through. During this interaction, some electrons are passed in a straight path without changing their trajectory (direct electrons), and some electrons that changed their trajectory (scattered electrons) are obtained for the formation of images. Both scattered and direct electrons do not lose energy during this interaction, and thus, their energy almost remains the same as the primary electrons (e.g., very high). However, the energy of the SE or BSE electrons is very low (~ maximum couple of 10 eV) as compared to TEM-transmitted electrons.

The operational voltage (V), the voltage that is used to accelerate the primary electrons (gun electrons) toward the sample, is very high in the case of TEM. In world laboratories, the routinely used TEMs are operated between 80 and 300 kV, which is much higher than the SEM, as SEMs are operated at a maximum of 30 kV. Due to a high working voltage and principle, the produced electronic data with TEMs are much better than SEMs in terms of resolution and quality. The better resolution of the TEM is linked with a shorter wavelength (λ) of the electrons, which is related to V according to the following relation:

$$\lambda = \frac{h}{(2m_0 eV)^{1/2}} \tag{5.1}$$

In this equation (5.1), m_0 is the rest mass of electrons, eV is the energy provided by V, and h is the Planck's constant ($6.62607015 \times 10^{-34}$ m^2 kgs^{-1}). The relation between λ and V is a great benefit for TEM operation. For example, by increasing V, one could shorten the λ of the electrons and, hence, improve the resolution. By operating TEM at 300 kV, λ of electrons is comparable to or smaller ($\lambda \sim 0.00197$ nm) than the size of the atom ($\sim$ 1–2 Å). It is advantageous to achieve the short λ in the TEM to obtain the ultrastructure of the samples that is near and to reveal the individual atoms and molecules (Williams and Crater, 2009).

The basic working principle (sample-electron interaction), along with the main unit of TEM is shown in Figure 5.9. In the TEM, different kinds of electrons are produced once the electron beam is transmitted through a thin sample (Figure 5.9A). These electrons include scattered and direct electrons. TEM consists of the following main parts (starting from the top of the photo): an electron gun, electron column, electromagnetic lenses, apertures, sample holder, screen and/or digital camera, vacuum pumps, and high-tension tank (not shown in this photo) (Figure 5.9B). A short

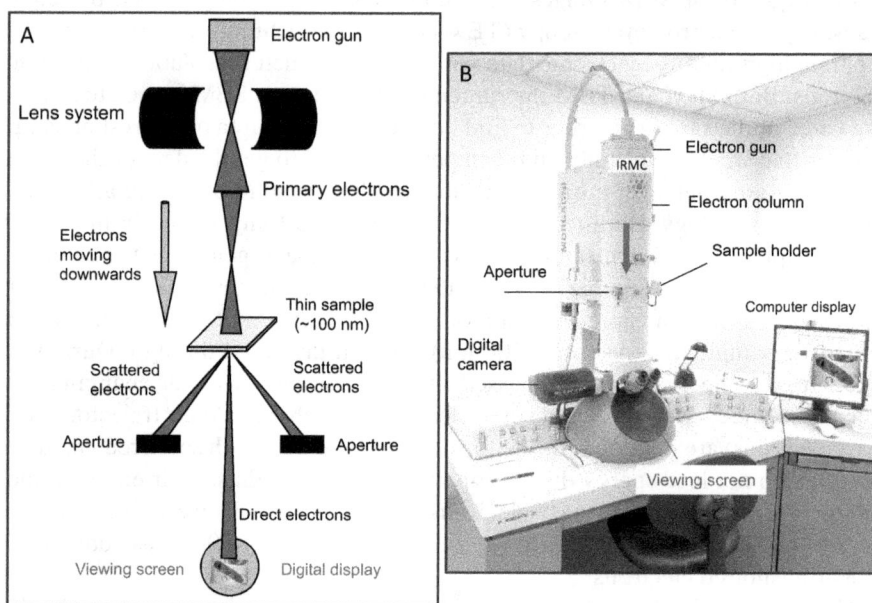

FIGURE 5.9 Schematic illustration of the transmission electron microscope (TEM) instrument, along with a digital photo of the main unit of the TEM instrument: (A) basic signals produced by the primary electron after interaction with the specimen, and direct or scattered electrons are utilized to form TEM images; and (B) photo of the TEM shows the main parts of the instrument (IRMC facility, January 2023).

description of the functions and uses of these parts is provided as follows. The electron gun is used to produce the primary electrons, the electron column is a path where electrons travel toward the sample, electromagnetic lenses are used to condense the electrons in the form of a narrow beam, apertures are used to select the particular electrons, the sample holder is used to mount the sample, the screen and digital camera are used to view and record the electronic data/images on a computer, vacuum pumps are used to produce the vacuum inside the TEM working parts, and a high tension is used to get the desired accelerating voltage (typically, up to 300 kV).

This section is about the working principle of TEM to form the electronic images of the samples (Figure 5.10). It is important to note that the working

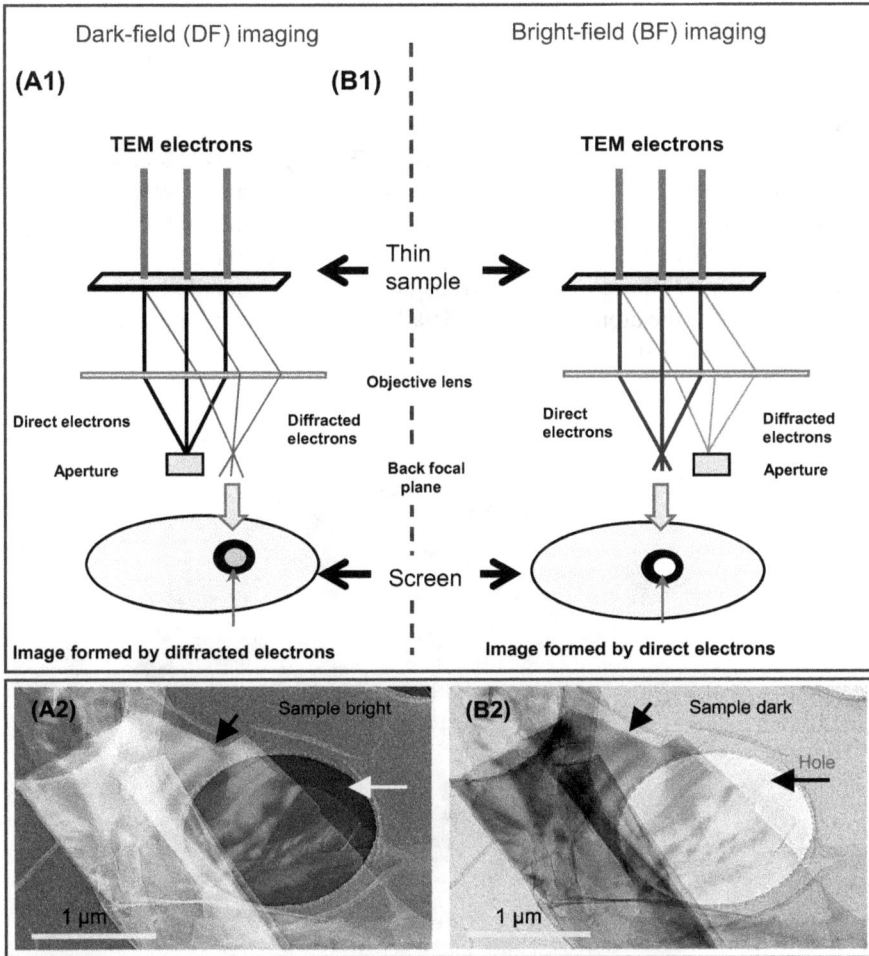

FIGURE 5.10 Working principle of TEM (modes of TEM), along with an example: (A1, A2) dark-field imaging (DF imaging); (B1, B2) bright-field imaging (BF imaging). In DF imaging mode, the sample appears in bright contrast and vice versa in BF imaging; follow the arrow in each image to understand the contrast. (TEM working voltage: 200 kV.) The scale bars are 2 μm.

principle of TEM is rely on the interaction between primary electrons and the sample. For example, a beam of electrons advances toward the sample in a TEM and strikes with high energy (80,000–300,000 eV). On the way toward the samples, the electrons are focused by a system of lenses. A fine beam is then transmitted through the thin sample, where the sample thickness is defined in the order of ~ 100 nm (materials science specimens) and ~ 200 nm (life science specimens). The transmitted electrons are categorized into two forms: the direct electrons that do not change their path and move in a straight path along the optical axis, while the other type of electrons is called scattered electrons, and they change their direction after passing through the sample. Both types of electrons are important, and they are utilized to form the images. The TEM instrument has more than one mode to collect information on the samples in terms of images (Figure 5.10). These imaging modes include dark-field (DF), bright-field (BF), and high-resolution (HR) imaging; they are commonly abbreviated simply as DF-TEM, BF-TEM, and HR-TEM, respectively. (Akhtar et al., 2019; Williams and Crater, 2009). For DF-TEM, the scattered electrons are utilized in order to form the images of the samples by blocking the direct electrons with the help of the aperture (Figure 5.10A). Meanwhile, direct electrons are used in BF imaging mode (Figure 5.10B). In this way, the contrast of these two images is opposite each other; for example, the features that appear bright in DF-TEM will be altered in BF-TEM (see Figure 5.11A2–B2). HR-TEM is performed using the phase of the electrons and acquires a detailed structure of the specimens down to the atomic level (the detail of this imaging mode is not provided) (Amenabar et al., 2013).

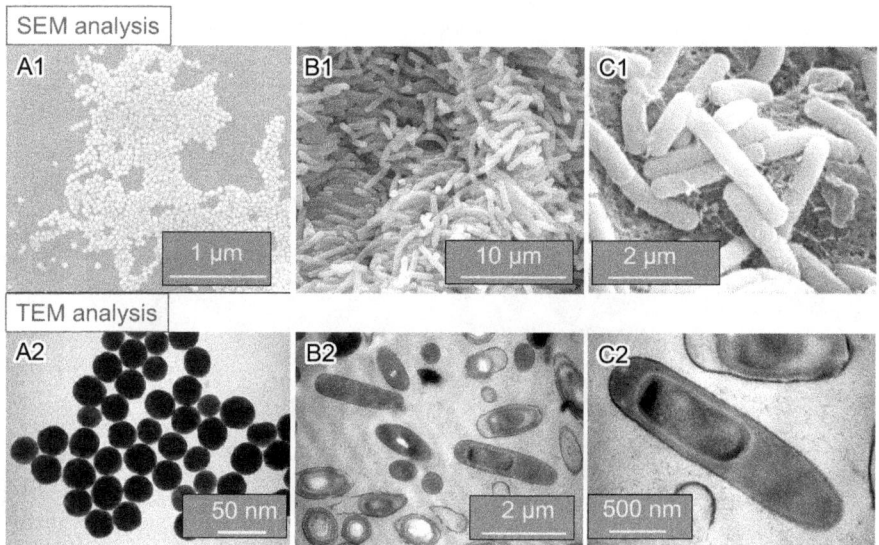

FIGURE 5.11 (A1–C1) TEM images of the gold nanoparticles and ultramicrotomy-prepared bacteria cells, and (A2–C2) the same specimens are examined by SEM for comparison. The acceleration voltage is 80 kV for TEM and 15 kV for SEM.

It is highlighted that TEM images have proven to provide better resolution and quality than SEM due to the working principle of TEM; that is, the process of transmission of high-energy electrons. To see the quality and resolution of both the microscopes, SEM and TEM, specimens from materials science (gold nanoparticles) and life science (bacteria) are taken for comparison. Both specimens are then examined under TEM and SEM; the data is displayed in Figure 5.12. It can be seen that the features that are not clear in SEM are much clearer in terms of particle size and structure. From the TEM image, it is possible to measure the size of the individual particle and to analyze the internal structure of the bacteria with high resolution.

5.5.1 Sample Preparation of Materials and Life Science Specimens (TEM)

Sample preparation is a key factor in generating high-quality data and images by utilizing electron microscopes. All TEM samples required preparation for their successful characterization before introducing into the TEM. TEM samples are categories based on their nature; either they fall under materials science specimens or life science specimens. In general, materials science specimens include powders of nanoparticles, thin films, plastics, and ceramics. Life science specimens are parts of plants, organs, or tissues of animals, and all kinds of bacteria and candida (Akhtar et al., 2019; Khan et al., 2018, 2019).

In general, TEM samples can be prepared by adopting three procedures as follows: (1) Powder samples: If the nanoparticles are in the form of a powder, then the nanoparticles are dispersed into the ethanol/water by using sonication. After well-dispersion, a droplet of dispersion is then picked by a pipette tip and deposited on the top of the TEM copper grid that has carbon support films. A digital photo and an SEM image of the TEM copper grid are shown in Figure 5.12A and Figure 5.12B in order to understand and realize the dimensions of the TEM grid. The maximum diameter of the TEM copper grid is about 3 mm. The prepared TEM grids are then dried and transferred into the TEM for examination (Akhtar et al., 2022). The whole process of sample preparation in the case of powders is described in Figure 5.12C and Figure 5.12D. (2) Bulk specimens: For the bulk samples, the procedure is slightly tedious and time-consuming. In this approach, bulk samples are prepared either by adopting the traditional way of preparation or using an advanced instrument, known as a dual-beam FIB/SEM. In FIB/SEM preparation, a rectangular portion ($25 \times 5 \times 0.1$ μm^3) of the sample, commonly known as lamella, is extracted from the bulk specimen for TEM. The detail of this preparation is provided in this report (Rubino et al., 2012). The prepared lamella is then introduced to the TEM for visualization. It is highlighted that the same procedure of FIB/SEM could be used for biological specimens with some additional steps. For example, the biological samples are first frozen in liquid nitrogen (LN_2) and then transferred into the cryo-FIB/SEM for further preparation, as given for bulk samples. (3) Biological samples are prepared by using chemical fixation and then cutting semi-thin and ultrathin sections of the samples by ultra-microtome (Figure 5.12E and Figure 5.12F). The chemical preparation of biological specimens is common in SEM and TEM up to step 5 (dehydration), as explained earlier in Figure 5.7. Thereafter, the samples are

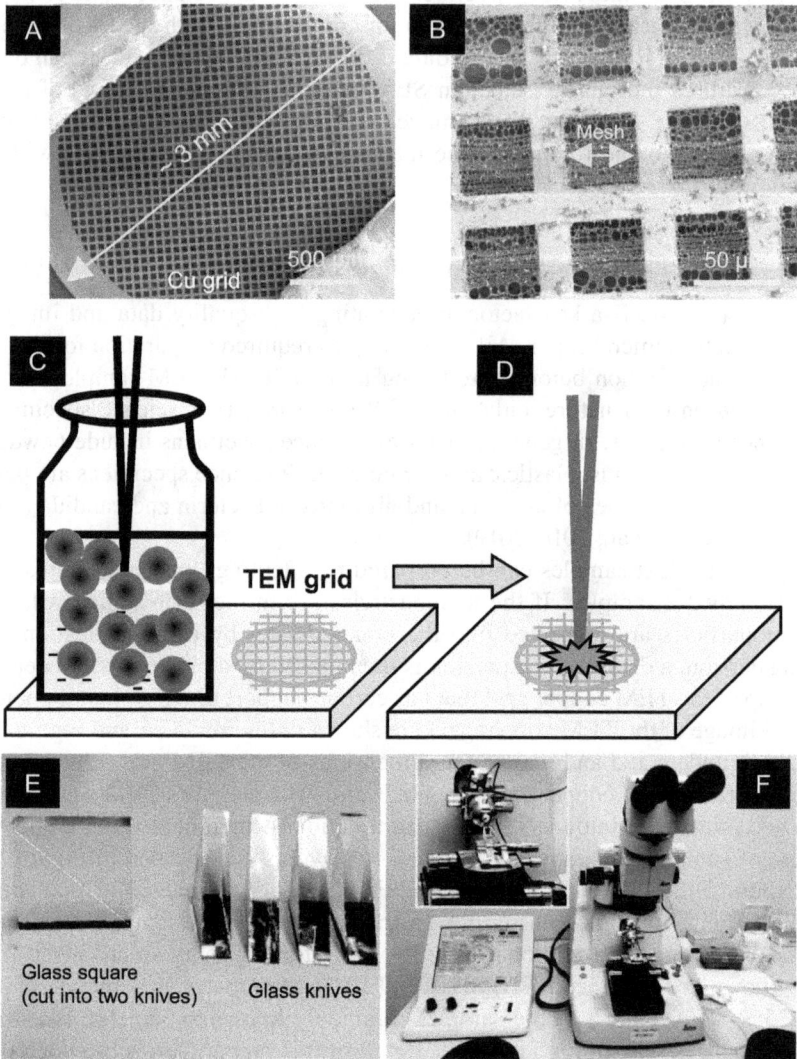

FIGURE 5.12 (A) A photo and (B) an SEM micrograph of the TEM copper grid having carbon support films. Sample preparation of (C, D) powder samples and (E, F) biological sample preparation using ultramicrotomy procedure. (F) A zoomed-in photo of the mounted sample and glass knife in a ready position to start sectioning.

immersed in a transitional solution (propylene oxide) and applied the steps for infiltration with propylene oxide and resin. Finally, samples are embedded in pure resin and cured in an oven for the ultramicrotomy procedure. The embedded samples are trimmed and sectioned using glass or diamond knives. The ultrathin sections are transferred into the TEM copper grid and stained with uranyl acetate and lead acetate. A detailed description of biological preparation is given elsewhere (Akhtar et al., 2012, 2019).

APPENDIX

CREDITS FOR USING THE PHOTOS OF INSTRUMENTAL FACILITIES AND SAMPLE IMAGES

Figure 5.2 (A, B): XRD instrumental facility (XRD lab) is available at Institute for Researcher and Medical Consultations (IRMC), Imam Abdulrahman Bin Faisal University, Dammam (16th January 2023).

Figure 5.3(A): FTIR instrumental facility is available at Institute for Researcher and Medical Consultations (IRMC), Imam Abdulrahman Bin Faisal University, Dammam (16th January 2023).

Figure 5.4: FTIR plots of the denture base resin materials (heat polymerized resin). The samples were provided by M. Gad, Dentist at college of dentistry at Imam Abdulrahman Bin Faisal University, Dammam (27th November 2022).

Figure 5.5(B, C): SEM and gold coating instrumental facilities are available at EM unit of Institute for Researcher and Medical Consultations (IRMC), Imam Abdulrahman Bin Faisal University, Dammam (16th January 2023).

Figure 5.8: Credit goes to Professor Ebtesam A. Al-Suhaimi and Dr. Hussain Alhawaj, Institute for Researcher and Medical Consultations (IRMC), Imam Abdulrahman Bin Faisal University, Dammam for Animal facility. The samples are mice bone and liver C57BL6; aged 4 months) (July 2022).

Figure 5.8: Credit goes to DR. Erika Widenkvist and Prof. Klaus Leifer, Uppsala University, Uppsala for graphene samples of sonochemically exfoliated graphene (2009).

Figure 5.9(B): TEM instrumental facility is available at Institute for Researcher and Medical Consultations (IRMC), Imam Abdulrahman Bin Faisal University, Dammam (16th January 2023).

Figure 5.11A1-A2: Credit goes to Prof. Ayhan Bozkurt and Prof Firdos Khan, Institute for Researcher and Medical Consultations (IRMC), Imam Abdulrahman Bin Faisal University, Dammam for Animal facility. The samples are commercially purchased gold nanoparticles (14th October 2014).

Figure 5.11B1-C1: Credit goes to DR. Francis Borgio and Dr. Abdul Azeez Sayed, Institute for Researcher and Medical Consultations (IRMC), Imam Abdulrahman Bin Faisal University, Dammam for samples of bacteria (ESH1) (29th December 2022).

Figure 5.11B1-C1: Credit goes to DR. Suriya Rehman, Institute for Researcher and Medical Consultations (IRMC), Imam Abdulrahman Bin Faisal University, Dammam for bacteria samples (CLD3C-37) (30th May 2018).

REFERENCES

Akhtar, S. (2012). *Transmission Electron Microscopy of Graphene and Hydrated Biomaterial Nanostructures: Novel Techniques and Analysis.* Uppsala University, urn: nbn:se: uu:diva:171991. https://dresden-technologieportal.de/en/equipment/view/id/1243.

Akhtar, S.; Ali, S. (2020). Characterization of nanomaterials: Techniques and tools. In: Khan, F. (ed.), *Applications of Nanomaterials in Human Health*. Springer, Singapore. https://doi.org/10.1007/978-981-15-4802-4_3.

Akhtar, S.; Asiri, S.M.; Alam Khan, F.; Gunday, S.T.; Iqbal, A.; Alrushaid, N.; Labib, O.A.; Deen, G.R.; Henari, F.Z. (2022). "Formulation of gold nanoparticles with hibiscus and curcumin extracts induced anti-cancer activity". *Arabian Journal of Chemistry*. 15 (2): 103594. https://doi.org/10.1016/j.arabjc.2021.103594

Akhtar, S. et al. (2019). "Functionalized magnetic nanoparticles attenuate cancer cells proliferation: Transmission electron microscopy analysis". *Microscopy Research and Technique*. 82: 983–992. doi:10.1002/jemt.23245.

Amenabar, I.; Poly, S.; Nuansing, W.; Hubrich, E.H.; Govyadinov, A.A.; Huth, F.; Krutokhvostov, R.; Zhang, L.; Knez, M. (04 December 2013). "Structural analysis and mapping of individual protein complexes by infrared nanospectroscopy". *Nature Communications*. 4: 2890. Bibcode:2013NatCo . . . 4E2890A. doi:10.1038/ncomms3890. ISSN 2041–1723. PMC 3863900. PMID 24301518.

Berne, B.J.; Pecora, R. (2000). *Dynamic Light Scattering*. Courier Dover Publications. ISBN 0-486-41155-9.

Fouda, S.M.; Gad, M.M.; Ellakany, P.; Al Ghamdi, M.A.; Khan, S.Q.; Akhtar, S.; Ali, M.S.; Al-Harbi, F.A. (2022). "Flexural properties, impact strength, and hardness of nanodiamond-modified PMMA denture base resin". *International Journal of Biomaterials*. 2022: Article ID 6583084. https://doi.org/10.1155/2022/6583084

Haris, P.; Severcan, F. (1999). "FTIR spectroscopic characterization of protein structure in aqueous and non-aqueous media". *Journal of Molecular Catalysis B: Enzymatic*. 7 (1–4): 207–221.

Khan, F.A.; Akhtar, S.; Almohazey, D.; Alomari, M.; Almofty, S.A. (2018). "Extracts of clove (*Syzygium aromaticum*) potentiate FMSP-nanoparticles induced cell death in MCF-7 cells". *International Journal of Biomaterials*. 2018: Article ID 8479439. https://doi.org/10.1155/2018/8479439.

Khan, F.A. et al. (2019). "Targeted delivery of poly (methyl methacrylate) particles in colon cancer cells selectively attenuates cancer cell proliferation". *Artificial Cells, Nanomedicine, and Biotechnology*. 47: 1533–1542.

Kumar, A.; Dixit, C.K. (2017). "Methods for characterization of nanoparticles". In *Advances in Nanomedicine for the Delivery of Therapeutic Nucleic Acids*, pp. 43–58. doi:10.1016/B978-0-08-100557-6.00003-1. ISBN 9780081005576.

Misture, S.T.; Snyder, R.L. (2001). "Chapter: X-ray diffraction". In *Encyclopedia of Materials: Science and Technology*. 1st edition.

Richard, A.D. (2009). "Chapter 2: X-ray diffraction techniques". Published November 2018. Morgan & Claypool Publishers, pp. 2–1 to 2–16.

Rubino, S.; Akhtar, S.; Melin, P.; Searle, A.; Spellward, P.; Leifer, K. (2012). "A site-specific focused-ion-beam lift-out method for cryo transmission electron microscopy". *Journal of Structural Biology*. 180: 572–576.

Slimani, Y.; Almessiere, M.A.; Baykal, A.; Gungunes, H.; Alsalem, Z.; Demir Korkmaz, A.; Akhtar, S.; Caliskan, S. (2023). "Impact of Er-Y co-doping on structure, magnetic features, and hyperfine interactions of NiCo nanospinel ferrites: Sonochemical synthesis". *Inorganic Chemistry Communications*. 152: 110719. https://doi.org/10.1016/j.inoche.2023.110719.

Talari, A.C.S.; Martinez, M.A.G.; Movasaghi, Z.; Rehman, S.; Rehman, I.U. (2017). "Advances in Fourier transform infrared (FTIR) spectroscopy of biological tissues". *Applied Spectroscopy Reviews*. 52 (5): 456–506. DOI: 10.1080/05704928.2016.1230863

Williams, D.B.; Crater, C.B. (2009). *Transmission Electron Microscopy: A Textbook for Materials Science*. Springer, The University of Alabama, Huntsville, AL, p. 14.

Zupančič, B.; Umek, N.; Ugwoke, CK.; Cvetko, E.; Horvat, S.; Grdadolnik, J. (2022). "Application of FTIR spectroscopy to detect changes in skeletal muscle composition due to obesity with insulin resistance and STZ-induced diabetes". *International Journal of Molecular Sciences*. 23 (20): 12498. https://doi.org/10.3390/ijms232012498.

6 In Vitro Testing of Materials for Medical Applications — In Vitro Testing of Materials for Toxicity, Disease Treatment, and Diagnosis

Vidhya Sunil

6.1 INTRODUCTION

Over the years, more importance is given to finding new materials with biological activity, rather than inert materials, in medical applications. The invention of new biomaterial compositions has changed the prime focus of research to ensure the safety of newly developed biomaterials. They are used to study the cell-material interactions to assess the safety of the biomaterials intended for human use. In vitro tests are gaining popularity worldwide in drug discovery and pharmacological research. In vitro testing allows us to test toxicity and efficacy, and validate the genetic differences that can cause sensitivity. Although they cannot be used as a substitute for animal models, they can be used as an adjunct to animal studies. They provide biochemical, morphological, and molecular information regarding the biocompatibility and toxicity of materials used in different medical applications. In vitro tests stimulate biological reactions in the cells they are in contact with. They allow control over the growth conditions of cells and make it easy to manipulate and assess metabolism. This makes it possible to test the conditions that cannot be done in in vivo conditions. These in vitro methods can be robust alternatives to using animals to evaluate materials in medical applications. In vitro methods are fast and can reduce the resources required and increase the efficacy of the evaluation of materials. Thus, in vitro tests make it possible to answer many questions that were not answerable due to constraints in whole animal or human studies.

DOI: 10.1201/9781003317715-6

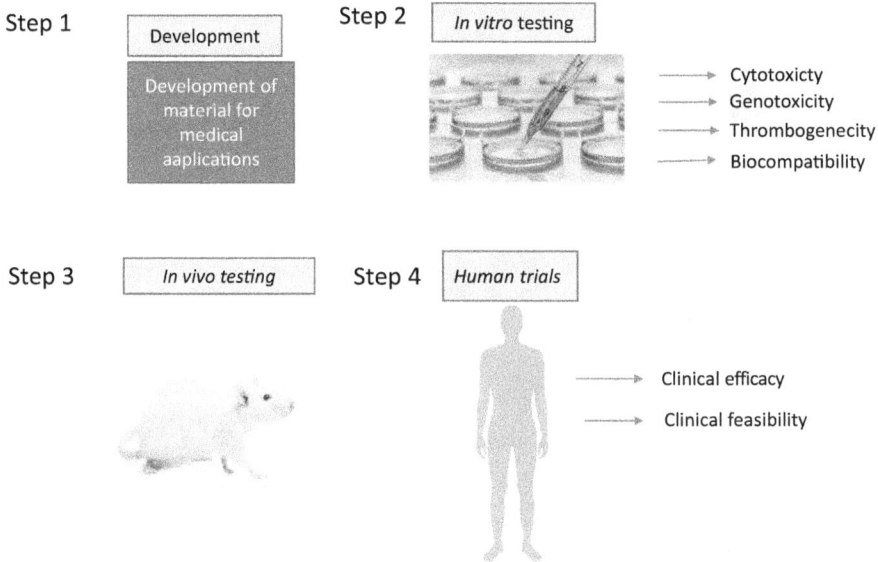

FIGURE 6.1 Testing of material-based product from bench side to bedside.

There are several validated in vitro tests in use for testing materials. These are often required for premarket approval of materials by a regulatory authority. These form an important established battery of tests that are useful in determining the possible adverse effects of materials. It has been stated that in vitro tests are always useful due to the shorter period for testing and low cost. In addition to that, they have high reproducibility and reliability (Russel, 1959). But the results of in vitro tests cannot be directly related to the results in living tissue, as in vitro tests only expose a single cell type in the culture (Rosengren et al., 2005). A poor correlation between in vitro and in vivo results has been reported by Hulsart-Billström et al. (2016). Therefore, an array of assessments—cytotoxicity, genotoxicity, and thrombogenicity assessments—is necessary to completely understand the nature of the materials used in medical applications (Figure 6.1).

6.2 IN VITRO MODELS

A wide variety of in vitro testing models are in use now. This includes 2D monolayers in well plates, 3D tissue cultures, and organ-on-chip (OOC) models that can mimic the organs, like lungs, liver, and gut (Mosig, 2016; Gröger et al., 2016; Jang et al., 2019; Benam et al., 2016; Deinhardt-Emmer et al., 2020; Shin and Kim, 2018; Maurer et al., 2019). Each model has specific advantages and disadvantages.

6.2.1 IN VITRO 2D AND 3D CELL CULTURE MODELS

In vitro cell culture models are used for studying the behavior of animal cells in controlled environments. The 2D and 3D in vitro cell culture models are used for testing

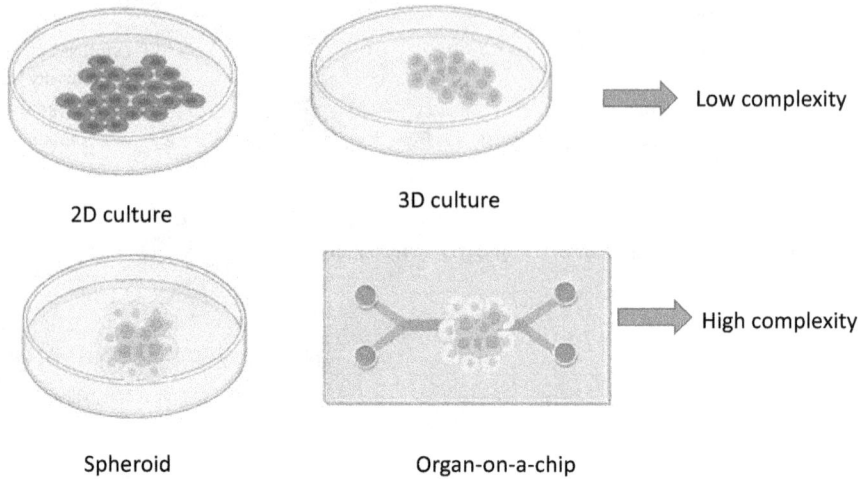

FIGURE 6.2   Development of in vitro models in 2D culture, 3D culture, spheroid, and organ-on-a-chip.

patient-derived cells in clinics. The advantages of these models are that it is possible to perform the test within 2 to 3 days and requires low cell numbers. But it has been stated that the 2D model represents cells inaccurately in in vitro (Costa et al., 2016). The 3D cultures have more potential in in vitro testing, and this will change the way in terms of disease modeling and organ transplantation (Figure 6.2).

6.2.2   SPHEROIDS

Spheroids are simple and reproducible in vitro 3D models compared to in vitro 2D models.

It mimics the cell aggregates or tumors, including in vivo characteristics, like cell morphology, production of extracellular matrix (ECM), and cell-cell interaction. It also exhibits protein and gene expression patterns in the cells (Hirschhaeuser et al., 2010). They take only a few days to form and can be a suitable model for the drug sensitivity and resistance test (DSRT) for cancer. In this test, spheroids from fresh patient-derived cells are tested against several anticancer compounds.

6.2.3   ORGAN-ON-A-CHIP

The organ-on-a-chip system, in which tissues are grown inside microfluidic chips, closely represents in vivo situations. This system is very useful in drug discovery for toxicity assessment of new materials in medical applications. But these systems are complex for clinical trials. So it is recommended that fast, simple, miniaturized systems are more promising for clinical trials (Popova and Levkin, 2020).

TABLE 6.1
Common Cytotoxicity Tests

Test	Principle
Cytotoxicity elution test	Examination of morphological changes, like lysis and deformity
MTT assay	Reduction of tetrazolium salts by succinate dehydrogenase
Neutral red uptake assay (NRU assay)	Uptake of neutral red dye by lysosomes in viable cells
Colony forming assay	Determination of cell viability by colony forming efficiency and colony size
Direct contact test	Measurement of the morphological changes of damaged cells
Agar diffusion test	Morphological signs of damaged cells
Lactate dehydrogenase assay (LDH cytotoxicity assay)	Detection of LDH released into the culture medium from cells
MTS assay	Reduction of (3-(4,5-dimethylthiazol-2-yl)-5-(3-carboxymethoxyphenyl)-2(4-sulfophenyl)2H-tetrazolium) to a formazan product

6.3   IN VITRO DIAGNOSTICS AND TREATMENT OF DISEASES USING MATERIALS THROUGH IN VITRO METHODS

In vitro diagnostics (IVD) are tests that analyze samples taken from the human body. They provide new tools to support disease diagnosis and treatment. There is a broad range of in vitro diagnostics used to treat and prevent diseases. In vitro diagnostic has become an important tool in clinical trials for detecting and monitoring diseases, providing prognosis, and determining responses to treatment (Raman et al., 2013; Billings, 2006). IVD testing allows early-stage and cost-effective interventions of diseases instead of advanced-staged therapy, which leads to worse prognosis and higher use of healthcare resources (Table 6.1) (Mignogna et al., 2002; Cressman et al., 2014).

6.3.1   CANCER

Generally, cancer is treated with chemotherapeutic agents. But these chemotherapeutic agents are toxic for all cells of the body, with most of the drugs affecting rapidly dividing cells and being more toxic for cancer cells than normal cells (Malhotra and Perry, 2003). In addition to this, the majority of the patients do not respond to standard therapies due to the high level of heterogeneity of cancer. It is very difficult to personalize cancer treatment, as it is difficult to test tumor cells from individual patients for sensitivity and resistance against anticancer drugs before starting treatment. But recent developments in in vitro testing help to determine personalized medicine for each patient.

6.3.1.1   Liquid Biopsy

In vitro diagnostics suggest liquid biopsy as a diagnostic tool for cancer. Liquid biopsy performed on peripheral blood is a non-invasive, real-time tool for the early diagnosis of cancers. It is considered a revolutionary tool for cancer screening as it searches for cancer cells or DNA pieces from tumor cells in a patient's sample. It avoids the complications of traditional biopsies, like the spreading of the tumor, injuries to surrounding cells, and bleeding. It saves time for diagnosis and treatment, improves efficiency, and is easy to perform. It provides a clearer genomic picture, as it can detect tumor DNA from numerous sites of the tumor.

6.3.1.2   Circular Tumor DNA (ctDNA) or Circulating Tumor Cells (CTCs)

In recent years, circular tumor DNA (ctDNA) from cancerous cells, tumors, or circulating tumor cells (CTCs)—cells that detach from the original solid tumor and enter the blood circulation—are used as markers for cancer screening and cancer treatment, and as a monitor for the response of tumor cells to treatments (Sorenson et al., 1994; Martignetti et al., 2014). They are very important for monitoring the sensitivity of a cancer drug toward a tumor as they represent the population of tumor cells that cause the majority of cancer deaths. ctDNA analysis reduces the need for tumor biopsy, which can be challenging when a tumor is difficult to access. Blood sampling for cDNA analysis is non-invasive, and this can be repeated during and after the treatment to monitor sensitivity and resistance to drugs. It is also possible to expand CTCs in vitro and establish a long-term cell culture (Popova and Levkin, 2020).

6.3.1.3   In Vitro Drug Sensitivity and Resistance Test (DSRT)

In vitro drug sensitivity and resistance test (DSRT) on cancer cells is used to define the sensitivity and resistance of cancer cells to different anticancer drugs. DSRT can be used to find more appropriate therapy in each case. The sensitivity of different tumor cells to new anticancer compounds can be identified by testing the tumor cells with a library of anticancer compounds (Maxson et al., 2016). After the therapy, repeated DSRT can identify the resistant cells and find the drugs effective against the tumor cells (Popova and Levkin, 2020). DSRT also elucidates the sensitivity and resistance of individual patients to different drugs that can help in determining suitable treatment for each patient. This decreases the risk of adverse effects and drug resistance. But still, this test is not recommended as a predictive test. It has been suggested that DSRT can be used as a test to identify the resistance of tumor cells to anticancer compounds before, during, and after therapy. It will increase the efficiency of therapy and reduce the side effects of therapy (Popova and Levkin, 2020).

An extended DSRT also tests the toxicity of anticancer drugs to normal healthy cells of the body. A therapeutic index (ratio of LC90—lethal concentration of drug killing 90% of the cell population—of normal cells to tumor cells) is used in drug development to determine the efficacy and safety of newly developed cancer drugs (Muller and Milton, 2012). DSRT can be done on tumor cells from blood or bone marrow or from pieces of solid tumors, which are disintegrated into a single-cell suspension for testing. It is essential to repeat the test during the disease course to identify the suitable chemotherapy for individual patients (Shah et al., 2003). The use of technology based on miniaturized platforms than microtiter plates alleviates the problem of the unavailability of required cells.

6.3.2 BACTERIAL INFECTIONS

Over the past few years, invasive bacterial infections have become more prevalent all over the world. This may be due to the rise in bacteria that are resistant to antibiotics, the use of immune suppressants, and the limited effectiveness of antibiotics in eradicating infections. This has led to the necessity for the development of alternative antibacterial treatments. Numerous bacterial species' antibiotic resistance has sparked efforts to develop novel materials with effective antibacterial properties. Antibiotic-resistant and recurrent infections are now more easily treated with the use of antibacterial biomaterials and biomaterial-assisted delivery of bacteriophages and antimicrobial compounds. Targeted delivery of antibacterial agents and prolonged release of these agents at the infection site are made possible by biomaterials. Thus, it lessens the possibility of systemic negative effects in the body.

Newly developed in vitro methods, like synthetic RNA-based and CRISPR (clustered regularly interspaced short palindromic repeats) based biosensors were reported remarkedly sensitive and specific in detecting the presence of pathogens. These methods are cheaper in developmental and operational costs compared to current antibody-based diagnostics (Geraldi and Giri-Rachman, 2018). A silicone-based biomaterial containing a novel polymeric imidazolium antibacterial compound, created using the organic polymer polydimethylsiloxane (PDMS), was found to completely remove microbe colonies even after many days in culture (Armugam et al., 2021). Recent research has shown that composite biomaterials can be created by casting a mixture of biomaterials and antibacterial agents (Thomé et al., 2012). Biomaterials that have been impregnated or cast with antimicrobials appear to have bactericidal capabilities, in contrast to surfaces that have been coated with antimicrobials that were only found to be bacteriostatic (Anjum and Gupta, 2018). It has been demonstrated that the controlled release of an antimicrobial agent from polymeric material is effective in inhibiting both planktonic and biofilm microbial development on biomaterials (Francolini et al., 2017; Dave et al., 2011; Liu et al., 2019; Schierholz et al., 1997; Riool et al., 2017).

Staphylococcus aureus and *Escherichia coli* co-cultured with copper sulfide nanoparticles (CuS NPs) fully destroyed the co-cultured bacteria in a matter of minutes upon near-infrared irradiation. Compared to natural healing, NP treatment accelerates wound healing by effectively eliminating bacteria. This is confirmed by the outstanding antibacterial performance of CuS nanoparticles against gram-positive and gram-negative bacteria (Wang et al., 2022). The most frequent issue when using external bone fixation pins is pin tract infections. Ti-ZrN/Ag coatings have shown antibacterial effectiveness and may lessen the viability of bacteria that cause pin tract infections (Slate et al., 2018). Hydroxyapatite (HA) modified with antibacterial ions can be used for the prevention and treatment of bone infections (Rajendran et al., 2014; Zhao et al., 2014; Shanmugam and Gopal, 2014; Kolmas et al., 2015). Zn-HA proved efficient in preventing the growth of pathogenic oral bacteria (Chen et al., 2012). *Porphyromonas gingivalis*, a significant contributor to chronic periodontitis, was successfully combated by the titanium implants' Zn-HA coating's antibacterial capabilities (Zhang, 2013).

6.3.3 FUNGAL INFECTIONS

Fungal infections are very common nowadays and lead to about 1.5 million deaths per year worldwide (Brown et al., 2012; Bongomin et al., 2017). Many of these are life-threatening for patients with compromised immune systems. Importantly, the number of cases continues to constantly rise (Houšť et al., 2020). Current antifungal treatments are limited to three distinct chemical classes—azoles, echinocandins, and polyenes (Houšť et al., 2020; Campoy and Adrio, 2017). It has been reported that yeast can develop resistance against these fungicidal agents both in in vitro and in vivo conditions (Pais et al., 2019). This highlights the need for novel approaches to treat fungal infections and the need for standardization of antifungal susceptibility testing (Van Dijck et al., 2018). It is important to find the optimal approach for the detection of antifungal resistance and treatment of fungal infection (Houšť et al., 2020). The use of appropriate models to study fungal infection is important for gaining insights into the development of the disease. In vitro models contribute more to the existing knowledge, as they can be used to mimic the infection routes and related immune responses under circumstances that are close to physiological. Fungal interactions with the host microbiota can be incorporated into models to replicate the in vivo environment on the skin and mucosal surfaces. An in vitro model can mimic the transmission route of fungal infections. The interaction of fungi with the immune system can be easily studied in vitro using cell lines and immune cells. Some of the antifungal drugs that target pathogens are proven to be the best treatments for most fungal infections in in vitro conditions. Ketoconazole is active against a wide range of fungi, including yeast, dimorphic fungi, and dermatocytes, in vitro. Luliconazol is active against *Candida albicans, Malassezia spp., Aspergillus fumigatus*, and *Trichophyton spp.* in vitro *(Khanna and Bharti, 2014)*. In vitro studies have shown significant antifungal effects of retinoids on a wide range of opportunistic fungi. All-trans retinoic acid (ATRA) is effective against *Candida sps.* and *Aspergillus*. Tazarotene is effective against *Candida sps.* and *Trichophyton belcosam* (Cosio et al., 2021). *Solanaceae* species and bitter orange oil have been shown to have antifungal effects in vitro (Martin and Ernst, 2004). Echinocandin exhibits potent in vitro antifungal activity against *Candida* species, including azole-resistant pathogens (Chen et al., 2011).

6.4 PREREQUISITES FOR RELIABLE IN VITRO TESTING

The choice of cell source for in vitro studies demands careful attention. The use of non-human animal tissue is easier, but the problem of species differences makes data interpretation difficult. Functional heterogenicity is very important for in vitro study systems. Endothelial cells (EC) are considered suitable cells for the study of vascularization of arterial stents. For the assessment of inflammation and repair, microvascular endothelial cells (MEC) are needed.

To avoid microbial contamination, working under clean room conditions and application of endotoxin-free materials are inevitable in in vitro studies. The presence of endotoxin can lead to aggregation, fusion, and fragmentation of platelets; activation of macrophages and neutrophils; and secretion of signaling molecules, like interleukins, serotonin, histamine, platelet factor, and tumor necrosis factor. Removal of chemical residues is another requirement to reduce cytotoxicity. All materials should undergo sterilization to avoid/limit the changes in functional properties due to changes in physical and chemical properties. Appropriate sterilization must be conducted before testing the sample.

6.5 MORPHOLOGICAL EVALUATION

Cell-material interaction on the surface of the material is a key determinant for assessing a new material (Lohmann et al., 1999). Morphology of the cells in contact with the material, adhesion of the material to the cells, and cell proliferation provide a clear indication of the behavior and response of cells to the tested material (Folkman and Moscona, 1978). Recent advances in microscopy and image analysis help in the systematic analysis of cell morphologies. Early-stage cell-biomaterial interaction can be evaluated using time-lapse microscopy (Rasekh et al., 2013). Image-based or morphological profiling provides quantitative information about cell state (Pennisi, 2016). It has been shown that fluorescence microscopy and bio-image analysis–based morphological evaluation help in the evaluation of cell morphology and cell-biomaterial interactions (Klußmann-Fricke et al., 2021).

6.6 BIOCOMPATIBILITY

Determining the biocompatibility of materials is essential, as new materials may cause harmful effects in the cells. In vitro biocompatibility testing has been widely used to screen materials.

Previous studies show that in vitro studies are in good correlation with in vivo studies in determining the biocompatibility of materials (Cenni et al., 1999). The first phase includes the physical, chemical, and biological characterization of biomaterials. Then biocompatibility is tested based on the guidelines of ISO 10993 (1999) and the US Food and Drug Administration (FDA). The test will be conducted based on the use of the material, the type of tissue that will be in contact with the material, and the duration of contact (Hermansky, 2001). The last stage is product validation. All components of the material should be tested individually and also the final product. Leachability and toxicity of the soluble components also contribute to biocompatibility.

6.7 IN VITRO TOXICITY TESTING

6.7.1 IN VITRO CYTOTOXICITY TESTING

Primary in vitro studies help to evaluate the behavior of materials in a biological environment. Cytotoxicity of materials can be determined by seeding the cells on the material or by exposing the cells to extraction fluids (Wang et al., 2013). In vitro cytotoxicity tests evaluate the ability of materials to inhibit cell proliferation in culture. A battery of tests is used in the cytotoxicity testing of materials. The selection of cell type is very crucial in determining the cytotoxicity of materials.

6.7.1.1 Cytotoxicity Elution Test

Cytotoxicity elution test (MEM elution test) is an in vitro qualitative assay. In this test, mouse fibroblast cells are incubated with test material extract for 48 hours. The cells are examined to determine morphological changes after incubation. The changes are scored on a scale of 0 to 4. If the score value is not greater than 2, the material is considered biocompatible (Assad and Jackson, 2019).

6.7.1.2 MTT Assay

MTT [3-(4,5-dimethylthiazol-2-yl)-2,5-diphenyltetrazolium bromide] assay is used to evaluate the viability and proliferation of cells. It relies on the reduction of MTT to formazan precipitates by cells. Formazan that accumulates in the cell is quantified by solubilizing in solvents like DMSO or isopropanol. The intensity of the color is proportional to the number of active cells. Absorbance can be measured at 570nm (Mosmann, 1983). This assay has been used in several studies to evaluate the cytotoxic effects of materials. Yang et al. (2002) demonstrated the cytotoxic effect of phytohaemagglutinin (PHA) against murine fibroblast cells using the MTT assay. This assay is sensitive in determining early toxicity (Fotakis and Timbrell, 2006). But the result of this assay may be modified by cell culture conditions and interaction between the material and MTT. The material is cytocompatible if the number of viable cells is equal to or greater than 70% (Assad and Jackson, 2019; Iqbal and Keshavarz, 2017).

6.7.1.3 Neutral Red Uptake Assay (NRU Assay)

The neutral red uptake assay by Finter (1969) has been frequently used in assessing cell viability and determining material cytotoxicity. It is a recommended method for biomaterial testing. Viable cells intake a neutral red dye by endocytosis and internalize it inside the lysosome. This process indicates cell integrity. Cytotoxic material can interfere with this process and reduce the number of viable cells. Thus, NRU correlates well with the number of viable cells. NRU assay is considered a more reliable assay than MTT assay, as it is not affected by microbial contamination, which often results in a wrong cell viability result (Ciapetti et al., 1996). They used NRU to evaluate the cytotoxicity of cement extracts on MG 63 osteoblast-like cells. This test is also used by NICEATM for cytotoxicity evaluation (2003).

6.7.1.4 Colony Forming Assay

Colony forming assay (CFA) introduced by Puck and Marcus (1956) has been one of the most reliable tests for cytotoxicity over the years (Sasaki and Tanaka, 1991). It is used to evaluate the action of different materials on the growth and proliferation of cells in vitro. It can be performed with any cells that can form colonies. It measures the fraction of cells that survive after treatment as plating efficiencies (PE).

6.7.1.5 Direct Contact Test

A direct contact test measures the morphological changes and the change in the number of cells according to ISO 10993-5 (1999) to evaluate the cytotoxicity of materials. It reflects the impact of biomaterials on cells. It shows the effect of materials on adjacent cells. This method is highly sensitive. Viable cells that adhere to the culture plate can be stained with cytochemical stain. Dead cells lose their adhering capacity and are lost during the fixation process. The difference between dead and live cells is shown by the intermediate zone of damaged cells.

6.7.1.6 Agar Diffusion Test

The agar diffusion test described by Schmalz (1988) has been used to assess cytotoxicity. It evaluates cytotoxicity by indirect contact qualitatively. A piece of material to be tested is placed on an agar layer covering a layer of cells, and it is removed after 24–72 hours of exposure. Toxic compounds from materials diffuse through the agar layer and damage the cells in the monolayer. The cells are exposed to neutral red staining. The zone of discoloration caused by damaged cells indicates the toxicity of the material. The lysis index shows the morphological signs of cell damage. Response index (zone index/lysis index) is used to evaluate cytotoxicity. Scoring of cell lysis indicates the toxicity of the material. This test is suitable for high-density biomaterials. But this test can be used only for acute cytotoxicity detection (Li et al., 2015; Assad and Jackson, 2019; Bruinink and Luginbuehl, 2012).

6.7.1.7 Lactate Dehydrogenase (LDH) Assay

This test has been used to assess the viable cells in a culture even though it is not a supersensitive assay. It reflects membrane integrity in cells. Cultured cells are incubated with LDH substrate, cofactor (NAD), and dye (tetrazolium salt) at 25°C for 30 minutes in the dark. After incubation, the reaction is quenched with 1N HCl, and the absorbance is read at 490nm. The amount of LDH produced from cells is determined by the amount of formazan produced. This is proportional to the number of viable cells in the culture (Ohno et al., 1995; Harbell et al., 1997).

6.7.1.8 MTS Assay

Intermittent steps in MTT assay can be omitted in MTS [3-(4,5-dimethylthiazol-2-yl)-5-(3-carboxymethoxyphenyl)-2-(4-sulfophenyl)2H tetrazolium)] assay, as the reagent can be directly added to the cell culture. In this one-step MTT assay, MTS is reduced by cells to a formazan compound in the presence of phenazine methosulfate (PMS). NADPH-dependent dehydrogenase enzymes present in active cells are carrying out this conversion. The amount of the formazan compound is determined by measuring the absorbance at 490–500nm (Cory et al., 1991).

6.7.2 IN VITRO GENOTOXICITY TESTING

The term "genotoxic" indicates substances that are capable of damaging DNA. The genotoxic effects of a material are an important aspect of the safety evaluation of

TABLE 6.2

Common Genotoxicity Tests

Test	Principle
Ames test	Reverse mutation at histidine locus
Cytogenetic analysis	Measurement of aneugenicity using staining techniques, like FISH or chromosome painting
Mammalian gene mutation assay	Measurement of thymidine kinase mutation
Micronucleus assay (MN assay)	Determination of the percentage of micronucleus per nucleus using flow cytometry
Alkaline comet assay	Detection of strand breaks in DNA by utilizing gel electrophoresis
Mouse lymphoma assay	Quantification of thymidine kinase expression alterations
Chromosomal aberration assay	Determination of chromosomal breaks and chromatid changes, and detection of polyploidy

materials for medical applications. Genotoxicity tests determine differences in chromosome structure and chromosome number and mutations. Genotoxic substances can interact with DNA, leading to alterations in DNA. These can result in carcinogenesis and alteration in reproductive function. Important genotoxic effects are mutations and chromosomal aberrations. A battery of tests is normally used to find out genotoxicity, as a single test cannot detect all these effects. A different family of gene regulatory proteins is being activated in genotoxicity. Different materials, like cadmium, cobalt, nickel, and aluminum alloy, are reported to induce carcinogenesis in animal models. Numerous medical metal implants have developed sarcoma in humans after implantation. It has been stated that the identification of carcinogenic effects is also required to be included in genotoxicity testing. Important genotoxicity endpoints include DNA damage, gene mutations, and chromosomal damage (Kohl et al., 2020; Raghavendra et al., 2015). Genotoxicity evaluation of materials is done in mammalian and non-mammalian systems (Table 6.2) (Assad and Jackson, 2019).

6.7.2.1 Ames Test

Ames test or reverse mutation assay is the most widely used in vitro genotoxicity assay, developed by Ames et al. (1975). It has been shown that this test can evaluate the mutagenic action of materials and chemicals (Siew et al., 2009; Kaplan et al., 2004). This assay is performed with *Salmonella typhimurium* and *Escherichia coli* with point mutations in the histidine gene and tryptophan operon, respectively. Bacterial cultures are exposed to test material at 37°C. Exposure of these cells to genotoxic cells leads to reverse mutation and makes the bacteria able to grow on histidine-lacking media. A number of revertant bacterial colonies indicates the mutagenicity of the material (Assad and Jackson, 2019; Jain et al., 2018; Guy, 2005).

6.7.2.2 Cytogenetic Analysis

In vitro cytogenetic assay can be used to screen materials for their potential to induce aneuploidy. Aneugenicity can be confirmed by using staining techniques, such as fluorescence in situ hybridization (FISH), to detect changes in chromosome number (Parry, 1996).

6.7.2.3 Mammalian Gene Mutation Assay

Gene mutations are determined by different mammalian gene mutation protocols (UKEMS, 1989). Among these, measuring mutation at thymidine kinase in mouse lymphoma cells is widely used, as it can detect various chromosome deletions in addition to gene mutations. Mouse lymphoma assay can identify materials that induce gene mutations and potential clastogens.

6.7.2.4 Micronucleus Assay (MN Assay)

Micronucleus assay (MN assay) is a genotoxicity assay conducted with flow cytometry (Sommer et al., 2020). In this highly sensitive assay, cultured cells are treated with material eluate. Then at the end of the treatment, using a flow cytometer, the suspension of nuclei and micronuclei are analyzed. The percentage of micronuclei per nucleus is quantified by dividing the number of micronuclei by the number of nuclei.

6.7.2.5 Alkaline Comet Assay

Alkaline comet assay or single-cell gel electrophoresis (SCGE) is another test for genotoxicity.

Comet assay can quantify DNA. Breaks in DNA strand is used to evaluate DNA damage (Collins et al., 1997; Rojas et al., 1999; Tice and Strauss, 1995). In this test, cells suspended in molten agar are layered on a microscope slide. The cells are lysed by detergent with high salt and liberated DNA electrophoreses. Cells with damage in the DNA strand display altered migration toward the anode, forming comets. Comets can be viewed after staining using fluorescent or non-fluorescent microscopy. Comet formation is increased by double-strand breaks in the DNA. The level of damage is evaluated by DNA tail length or tail moment values. Comet assay evaluates the interaction between materials and living cells.

6.7.2.6 Mouse Lymphoma Assay

Mouse lymphoma assay (MLN) is used to detect gene mutations, like point mutations, deletions, translocations, and aneuploidy. This test quantifies alterations in thymidine kinase gene expression on chromosome 11. A mouse lymphoma cell line is used for the assay. The cells that lack TK genes are resistant to the cytostatic activity of trifluorothymidine (TFT)–pyrimidine analog. Mutant cells can survive in the presence of TFT, whereas normal cell scans do not. Cells are incubated with test material for a period of three to four hours. After incubation, cells are subcultured to allow the expression of the mutant phenotype. The cells are then seeded on the cell plate to detect the mutant cells. The mutagenicity of the material is evaluated by the presence of colonies, size of the colonies, and mutant frequency. The factors influencing the result of the test include solubilization of the material, changes in pH, osmolality, and cell line viability (Assad and Jackson, 2019; Moore et al., 2006; OECD Guideline for the Testing of Chemicals. In vitro mammalian cell gene mutation assays using the thymidine kinase gene, 2014).

6.7.2.7 In Vitro Chromosomal Aberration Assay

In vitro chromosomal aberration assay is used to determine structural changes, like chromosome breaks, chromatid exchanges, polyploidy, and endoreduplication. Primary human peripheral blood lymphocytes or cell lines, like Chinese hamster ovary cells and Chinese hamster fibroblasts, are used to perform this test. Proliferating cells are exposed to the extract test dilutions for three to six hours.

After exposure, cell cultures are treated with metaphase-arresting compound at intervals for one to three hours, per the cell cycle length. Cells are harvested by hypotonic treatment, fixation, and staining with Giesma. The type and number of chromosomal aberrations are scored. The percentage of cells with chromosome aberration is determined, compared with the controls. Results may be influenced by the solvent used, pH changes, and other test conditions (Assad and Jackson, 2019).

6.7.3   IN VITRO THROMBOGENICITY TEST

Thrombogenicity is the tendency of a material to form a blood clot or thrombus when in contact with the blood. Blood-contacting medical devices are used in the treatment of a number of diseases. Failure of the blood-contacting devices occurs mainly due to the thrombogenicity of a material surface (Gorbet and Sefton, 2004; Jaffer et al., 2015; Salacinski et al., 2001). Thrombogenicity testing is important for materials used in artificial organs, like heart valves, blood pumps, and others, which are in direct contact with blood.

Thrombogenic toxicity evaluation is difficult due to the complexity of the blood coagulation system. Thrombogenicity testing helps to improve material selection and device design in medical implants. It also provides a more reliable prediction of device safety. A thorough investigation of thrombosis is rarely done in vitro. Most studies are to measure hemolysis. It has been reported that studies that use in vivo models failed to correlate in vivo thrombosis testing with in vitro results (Amoako et al., 2013; Goudie et al., 2017). The requirement for anticoagulants is the most important limitation of in vitro systems. Thrombogenicity testing includes coagulation, hemolysis, hematology, and platelet and the complement system. Before and after incubation, hemocompatibility markers are determined (Weber et al., 2018). It is done using static, agitated, or shear flow in vitro models for the incubation of human blood with biomaterials. Although there are many in vitro tests available for thrombogenicity testing, there is no clear recommendation due to the unavailability of comparative studies (Table 6.3).

6.7.3.1   Hemolysis

Hemolysis is a measure of hemoglobin release in plasma as an indicator of red blood cell lysis. It occurs due to the rupture of red blood cells after contacting the materials. This hemoglobin is released either by leaking through the RBC membrane or by the destruction of RBCs. Mechanical and non-mechanical factors can lead to hemolysis. But the focus is on the damage caused by the mechanical stress of materials used.

6.7.3.2   Coagulation

Coagulation is evaluated by measuring the rate of clot formation or partial thromboplastin time (PTT) of plasma exposed to materials during incubation with materials in vitro. Internal coagulation pathway activation is assessed by comparing the PTT shortening with negative controls. Key coagulation proteins TAT, F1.2, and beta-thromboglobulin are measured using ELISA assays as indicators of

TABLE 6.3
Common Thrombogenicity Tests

Test	Principle
Hemolysis	Rupture of blood cells and subsequent release of intracellular molecules
Coagulation	Measurement of the rate of clot formation
Partial thromboplastin time (PTT) assay	Determination of coagulation induced by materials
Fibrinogen binding	Labeling of antibody binding to detect fibrin/fibrinogen on the surface
Complement system activation	Determination of activation of a complementary pathway
Accelerated clotting test	Measurement of the thrombus formation
Leucocyte and platelet count	Indirect quantification of the retention of leucocyte and platelet on the material surface
Platelet activation	Determination of platelet thrombin receptor PAR 1 cleavage, which leads to increased adhesion

platelet activation. The main enzyme of the coagulation, thrombin, is also determined by measuring the thrombin-antithrombin complex (TAA) and prothrombin fragments using ELISA techniques. The formation of the TAA complex indicates coagulation. Thrombin formation results in the release of prothrombin fragments. Thromboelastography, an in vitro whole blood–based test, gives an overall picture of the clotting processing (Nalezinková, 2020; Weber et al., 2018).

6.7.3.3   Partial Thromboplastin Time (PTT) Assay

The thrombogenic property of biomaterials can be also assessed by measuring partial thromboplastin time (PTT). This assay is the most used assay to determine the coagulation induced by materials. But as reported by Prince et al. (1988), this test lacks reproducibility due to the relative insensitivity of the test for different biomaterials. PTT can be used to determine large deviations in material characteristics. But it is not suitable for the fine selection of material for the long term, like implants.

6.7.3.4   Fibrinogen Binding

Fibrinogen binding is another method used to determine the hemocompatibility of materials in medical applications (Bailly et al., 1996). Labeled antibody binding or labeled fibrinogen method or microscopic techniques or a combination of these methods can be used to detect fibrin/fibrinogen on the surface (van Oeveren et al., 2002).

6.7.3.5   Complement System Activation

The complement system is an important component of the immune response. Materials used in medical applications act on the alternative pathway of the complement and lead to the formation of complement proteins, like C3, C5b, C7, C8, and C9. Complement cascade activation is associated with conformational changes in the components involved in the different activation pathways (Nilsson et al., 2007;

Engberg et al., 2015; Markiewski et al., 2007). Hydrophobic surfaces and materials with amine or hydroxyl groups were shown to activate the alternative pathway (van Oeveren et al., 2002; DeHeer et al., 2001). These processes involve the covalent binding of complement component C3 and its conversion to molecules like C3b. Interactions of non-antigen bound IgG and C1(q) with material surfaces induce activation of the classical pathway. Hydrophobic surfaces of materials cause increased complement activation than hydrophilic surfaces. But binding of complement components to the material alters the result (Nalezinková, 2020; Weber et al., 2018).

6.7.3.6 Leucocytes and Platelet Count

Thrombosis can also be determined by counting the platelets and leukocytes. As they are involved in clot formation, they are depleted from serum. It can provide insight into the material's thrombogenicity.

The interaction of leukocytes with material surfaces is determined directly by visualizing adhesion and activation-induced morphological changes at the material's surface (Klopfleisch and Jung, 2017; Franke and Jung, 2012; Anderson et al., 2008). The counting of nonadherent leukocytes indicates an indirect quantification of the retention of these cells on the material's surface (Anderson et al., 2008). Activation of leukocytes and their contribution to thrombus formation can be measured. Complete blood counts (CBCs) by routine electronic methods are used to determine plate counts before and after material-blood exposure. Platelet counts will decrease with time if the material is highly thrombogenic. Platelet function is assessed using colorimetric assays or automated image-based analysis, as outlined in the ASTM-F2888 Standard Test Method for Platelet Leukocyte Count—An In Vitro Measure for Hemocompatibility Assessment of Cardiovascular Materials (ASTM International, 2016).

6.7.3.7 Platelet Activation

Platelet activation level is another indicator of thrombogenicity. It can take place when blood comes in contact with biomaterials. Platelet activation is measured by determining the platelet thrombin receptor PAR 1 cleavage. Cleavage of this receptor by thrombin leads to platelet activation and leads to several reactions in the thrombocytes, like increased adhesion. PAR 1 antibody binds only to uncleaved receptors. So a reduction in antibody binding indicates platelet activation. The formation of platelet-derived microparticles (PMPs) is another indicator of platelet activation. They play a role in blood clotting and thrombus formation. The evaluation of material-induced platelet activation and the formation of thrombin help in understanding the thrombogenicity of the material (Jung and Braune, 2016; Gorbet and Sefton, 2004). Assessment of degranulated proteins released after activation of platelets and detection of P selectin CD62P or selectin CD62P or activated GPIIB/IIIa also used to evaluate undesired platelet activation (Nalezinková, 2020; Weber et al., 2018).

6.7.3.8 Accelerated Clotting Test

Studies indicate that the accelerated clotting test is very useful and reliable in testing mechanical heart valves and blood pumps (Paul et al., 1998). It allows studies of early-stage thrombus formation. It has been reported that the in vitro test results are well correlated with in vivo test results, and it is a cost-effective method (Kim et al., 2020).

6.8 MECHANICAL PROPERTY EVALUATION

Mechanical evaluation of materials is very important in medical applications, like transplants. In in vitro fatigue, performance assessment using the fatigue-wear approach helps to determine fatigue performance (Teoh, 2000). Recently, simulators have been developed to determine fatigue and wear behavior in clinical situations (Benazzo et al., 2006; Nevelos et al., 2000).

6.9 FUTURE TRENDS

There has been a tremendous increase in in vitro testing of materials for medical applications. In vitro testing results need to be proved in animal models to determine whether the material should be carried out in clinical trials. The ability of in vitro systems to mimic physiological conditions helps to evaluate the therapeutic strategies addressing different diseases. But it is always criticized due to its lack of reproducibility. The poor correlation between in vivo and in vitro results calls for further studies in this area. In a human-based screening study, Jannasch et al. (2017) explained how sensitive in vitro biomaterial assessments rely on test conditions and influence the outcome of biomaterial ranking. They also proposed the use of human cell–based in vitro test systems for material assessment. The tissue response to materials in vascular areas and avascular areas may be different. In vitro testing can serve as a screening platform that helps to identify the properties of materials before in vivo testing. Every in vitro model represents a system with specific physiological functions. The selection of a suitable in vitro test system to solve a particular problem is a promising approach. High throughput screening (HTS) can be used to evaluate new biomaterials for medical applications. To study diseases of high-level complexity, expertise in that area needs to be combined with new in vitro system models. For example, 3D intestine-on-chip models help to understand the host immune response to fungi and the effects of microbes and their products in the body.

Even though ISP guidelines provide many choices of molecular markers, they are not used in the in vitro testing for materials for medical applications. A thorough investigation of all these markers can provide a base for updating in vitro testing guidance documents for medical applications. Identifying an appropriate marker for in vitro models is important in designing in vitro tests for materials for medical applications. It has been proposed that researchers should test combinations of markers that assess different components of the coagulation system and general measures of coagulation to assess the thrombogenicity of materials (Sarode and Roy, 2019). The type of system should be considered. An ideal system should identify toxicity early in the development process so that we can reduce the unnecessary use of valuable resources in in vivo tests. Appropriate steps taken to evaluate and understand cell-material interactions in each medical application lead to effective and safe use in humans. Performing in vitro tests as a part of the routine analysis in clinics will help in precision medicine in oncology and will help to provide successful therapy for each patient.

REFERENCES

Ames, B. N., McCann, J., & Yamasaki, E. (1975). Methods for detecting carcinogens and mutagens with the *Salmonella*/mammalian-microsome mutagenicity test. *Mutation Research*, *31*(6), 347–364.

Amoako, K. A., Montoya, P. J., Major, T. C., Suhaib, A. B., Handa, H., Brant, D. O., Meyerhoff, M. E., Bartlett, R. H., & Cook, K. E. (2013). Fabrication and *in vivo* thrombogenicity testing of nitric oxide generating artificial lungs. *Journal of Biomedical Materials Research Part A*, *101*(1 2), 3511–3519. https://doi.org/10.1002/jbm.a.34655.

Anderson, J. M., Rodriguez, A., & Chang, D. T. (2008). Foreign body reaction to biomaterials. *Seminars in Immunology*, *20*(2), 86–100. https://doi.org/10.1016/j.smim.2007.11.004.

Anjum, S., & Gupta, B. (2018). Bioengineering of functional nanosilver nanogels for smart healthcare systems. *Global Challenges*, *40*(10), 1800044. https://doi.org/10.1002/gch2.201800044.

Armugam, A., Teong, S. P., Lim, D., Chan, S. P., Yi, G., Yew, D. S., Beh, C. W., & Zhang, Y. (2021). Broad spectrum antimicrobial PDMS-based biomaterial for catheter fabrication. *Biomaterials Resear ch*, *25*(1), 33. https://doi.org/10.1186/s40824-021-00235-5.

Assad, M., & Jackson, N. D. (2019). Biocompatibility evaluation of orthopedic biomaterials and medical devices: A review of safety and efficacy models. In: *Encyclopedia of Biomedical Engineering*. Kaminski, D. B. (ed.). Elsevier, pp. 322–330. https://doi.org/10.1016/B978-0-12-801238-3.65085-8.

ASTM International. (2016). *ASTM F2888-16: Standard Test Method for Platelet Leukocyte Count—An In Vitro Measure for Hemocompatibility Assessment of Cardiovascular Materials*. ASTM International, West Conshohocken, PA. https://doi.org/10.1520/F2888-16.

Bailly, A. L., Laurent, A., Lu, H., Elalami, I., Jacob, P., Mundler, O., Merland, J. J., Lautier, A., Soria, J., & Soria, C. (1996). Fibrinogen binding and platelet retention: Relationship with the thrombogenicity of catheters. *Journal of Biomedical Materials Research*, *30*(1), 101–108. https://doi.org/10.1002/(SICI)1097-4636(199601)30:1<101::AID-JBM13>3.0.CO;2-R.

Benam, K. H., Villenave, R., Lucchesi, C., Varone, A., Hubeau, C., Lee, H. H., Alves, S. E., Salmon, M., Ferrante, T. C., Weaver, J. C., Bahinski, A., Hamilton, G. A., & Ingber, D. E. (2016). Small airway-on-a-chip enables analysis of human lung inflammation and drug responses in vitro. *Nature Methods*, *13*(2), 151–157. https://doi.org/10.1038/nmeth.3697.

Benazzo, F., Falez, F., & Dietrich, M. (2006). *Bioceramics and Alternative Bearings in Joint Arthroplasty*. 11th BIOLOX® Symposium Rome, 2006 Proceedings, June 30–July 1. 10.1007/978-3-7985-1635-9.

Billings, P. R. (2006). Three barriers to innovative diagnostics. *Nature Biotechnology*, *24*(8), 917–918. https://doi.org/10.1038/nbt0806-917.

Bongomin, F., Gago, S., Oladele, R. O., & Denning, D. W. (2017). Global and multi-national prevalence of fungal diseases-estimate precision. *Journal of Fungi (Basel, Switzerla nd)*, *3*(4), 57. https://doi.org/10.3390/jof3040057.

Brown, G. D., Denning, D. W., Gow, N. A., Levitz, S. M., Netea, M. G., & White, T. C. (2012). Hidden killers: Human fungal infections. *Science Translational Medicine*, *4* (165), 165rv13. https://doi.org/10.1126/scitranslmed.3004404.

Bruinink, A., & Luginbuehl, R. (2012). Evaluation of biocompatibility using in vitro methods: Interpretation and limitations. *Advances in Biochemical Engineering/Biotechnology*, *126*, 117–152. https://doi.org/10.1007/10_2011_111.

Campoy, S., & Adrio, J. L. (2017). Antifungals. *Biochemical Pharmacolog y*, *133*, 86–96. https://doi.org/10.1016/j.bcp.2016.11.019.

Cenni, E., Ciapetti, G., Granchi, D., Arciola, C. R., Savaring, L., Stea, S., Montanaro, L., & Pizzoferrato, A. (1999). Established cell lines and primary cultures in testing medical devices in vitro. *Toxicology in Vitro*, *13*, 801–810.

Chen, S. C. A., Slavin, M. A., & Sorrell, T. C. (2011). Echinocandin antifungal drugs in fungal infections. *Dru gs*, *71*, 11–41. https://doi.org/10.2165/11585270-000000000-00000.

Chen, X., Tang, Q. L., Zhu, Y. J, Zhu, C. L., & Feng, X. P. (2012). Synthesis and antibacterial property of zinc loaded hydroxyapatite nanorods. *Materials Letters*, *89*, 233–235. https://doi.org/10.1016/j.matlet.2012.08.115.

Ciapetti, G., Granchi, D., Verri, E., Savarino, L., Cavedagna, D., & Pizzoferrato, A. (1996). Application of a combination of neutral red and amido black staining for rapid, reliable cytotoxicity testing of biomaterials. *Biomaterials*, *17*(13), 1259–1264.

Collins, A. R., Dobson, V. L., Dusinska, M., Kennedy, G., & Stetina, R. (1997). The comet assay: What can it really tell us? *Mutation Research*, *375*, 183–193.

Cory, A. H., Owen, T. C., Barltrop, J. A., & Cory, J. G. (1991). Use of an aqueous soluble tetrazolium/formazan assay for cell growth assays in culture. *Cancer Communications*, *3*(7), 207–212. https://doi.org/10.3727/095535491820873191.

Cosio, T., Gaziano, R., Zuccari, G., Costanza, G., Grelli, S., Di Francesco, P., Bianchi, L., & Campione, E. (2021). Retinoids in fungal infections: From bench to bedside. *Pharmaceuticals*, *14*(10), 962. https://doi.org/10.3390/ph14100962.

Costa, E. C., Moreira, A. F., de Melo-Diogo, D., Gaspar, V. M., Carvalho, M. P., & Correia, I. J. (2016). 3D tumor spheroids: An overview on the tools and techniques used for their analysis. *Biotechnology Advances*, *34*(8), 1427–1441.

Cressman, S., Lam, S., Tammemagi, M. C., Evans, W. K., Leighl, N. B., Regier, D. A., Bolbocean, C., Shepherd, F. A., Tsao, M. S., Manos, D., Liu, G., Atkar-Khattra, S., Cromwell, I., Johnston, M. R., Mayo, J. R., McWilliams, A., Couture, C., English, J. C., Goffin, J., Hwang, D. M., . . . Pan-Canadian Early Detection of Lung Cancer Study Team. (2014). Resource utilization and costs during the initial years of lung cancer screening with computed tomography in Canada. *Journal of Thoracic Oncology: Official Publication of the International Association for the Study of Lung Cancer*, *9*(10), 1449–1458. https://doi.org/10.1097/JTO.0000000000000283.

Dave, R. N., Joshi, H. M., & Venugopalan, V. P. (2011). Novel biocatalytic polymer-based antimicrobial coatings as potential ureteral biomaterial: Preparation and *in vitro* performance evaluation. *Antimicrob Agents Chemother*, *5 5*(2), 845–853. https://doi.org/10.1128/AAC.00477-10.

DeHeer, D. H., Engels, J. A., DeVries, A. S., Knapp, R. H., & Beebe, J. D. (2001). In situ complement activation by polyethylene wear debris. *Journal of Biomedical Materials Research*, *54*(1), 12–19. doi:10.1002/1097-4636(200101)54:1<12::aid-jbm2>3.0.co;2-x. PMID: 11077398.

Deinhardt-Emmer, S., Rennert, K., Schicke, E., Cseresnyés, Z., Windolph, M., Nietzsche, S., Heller, R., Siwczak, F., Haupt, K. F., Carlstedt, S., Schacke, M., Figge, M. T., Ehrhardt, C., Löffler, B., & Mosig, A. S. (2020). Co-infection with Staphylococcus aureus after primary influenza virus infection leads to damage of the endothelium in a human alveolus-on-a-chip model. *Biofabrication*, *12*(2), 025012. https://doi.org/10.1088/1758-5090/ab7073.

Engberg, A. E., Nilsson, P. H., Huang, S., Fromell, K., Hamad, O. A., Mollnes, T. E., Rosengren-Holmberg, J. P., Sandholm, K., Teramura, Y., Nicholls, I. A., Nilsson, B., & Ekdahl, K. N. (2015). Prediction of inflammatory responses induced by biomaterials in contact with human blood using protein fingerprint from plasma. *Biomateria ls, 36*, 55–65. https://doi.org/10.1016/j.biomaterials.2014.09.011.

Finter, N. B. (1969). Dye uptake methods for assessing vital cytopathogenicity and their application to interferon assays. *Journal of General Virology, 5*, 419–427.

Folkman, J., & Moscona, A. (1978). Role of cell shape in growth control. *Nature, 273*, 345–349. https://doi.org/10.1038/273345a0.

Fotakis, G., & Timbrell, J. A. (2006). In vitro cytotoxicity assays: Comparison of LDH, neutral red, MTT and protein assay in hepatoma cell lines following exposure to cadmium chloride. *Toxicology Letters, 160*, 171–177. doi:10.1016/j.toxlet.2005.07.001.

Francolini, I., Vuotto, C., Piozzi, A., & Donelli, G. (2017). Antifouling and antimicrobial biomaterials: An overview. *APMIS, 12 5*(4), 392–417. https://doi.org/10.1111/apm.12675.

Franke, R., & Jung, F. (2012). Interaction of blood components and blood cells with body foreign surfaces. *Series on Biomechanics, 27*(1), 51–58.

Geraldi, A., & Giri-Rachman, E. A. (2018). Synthetic biology-based portable in vitro diagnostic platforms. *Alexandria Journal of Medicine, 54* (4), 423–428. https://doi.org/10.1016/j.ajme.2018.11.003.

Gorbet, M. B., & Sefton, M. V. (2004). Biomaterial-associated thrombosis: Roles of coagulation factors, complement, platelets and leukocytes. *Biomaterials, 25*(26), 5681–5703. doi:10.1016/j.biomaterials.2004.01.023.

Goudie, M. J., Brainard, B. M., Schmiedt, C. W., & Handa, H. (2017). Characterization and in vivo performance of nitric oxide-releasing extracorporeal circuits in a feline model of thrombogenicity. *Journal of Biomedical Materials Research. Part A, 10 5*(2), 539–546. https://doi.org/10.1002/jbm.a.35932.

Gröger, M., Rennert, K., Giszas, B., Weiß, E., Dinger, J., Funke, H., Kiehntopf, M., Peters, F. T., Lupp, A., Bauer, M., Claus, R. A., Huber, O., & Mosig, A. S. (2016). Monocyte-induced recovery of inflammation-associated hepatocellular dysfunction in a biochip-based human liver model. *Scientific Repo rts, 6*, 21868. https://doi.org/10.1038/srep21868.

Guy, R. C. (2005). Ames test. In: *Encyclopedia of Toxicology*, 2nd edition. Wexler, P. (ed.). Elsevier, Amsterdam, pp. 88–91.

Harbell, J. W., Kootnz, S. W., Lewis, R. W., Lovell, D., & Acosta, D. (1997). Cell cytotoxicity assays. *Food and Chemical Toxicology, 35*, 79–126.

Hermansky, S. J. (2001). Regulatory toxicology: Medical devices. In: *Handbook of Toxicology*, 2nd edition. Derelanko, M. J., & Hollinder, M. A. (eds.). CRC Press, Boca Raton, pp. 1173–1233.

Hirschhaeuser, F., Menne, H., Dittfeld, C., West, J., Mueller-Klieser, W., & Kunz-Schughart, L. A. (2010). Multicellular tumor spheroids: An underestimated tool is catching up again. *Journal of Biotechnology, 148*(1), 3–15. https://doi.org/10.1016/j.jbiotec.2010.01.012.

Houšť, J., Spížek, J., & Havlíček, V. (2020). Antifungal drugs. *Metabolites , 10*(3), E106. https://doi.org/10.3390/metabo10030106.

Hulsart-Billström, G., Dawson, J. I., Hofmann, S., Müller, R., Stoddart, M. J., Alini, M., Redl, H., El Haj, A., Brown, R., Salih, V., Hilborn, J., Larsson, S., & Oreffo, R. O. (2016). A surprisingly poor correlation between in vitro and in vivo testing of biomaterials for bone regeneration: Results of a multicentre analysis. *European Cells & Materials , 31*, 312–322. https://doi.org/10.22203/ecm.v031a20.

Iqbal, H. M. N., & Keshavarz, T. (2017). The challenge of biocompatibility evaluation of biocomposites. In: *Woodhead Publishing Series in Biomaterials, Biomedical Composites*, 2nd edition. Ambrosio, L. (ed.). Woodhead Publishing, Cambridge, pp. 303–334,

ISO10993–5. (1999). International standards: Biological evaluation of medical device. Test for in vitro cytotoxicity.

Jaffer, I. H., Fredenburgh, J. C., Hirsh, J., & Weitz, J. I. (2015). Medical device-induced thrombosis: What causes it and how can we prevent it? *Journal of Thrombosis and Haemostasis*, 13(Suppl 1), S72–S81. https://doi.org/10.1111/jth.12961. PMID: 26149053.

Jain, A. K., Singh, D., Dubey, K., Maurya, R., Mittal, S., & Pandey, A. K. (2018). Models and methods for in vitro toxicity. In: *In vitro Toxicology*. Dhawan, A., & Kwon, S. (eds.). Academic Press, Amsterdam, pp. 45–65.

Jang, K. J., Otieno, M. A., Ronxhi, J., Lim, H. K., Ewart, L., Kodella, K. R., Petropolis, D. B., Kulkarni, G., Rubins, J. E., Conegliano, D., Nawroth, J., Simic, D., Lam, W., Singer, M., Barale, E., Singh, B., Sonee, M., Streeter, A. J., Manthey, C., Jones, B., . . . Hamilton, G. A. (2019). Reproducing human and cross-species drug toxicities using a Liver-Chip. *Science Translational Medicine*, *11*(5 17), eaax5516. https://doi.org/10.1126/scitranslmed.aax5516.

Jannasch, M., Gaetzner, S., Weigel, T., Walles, H., Schmitz, T., & Hansmann, J. (2017). A comparative multi-parametric *in vitro* model identifies the power of test conditions to predict the fibrotic tendency of a biomaterial. *Scientific Reports*, 7(1), 1689. https://doi.org/10.1038/s41598-017-01584-9.

Jung, F., & Braune, S. (2016). Thrombogenicity and hemocompatibility of biomaterials. *Biointerphases*, *11*(2), 029601.

Kaplan, C., Diril, N., Şahin, S., & Cehreli, M. C. (2004). Mutagenic potentials of dental cements as detected by the Salmonella/microsome test. *Biomaterials*, 25, 4019–4027.

Khanna, D., & Bharti, S. (2014). Luliconazole for the treatment of fungal infections: An evidence-based review. *Core Evidenc e*, 9, 113–124. https://doi.org/10.2147/CE.S49629.

Kim, C. H., Steinseifer, U., & Schmitz-Rode, T. (2020). Thrombogenic evaluation of two mechanical heart valve prostheses using a new in-vitro test system. *Journal of Heart Valve Disease,* *18*(2), 207–213. PMID: 19455896.

Klopfleisch, R., & Jung, F. (2017). The pathology of the foreign body reaction against biomaterials. *Journal of Biomedical Materials Research. Part A*, 10 5(3), 927–940. https://doi.org/10.1002/jbm.a.35958.

Klußmann-Fricke, B., Reske, T., Schmitz, K., Siewert, S., & Khaimov, V. (2021). Quantitative evaluation of cell morphology and material interactions on opaque biomaterials. *Current Directions in Biomedical Engineering*, 7(2), 664–667. https://doi.org/10.1515/cdbme-2021-2169.

Kohl, Y., Rundén-Pran, E., Mariussen, E., Hesler, M., El Yamani, N., Longhin, E. M., & Dusinska, M. (2020). Genotoxicity of nanomaterials: Advances in vitro models and high throughput methods for human hazard assessment-a review. *Nanomaterials (Base l)*, *10*(1911). https://doi.org/10.3390/nano10101911.

Kolmas, J., Groszyk, E., & Piotrowska, U. (2015). Nanocrystalline hydroxyapatite enriched in selenite and manganese ions: Physicochemical and antibacterial properties. *Nanoscale Research Let ters*, *10*, 278. https://doi.org/10.1186/s11671–015–0989-x.

Li, W., Zhou, J., & Xu, Y. (2015). Study of the in vitro cytotoxicity testing of medical devices. *Biomedical Reports*, 3, 617–620. https://doi.org/10.3892/br.2015.481.

Liu, H., Shukla, S., Vera-González, N., Tharmalingam, N., Mylonakis, E., Fuchs, B. B., & Shukla, A. (2019). Auranofin releasing antibacterial and antibiofilm polyurethane intravascular catheter coatings. *Frontiers in Cellular and Infection Microbiology*, 9, 37. https://doi.org/10.3389/fcimb.2019.00037.

Lohmann, C. H., Dean, D. D., & Schwartz, Z. (1999). Surface roughness mediates its effects on osteoblasts via protein kinase A and phospholipase A2. *Biomaterials*, *20*(23–24), 2305–2310.

Malhotra, V., & Perry, M. C. (2003). Classical chemotherapy: Mechanisms, toxicities and the therapeutic window. *Cancer Biology & Therapy*, *2*(Suppl 1), 1–3. https://doi.org/10.4161/cbt.199.

Markiewski, M. M., Nilsson, B., Ekdahl, K. N., Mollnes, T. E., & Lambris, J. D. (2007). Complement and coagulation: Strangers or partners in crime? *Trends in Immunology*, *28*(4), 184–192. https://doi.org/10.1016/j.it.2007.02.006. Epub 2007 Mar 1. PMID: 17336159.

Martignetti, J. A., Camacho-Vanegas, O., Priedigkeit, N., Camacho, C., Pereira, E., Lin, L., Garnar-Wortzel, L., Miller, D., Losic, B., Shah, H., Liao, J., Ma, J., Lahiri, P., Chee, M., Schadt, E., & Dottino, P. (2014). Personalized ovarian cancer disease surveillance and detection of candidate therapeutic drug target in circulating tumor DNA. *Neoplasia*, *16*, 97–103. https://doi.org/10.1593/neo.131900.

Martin, K. W., & Ernst, E. (2004). Herbal medicines for treatment of fungal infections: A systematic review of controlled clinical trials. *Mycoses*, *47*(3–4), 87–92. https://doi.org/10.1046/j.1439-0507.2003.00951.x.

Maurer, M., Gresnigt, M. S., Last, A., Wollny, T., Berlinghof, F., Pospich, R., Cseresnyes, Z., Medyukhina, A., Graf, K., Gröger, M., Raasch, M., Siwczak, F., Nietzsche, S., Jacobsen, I. D., Figge, M. T., Hube, B., Huber, O., & Mosig, A. S. (2019). A three-dimensional immunocompetent intestine-on-chip model as in vitro platform for functional and microbial interaction studies. *Biomaterials*, *220*, 119396. https://doi.org/10.1016/j.biomaterials.2019.119396.

Maxson, J. E., Abel, M. L., Wang, J., Deng, X., Reckel, S., Luty, S. B., Sun, H., Gorenstein, J., Hughes, S. B., Bottomly, D., Wilmot, B., McWeeney, S. K., Radich, J., Hantschel, O., Middleton, R. E., Gray, N. S., Druker, B. J., & Tyner, J. W. (2016). Identification and characterization of tyrosine kinase nonreceptor 2 mutations in leukemia through integration of kinase inhibitor screening and genomic analysis. *Cancer Research*, *76*(1), 127–138. DOI: 10.1158/0008-5472.can-15-0817. PMID: 26677978; PMCID: PMC4703549.

Mignogna, M. D., Fedele, S., Lo Russo, L., Ruoppo, E., & Lo Muzio, L. (2002). Costs and effectiveness in the care of patients with oral and pharyngeal cancer: Analysis of a paradox. *European Journal of Cancer Prevention*, *11*, 205–208. pmid:12131652.

Moore, M. M., Honma, M., Clements, J., Bolcsfoldi, G., Burlinson, B., Cifone, M., Clarke, J., Delongchamp, R., Durward, R., Fellows, M., Gollapudi, B., Hou, S., Jenkinson, P., Muster, W., Pant, K., Kidd, D. A., Lorge, E., Lloyd, M. et al. (2006). Mouse lymphoma thymidine kinase gene mutation assay: Follow-up meeting of the international workshop on genotoxicity testing-Aberdeen, Scotland, 2003-assay acceptance criteria, positive controls, and data evaluation. *Environmental and Molecular Mutagenesis*, *47*, 1–5. https://doi.org/10.1002/em.20159.

Mosig, A. S. (2016). Organ-on-chip models: New opportunities for biomedical research. *Future Science OA*, *3*(2), FSO130. https://doi.org/10.4155/fsoa-2016-0038.

Mosmann, T. (1983). Rapid colorimetric assay for cellular growth and survival: Application to proliferation and cytotoxicity assays. *Journal of Immunological Methods*, *65*(1–2), 55–63. https://doi.org/10.1016/0022-1759(83)90303-4.

Muller, P. Y., & Milton, M. N. (2012). The determination and interpretation of the therapeutic index in drug development. *Nature Reviews Drug Discovery*, *11* (10), 751–761. https://doi.org/10.1038/nrd3801. Epub 2012 Aug 31. PMID: 22935759.

Nalezinková, M. (2020). *In vitro* hemocompatibility testing of medical devices. *Thrombosis Research*, *195*, 145–190. https://doi.org/10.1016/j.thromres.2020.07.027.

National Toxicology Program (NTP) Interagency Center for the Evaluation of Alternative Toxicological Methods (NICEATM). (2003). *Test Method Protocol for NHK Neutral Red Uptake Cytotoxicity Test*. Retrieved from https://www.niehs.nih.gov/research/atniehs/labs/ptb/niceatm/index.cfm

Nevelos, J., Ingham, E., Doyle, C., Streicher, R., Nevelos, A., Walter, W., & Fisher, J. (2000). Microseparation of the centers of alumina-alumina artificial hip joints during simulator testing produces clinically relevant wear rates and patterns. *The Journal of Arthroplasty*, *15*(6), 793–795. https://doi.org/10.1054/arth.2000.8100.

Nilsson, B., Ekdahl, K. N., Mollnes, T. E., & Lambris, J. D. (2007). The role of complement in biomaterial-induced inflammation. *Molecular Immunology, 44*(1–3), 82–94. https://doi. org/10.1016/j.molimm.2006.06.020. Epub 2006 Aug 14. PMID: 16905192.

OECD. (2014). *Test No. 476: In Vitro Mammalian Cell Gene Mutation Tests Using the Thymidine Kinase Gene.* OECD Publishing. https://www.oecd.org/publications/test-no-490-in-vitro-mammalian-cell-gene-mutation-tests-using-the-thymidine-kinase-gene-9789264264908-en.htm

Ohno, T., Itagaki, H., Tanaka, N., & Ono, H. (1995). Validation study on five cytotoxicity assays in Japan-an intermediate report. *Toxicology in Vitro, 4*, 571–576.

Pais, P., Galocha, M., Viana, M., Cavalheiro, M., Pereira, D., & Teixeira, M. C. (2019). Microevolution of the pathogenic yeasts *Candida albicans* and *Candida glabrata* during antifungal therapy and host infection. *Microbial Cell, 6*(3), 142–159. https://doi. org/10.15698/mic2019.03.670.

Parry, J. M., Parry, E. M., Bourner, R., Doherty, A., Ellard, S., O'Donovan, J., Hoebee, B., de Stoppelaar, J. M., Mohn, G. R., Onfelt, A. et al. (1996). The detection and evaluation of aneugenic chemicals. *Mutation Research, 35*, 11–46.

Paul, R., Marseille, O., Hintze, E., Huber, L., Schima, H., Reul, H., & Rau, G. (1998). *In vitro* thrombogenicity testing of artificial organs. *International Journal of Artificial Organs, 21*(9), 548–552. PMID: 9828061.

Pennisi, E. (2016). IMAGING. 'Cell painting' highlights responses to drugs and toxins. *Science (New York, N.Y.), 352*(6 288), 877–878. https://doi.org/10.1126/science.352.6288.877.

Popova, A. A., & Levkin, P. A. (2020). Precision medicine in oncology: In vitro drug sensitivity and resistance test (DSRT) for selection of personalized anticancer therapy. *Advanced Therapeutics, 3*(2).

Prince, M. R., Salzman, E. W., Schoen, F. J., Palestrant, A. M., & Simon, M. (1988). Local intravascular effects of the nitinol wire blood clot filter. *Investigative Radiology, 23*, 294–300.

Puck, T. T., & Marcus, P. I. (1956). Action of x-rays on mammalian cells. Journal of Experimental Medicine, *103*(5), 653–666.

Raghavendra, G. M., Varaprasad, K., & Jayaramudu, T. (2015). Biomaterials: Design, development and biomedical applications. In: *Nanotechnology Applications for Tissue Engineering*. Thomas, S., Grohens, Y., & Ninan, N. (eds.). Elsevier, Amsterdam, pp. 21–44.

Rajendran, A., Barik, R. C., Natarajan, D., Kiran, M. S., & Pattanayak, D. K. (2014). Synthesis, phase stability of hydroxyapatite-silver composite with antimicrobial activity and cytocompatability. *Ceramics International, 40*, 10831–10838. https://doi.org/10.1016/j. ceramint.2014.03.075.

Raman, G., Avendano, E., & Chen, M. (2013). *Update on Emerging Genetic Tests Currently Available for Clinical Use in Common Cancers, in Technology Assessment Report.* Agency for Healthcare Research and Quality, Rockville, MD.

Rasekh, M., Ahmad, Z., Frangos, C. C., Bozec, L., Edirisinghe, M., & Day, R. M. (2013). Spatial and temporal evaluation of cell attachment to printed polycaprolactone microfibres. *Acta Biomater, 9*(2), 5052–5062.

Riool, M., de Breij, A., Drijfhout, J. W., Nibbering, P. H., & Zaat, S. A. J. (2017). Antimicrobial peptides in biomedical device manufacturing. *Frontiers in Chemistry , 5*, 63. https:// doi.org/10.3389/fchem.2017.00063.

Rojas, E., Lopez, M. C., &Valverde, M. (1999). Single cell gel electrophoresis assay: Methodology and applications. *Journal of Chromatography B, 722*, 225–254.

Rosengren, A., Faxius, L., Tanaka, N., Watanabe, M., & Bjursten, L. M. (2005). Comparison of implantation and cytotoxicity testing for initially toxic biomaterials. *Journal of Biomedical Materials Research. Part A, 7 5*(1), 115–122. https://doi.org/10.1002/jbm.a.30431.

Russell, W. B. R. (1959). *The Principles of Humane Experimental Technique.* Methuen & Co. Ltd, London.

Salacinski, H. J., Tiwari, A., Hamilton, G., & Seifalian, A. M. (2001). Cellular engineering of vascular bypass grafts: Role of chemical coatings for enhancing endothelial cell attachment. *Medical & Biological Engineering & Computing, 3 9*(6), 609–618. https://doi.org/10.1007/BF02345431. PMID: 11804165.

Sarode, D. N., & Roy, S. (2019). *In vitro* models for thrombogenicity testing of blood-recirculating medical devices. *Expert Review of Medical Devices, 1 6*(7), 603–616. https://doi.org/10.1080/17434440.2019.1627199. Epub 2019 Jun 10. PMID: 31154869; PMCID: PMC6660015.

Sasaki, K., & Tanaka, N. (1991). Chemical contamination suspected in cytotoxic effects of incubators on BALB 3T3 cells. *Alternatives to Laboratory Animals, 19*(4), 421–427. doi:10.1177/026119299101900405.

Schierholz, J. M., Steinhauser, H., Rump, A. F., Berkels, R., & Pulverer, G. (1997). Controlled release of antibiotics from biomedical polyurethanes: Morphological and structural features. *Biomaterials, 18* (12), 839–844. https://doi.org/10.1016/S0142-9612(96)00199-8.

Schmalz, G. (1988). Agar overlay method. *International Endodontic Journal, 21*(2), 59–66. https://doi.org/10.1111/j.1365-2591.1988.tb00956.x.

Shah, S. R., Walsh, T. L., Williams, C. B., & Soefje, S. A. (2003). Gefitinib a selective epidermal growth factor receptor-tyrosine kinase inhibitor. *Journal of Oncology Pharmacy Practice , 9*, 151–160. https://doi.org/10.1191/1078155203jp115oa.

Shanmugam, S., & Gopal, B. (2014). Copper substituted hydroxyapatite and fluorapatite: Synthesis, characterization and antimicrobial properties. *Ceramics International, 40* , 15655–15662. https://doi.org/10.1016/j.ceramint.2014.07.086.

Shin, W., & Kim, H. J. (2018). Pathomimetic modeling of human intestinal diseases and underlying host–gut microbiome interactions in a gut-on-a-chip. *Methods in Cell Biology, 146*, 135–148.

Siew, E. L., Rajab, N. F., Osman, A. B., Sudesh, K., & Inayat-Hussain, S. H. (2009). Mutagenic and clastogenic characterization of poststerilized poly(3-hydroxybutyrate-co-4-hydroxybutyrate) copolymer biosynthesized by Delftia acidovorans. *Journal of Biomedical Materials Research. Part A, 9 1*(3), 786–794. https://doi.org/10.1002/jbm.a.32290.

Slate, A. J., Wickens, D. J., El Mohtadi, M., Dempsey-Hibbert, N., West, G., Banks, C. E., & Whitehead, K. A. (2018). Antimicrobial activity of Ti-ZrN/Ag coatings for use in biomaterial applications. *Scientific Reports , 8*, 1497. https://doi.org/10.1038/s41598-018-20013-z.

Sommer, S., Buraczewska, I., & Kruszewski, M. (2020). Micronucleus assay: The state of art, and future directions. *International Journal of Molecular Sciences, 21*(4), 1534. Publishe d 2020 Feb 24. https://doi.org/10.3390/ijms21041534.

Sorenson, G. D., Pribish, D. M., Valone, F. H., Memoli, V. A., Bzik, D. J., & Yao, S. L. (1994). Soluble normal and mutated DNA sequences from single-copy genes in human blood. *Cancer Epidemiology Biomarkers and Prevention, 3*, 67–71.

Teoh, S. H. (2000). Fatigue of biomaterials: A review. *International Journal of Fatigue, 22*(10), 825–837, ISSN 0142–1123.

Thomé, I. P. S., Dagostin, V. S., Piletti, R., Pich, C. T., Riella, H. G., Angioletto, E., & Fiori, M. A. (2012). Bactericidal low-density polyethylene (LDPE) urinary catheters: Microbiological characterization and effectiveness. *Materials Science and Engineering C, 3 2*(2), 263–268. https://doi.org/10.1016/j.msec.2011.10.027.

Tice, R. R., & Strauss, G. H. S. (1995). The single cell gel electrophoresis/comet assay: A potential tool for detecting radiation-induced DNA damage in humans. *Stem Cells, 13*, 207S–214S.

UKEMS. (1989). *UKEMS Sub-Committee on Guidelines for Mutagenicity Testing. Part III. Statistical Evaluation of Mutagenicity Test Data*. Kirkland, D. J. (ed.). Cambridge University Press, Cambridge, UK.

Van Dijck, P., Jsjollema, J., Cammue, B. P., Lagrou, K., Berman, J., d'Enfert, C., Andes, D. R., Arendrup, M. C., Brakhage, A. A., Calderone, R., Cantón, E., Coenye, T., Cos, P., Cowen, L. E., Edgerton, M., Espinel-Ingroff, A., Filler, S. G., Ghannoum, M., Gow, N. A. R., Haas, H., Jabra-Rizk, M. A., Johnson, E. M., Lockhart, S. R., Lopez-Ribot, J. L., Maertens, J., Munro, C. A., Nett, J. E., Nobile, C. J., Pfaller, M. A., Ramage, G., Sanglard, D., Sanguinetti, M., Spriet, I., Verweij, P. E., Warris, A., Wauters, J., Yeaman, M. R., Zaat, S. A. J., & Thevissen, K. (2018). Methodologies for *in vitro* and *in vivo* evaluation of efficacy of antifungal and antibiofilm agents and surface coatings against fungal biofilms. *Microbial Cell*, 5(7), 300–326. https://doi.org/10.15698/mic2018.07.638.

van Oeveren, W., Haan, J., Lagerman, P., & Schoen, P. (2002). Comparison of coagulation activity tests in vitro for selected biomaterials. *Artificial Organs*, 26(6), 506–511. https://doi.org/10.1046/j.1525-1594.2002.06872.x. PMID: 12072106.

Wang, M. O., Etheridge, J. M., Thompson, J. A., Vorwald, C. E., Dean, D., & Fisher, J. P. (2013). Evaluation of the in vitro cytotoxicity of cross-linked biomaterials. *Biomacromolecules*, 14 (5), 1321–1329. https://doi.org/10.1021/bm301962f.

Wang, Z., Hou, Z., Wang, P., Chen, F., & Luo, X. (2022). CuS-PNIPAm nanoparticles with the ability to initiatively capture bacteria for photothermal treatment of infected skin. *Regenerative Biomaterials*, 9, rbac026. https://doi.org/10.1093/rb/rbac026.

Weber, M., Steinle, H., Golombek, S., Hann, L., Schlensak, C., Wendel, H. P., & Avci-Adali, M. (2018). Blood-contacting biomaterials: In vitro evaluation of the hemocompatibility. *Front Bioeng Biote chnol*, 6(99). https://doi.org/10.3389/fbioe.2018.00099.

Yang, X., Zhao, K., & Chen, G. Q. (2002). Effect of surface treatment on the biocompatibility of microbial polyhydroxyalkanoates. *Biomaterials*, 23(5), 1391–1397.

Zhang, J. (2013). Biocompatibility and anti-bacterial activity of Zn-containing HA/TiO$_2$ hybrid coatings on Ti substrate. *Journal of Hard Tissue Biology*, 22, 311–318.

Zhao, J., Sun, Y., Ma, H., Yu, X., Ma, Y., Ni, Y., Zheng, L., & Zhou, Y. (2014). Biocompatibility and antibacterial properties of zinc-ion implantation on titanium. *Journal of Hard Tissue Biology*, 23, 5–44.

7 Materials Testing for Toxicity, Efficacy, Disease Treatment, and Testing for Disease Diagnosis in the Animal Models

Rashi Sharma, Faizan Ahmad, Meghna Ghosal, Kamakshi Naik, Juweiriya, Manisha Lanka, Punya Sachdeva, Gagandeep Singh, and Firdos Alam Khan

7.1 INTRODUCTION

With its basis from the Latin word that is translated to "within the living", in vivo testing, in particular, has made its mark in the biomedical research field for the development of tools and techniques to reverse errors made by mankind or even due to fate. In a broader sense, in vivo refers to the procedures and various protocols performed by the researchers for the procurement of their results on or in a living being. It plays a significant role in the evaluation of the safety of biomaterials developed from emerging techniques. Animal models are used to act as a middle ground between the actual experimentation on humans and research trials. The similarity in the animals used for research is that they're genetically identical and laboratory-bred (Jamie Eske, 2020). These experiments occur with the protocols of the Principles of Humane Experimental Technique followed throughout the process (Alan M. Goldberg, 2010). The in vivo use of biomaterials in particular has advanced in the medical field, where even the functioning of organs can be replaced by synthetic or natural grafts, in the field of orthopedics, ophthalmic, cardiovascular surgeries, and dental applications. However, before the use of these biomaterials can be applied in experimental research, they undergo a safety evaluation. Using the global principles of the ISO 10993 series for evaluating medical devices' biological domain, safety concerns in regard to toxicity are gauged (W.H. De Jong et al., 2012; Anderson, n.d.). The toxicity studies also include research on genotoxicity, reproductive toxicity, carcinogenicity, and toxicokinetics in addition to acute, subacute, or sub-chronic, chronic, and special toxicity investigations (W.H. De Jong et al., 2012).

DOI: 10.1201/9781003317715-7

FDA G-95 Memorandum requirements, the ISO 10993 advice, are taken into account when evaluating the biocompatibility of medical devices and biomaterials to meet regulatory standards (Gad, 2013; Chen and Liu, 2016). The other category that falls under in vivo testing involves implantation. Implantation of biomaterials has solved many problems in the modern-day improvement of the human condition and the quality of life. Biomaterials are heavily in use for the last few decades and have a broad range of applications for medical purposes. They play a crucial role in the regeneration of tissue and the healing of wounds. The shape of the biomaterial should be considered for the implantation, as the shape mainly helps in the binding of the material to the tissues (Chen and Liu, 2016). Along with the shape of the biomaterial, bioactivity, biocompatibility, and mechanical properties are also considered for the better improvement of the implantation (Ben Arnold, 2019). Although the biomaterials are selected based on the aforementioned properties, an irritation reaction might occur that can cause adverse reactions (Tang and Eaton, 1995). Various irritation tests will provide information about the reactions occurring due to biomaterials and how to encounter them. Some materials were shown to have less irritable reactions when compared to others. Overall, the material selected should last for longer periods without side effects. Biomaterial, when induced in the host, can cause an immunogenic reaction and foreign body reaction, including hypersensitivity; skin, ocular, and mucosal irritation; and intracutaneous reactivity (Remes and Williams, 1992). The presence or absence and the severity of these hypersensitivity and immunogenic reactions depend on the duration for which the biomaterial is administered, along with other factors such as the route of exposure, its target vital organ, the temperature of the host and the environment, the nature of the biomaterial, the degree of the exposure, the frequency, and the dose of the biomaterial (James M. Anderson, 2001). Based on the duration, there are three systemic toxicity tests, which include acute systemic toxicity, subchronic/subacute systemic toxicity, and chronic toxicity. The biomaterial is first administered for 24 hours, and changes are noted. This is followed by the next dose of biomaterial being administered for a longer period, and further responses, such as tissue, blood, cellular, and long-term responses, are observed for the result (Li-Xia Hu et al., 2018).

7.2 PRETESTING CONSIDERATIONS

Before the implementation of a particular scheme curated for a biomaterial to be utilized on humans for their welfare, a series of step-by-step procedures are followed to rule out risks of hazard so that they may be controlled and evaluated in accordance with their risk level (Figure 7.1) (De Jong et al., 2012). After a safety evaluation by putting the biomaterial through different tests and assessing the biological effects, like cytotoxicity, sensitization, genotoxicity, implantation, or hemocompatibility, due to the contact duration of varied parameters on surfaces like skin, mucosal membrane, blood, tissue, and bone, the biomaterial is finally regarded as a safe device to use if provided with least identified potential side effects (De Jong et al., 2012). In order to determine if a medical device or biomaterial is safe, ISO 10993-1 provides guidelines for any additional testing that may be necessary. The equipment

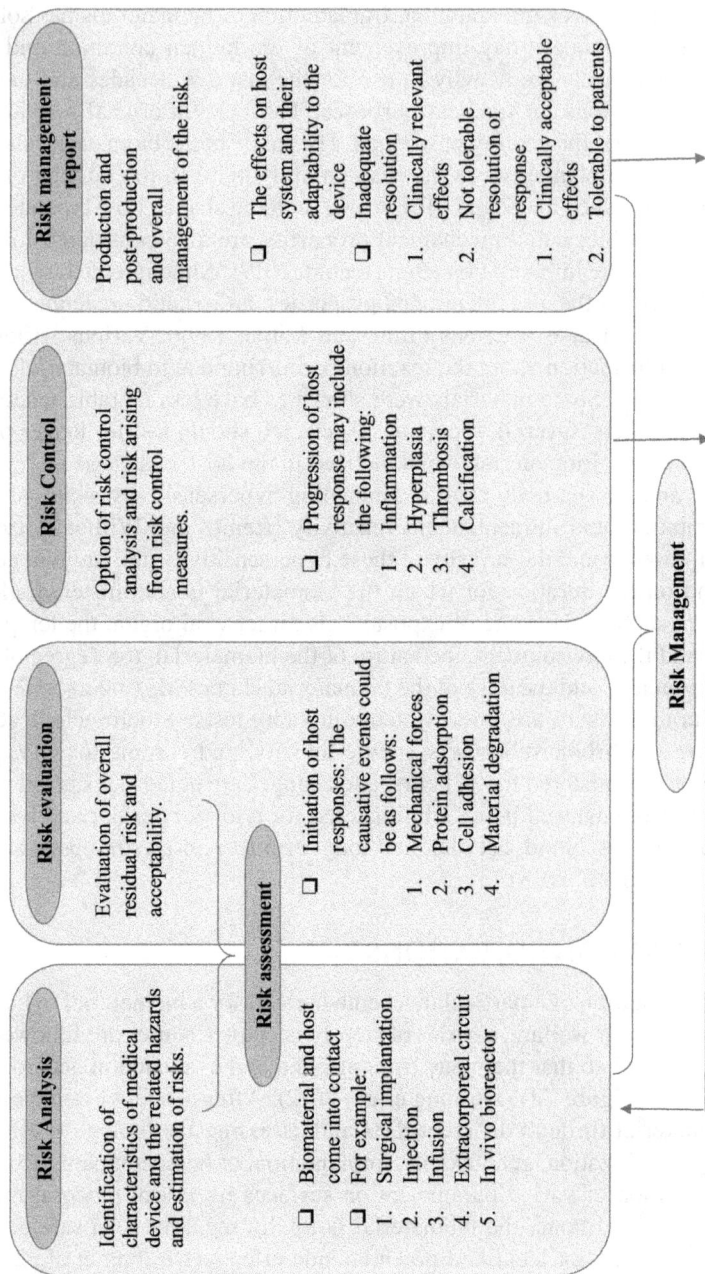

FIGURE 7.1 Schematic representation of risk management of medical devices and their host immune response. The figure describes various risks involved post-implantation of medical devices and the extent of their acceptability. It also describes the control measures to reduce the risk and the overall risk management.

specifications and contingency planning stages of the design process are essential in determining the biological hazard of medical devices. As crucial as testing, the biosafety assessment process needs to be developed and used to show that specific safety requirements are met (D.E. Albert, 2012).

7.3   TESTING: TYPES, COMPARISONS, AND DIFFERENCES

The two main assessments that are used for the evaluation of the safety of biomaterials are broadly classified into in vivo and in vitro testing methods. In vitro, in particular, refers to something "in glass" (for instance, a glass jar or a petri dish), whereas in vivo refers to something "inside a living organism." Both these terms have Latin etymological roots. Both these studies have been used for the testing of drugs and biomaterials before their application for human welfare. In vivo studies, however, are used for clinical trials and animal studies, whereas in vitro studies are utilized for microphysiological systems, cell-based screening, and diagnostic tests (Jonathan Dornell, 2022). Biomedical researchers use a variety of techniques to develop treatments for human diseases and disorders, including computer analysis, tissue and cell cultures, experimental animals (Figure 7.2), and clinical studies. Each of the aforementioned methods has pros and cons of its own (Saeidnia et al., 2016). Animal models are more reliable as compared to in vitro testing; however, they do have some limitations, such as using different biokinetics parameters or parameterization of results for human subjects (Saeidnia et al., 2016). The disadvantage of in vitro treatments is that they are typically performed on cancer cell lines with clearly abnormal functions. The biological sciences can also benefit from in vitro models, but there are some significant downsides, such as the challenge of predicting when a chemical attack will be most potent and extrapolating its consequences to people (Saeidnia et al., 2016). Both in vitro and in vivo research are vital to comprehending the pharmacokinetic or pharmacodynamic characteristics of a medicine. Each has advantages and drawbacks. In conclusion, these trials contribute to the development of safer and more potent medications for individuals who require them (Tang, n.d.).

7.4   IN VIVO TESTING CONSIDERATIONS

7.4.1   IN VIVO GENOTOXICITY

The genotoxicity tests assess gene mutations, modifications to DNA or chromosomes, and gene toxicities brought on by substances for a prolonged period. The evaluations of reproductive, carcinogenic, and genotoxic effects are described in great detail in the International Organization for Standardization (ISO) standard 10993-3 (W.J. Roger, 2012). In vivo testing of biomaterial for genotoxicity encompasses chromosomal analysis, rodent dominant lethal tests, mice spot test, mouse heritable translocation assay, mammalian bone marrow cytogenetic testing, micronucleus test, and rodent dominant lethal tests (Thomas et al., 2015). The manufacturing method and indication for use differ from product to product; therefore, each combination of products must be reviewed and evaluated for genotoxicity tests (Khamar and Richmond, 2018). The animal studies for the currently available mechanism reveal a

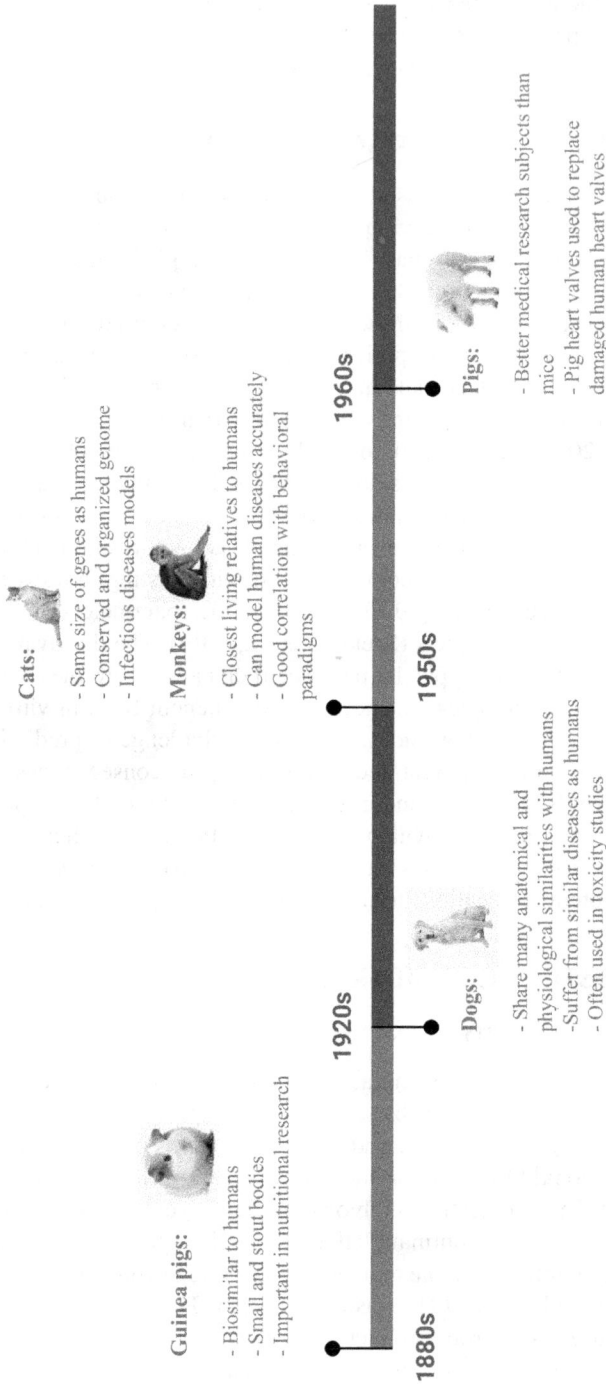

FIGURE 7.2 Timeline of animals used in testing for evaluation of biomaterials. The figure describes the timeline of animals that have been used for testing since the beginning of biomedical research and the benefits of using the aforementioned animals (guinea pigs, dogs, cats, monkeys, and pigs) for biomedical research.

different genotoxic scenario exhibited in the case of nanoparticles, depending on the basis of length of exposure (Klien and Godnić-Cvar, 2012). Genotoxicity tests have been proven to be a critical tool to measure the damage caused to the DNA and to determine the possibility of developing cancer (R.M. Santella, 1997; Vasavi Mohan, 2007; Kang et al., 2013).

7.4.2   In Vivo Mouse Micronucleus Assays

In vivo mouse micronucleus assays, when performed in an ethical manner, aid in the detection of aneugenicity and clastogenicity, which are categorized under the tests of genotoxicity. It is also one of the important tests recommended for the safety assessment of products used for the making of biomaterials in particular (Krishna and Hayashi, 2000). The protocol followed for these tests includes the principle of application of uniform criteria to the in vivo assays, identification of hazards, and consideration of the minimal requirement to produce an authentic and definable result. However, instead of depending on theoretical predictions, these criteria must be established on experimental facts (Hayashi et al., 1994).

7.4.3   In Vivo Chromosomal Aberration Assay

Chromosomal aberrations can be examined under the microscope with suitable staining. These aberrations may be produced in vitro following experimentally regulated interventions to identify or assess the mutagenic potential of particular substances, or they may be produced in vivo as a result of environmental or industrial factors (Johannes and Obe, 2019). To determine the degree of chromosome aberrations caused by model drugs in the bone marrow cells of animals, usually rodents that are considered as the test subjects (rats, mice, and Chinese hamsters), the mammalian in vivo chromosome aberration test is used. Two different forms of structural chromosomal aberrations are known to exist; namely, chromatid or chromosome (OECD Guidelines, 2016). In mammalian systems, the metaphase chromosomal aberration (CAb) assay has been frequently used to check substances for genotoxicity (Cheung et al., 2006). Animals are subjected to the test drug (liquid or solid) via a suitable method of exposure (typically through a stomach tube or an appropriate intubation cannula, intraperitoneal injection, or by sacrifice) and are prepared to be sacrificed at the appropriate intervals after medication. Animals are given a metaphase-arresting treatment (colchicine) before being sacrificed. The next step is to prepare and stain chromosome preparations from bone marrow cells; after which metaphase cells are examined for chromosome abnormalities (OECD Guidelines, 2016).

7.4.4   Carcinogenicity

Through single or repeated exposure or contact over the course of the majority of the model—animal's lifespan—the evaluation of medical products, materials, and their extracts for their tendency to induce malignancies in test animals is shown by carcinogenicity studies (Moeller and Matyjaszewski, 2012). When concerned with the case of biomaterials, the studies focus on solid-state carcinogenicity, also known as the Oppenheimer effect (Anderson, 2012). The International Organization for Standardization (ISO) has established a set of biocompatibility norms that address several topics, including the potential of a device material to induce or encourage the formation of malignant cells or its carcinogenicity when it comes in contact with a patient (Richard F. Wallin, 2017).

7.4.5 HEMOCOMPATIBILITY

The use of blood-compatible biomaterials—materials that can come into touch with blood without endangering the body—has been taken into consideration for use in medical devices (Xiaoli Liu et al., 2014). The endothelial cells that line the innermost layer of vasculature play a role in mediating the blood vessel wall's exceptional hemocompatibility (F. Jung et al., 2013; Pries and Kuebler, 2006). Since these materials come in close proximity with the blood, which compromises 1% leukocytes and platelets, 44% erythrocytes, and 55% plasma, any adverse effect that is triggered by the contiguity of blood with an unknown object leads to a cascade of events, which includes the adsorption of protein and adhesion of platelets to a foreign object, and finally, results in the stabilization of thrombosis by fibrin, which must be prevented. As a result of this, the consequence is followed by a decline in the number of blood cells, ensuing in the formation of a thrombus (Weber et al., 2018). When establishing blood compatibility, the three elements of Virchow's triad—blood, surface, and flow—must be taken into consideration. It is necessary to determine the characteristic impact of fluid dynamics and hemorheological attributes; the physical, chemical, viscoelastic, and morphological surface characteristics; as well as the hindered function of blood and its components, in order to effectively and adequately assess the degree and extent of the contact of blood and its constituents with surfaces (Anderson, 1988). Hemocompatibility is a major issue that limits the clinical applicability of blood-contacting biomaterials. To avoid the activation and annihilation of blood components, detrimental interactions between newly discovered biomaterials and blood should be amply researched (Weber et al., 2018).

7.4.6 IN VIVO THROMBOSIS TESTING

Blood coagulation proteins were discovered after the initial research of thrombus formation and pathology based on the characteristics of patients who inherited clotting disorders. For the study of thrombosis in vivo, the laser-injury thrombosis model offers several benefits. It is necessary to examine the conventional protocol that activated the platelets supply. The membrane surface is for thrombin production, so identify the crucial membrane surfaces in vivo. This model enables the study of thrombus development in a living animal with an intact vascular wall while having the circulating cellular components and the circulating plasma proteins that are not anticoagulated (B. Furie, 2005). Device-related thrombosis and thromboembolic consequences frequently affect patient morbidity and mortality and persist to be a therapeutic issue. Improved preclinical thrombogenicity evaluation techniques are, therefore, required to increase patient safety and more accurately anticipate clinical outcomes. However, there are a number of difficulties and restrictions related to carrying out preclinical thrombogenicity tests in animals (Figure 7.3) (Jamiolkowski et al., 2020). The genetically modified mice used for in vivo thrombosis testing provide a wide variety of rodent models for exploring the mechanism of blood coagulation. Analysis by tail breeding time followed by a particular protocol is used as a primary assessment for in vivo thrombosis (Marisa A. Brake et al., 2019). The probe in the in vivo thrombus formation has been on the rise due to the discovery of different factors that influence the interaction of platelets with walls of the vessels during normal homeostasis. The role of clotting factors, platelets, prostaglandins in thromboembolic diseases, and atherosclerosis have also played a crucial part in this domain (Dewanjee, 2017).

7.4.7 COMPLEMENT ACTIVATION

The complement activation test is used to assess whether a medical device has the ability to activate the complement system. This humoral immune response may be brought on by the administration of a foreign substance and can have negative outcomes, like tissue inflammation and damage (Ann Robinson, 2022). One important aspect of innate immunity is the complement system, which is extensively researched in relation to blood-contacting medical devices because it is quickly triggered by the insertion of a foreign object in the human body. The complement system is a humoral defensive mechanism of innate immunity that detects hazardous signals elicited by invading infectious agents or intrinsically dangerous chemical patterns in the body (DAMPs). The complement system can be triggered by using the alternate pathway, the lectin pathway, or the conventional pathway. Because they are foreign substances and, in theory, every substance that is foreign to the body can be used to trigger the complement system, as a consequence, biomaterials are recognized as complement activators. The biocompatibility of synthetic biomaterials is thought to be significantly influenced by complement activation. Furthermore, it was also proven that the complement altered the response to the implant by interacting with other biological mechanisms, such as platelet activation and coagulation factors (Daniel Ricklin et al., 2010; John D. Lambris et al., 1999; Kristina N. Ekdahl et al., 2011; Nilsson et al., 2007; Gorbet and Sefton, 2004; Shan Huang et al., 2016; Yvonne Mödinger et al., 2018).

7.4.8 IMPLANTATION

According to the ISO 10993-1 standard, biomaterial implantation is assessed based on the local effects. Biomaterials implantation is now used in various fields of biomedical sciences, such as dental implants, orthopedic prostheses, skin grafts, and medical implants, such as heart valves and stents. The implanted biomaterials react with the injured tissue and induce host response interactions and aid in tissue repair. The reaction varies depending on the type of biomaterial and the location of the injury. The biomaterial selected for implantation is very important for long-term results.

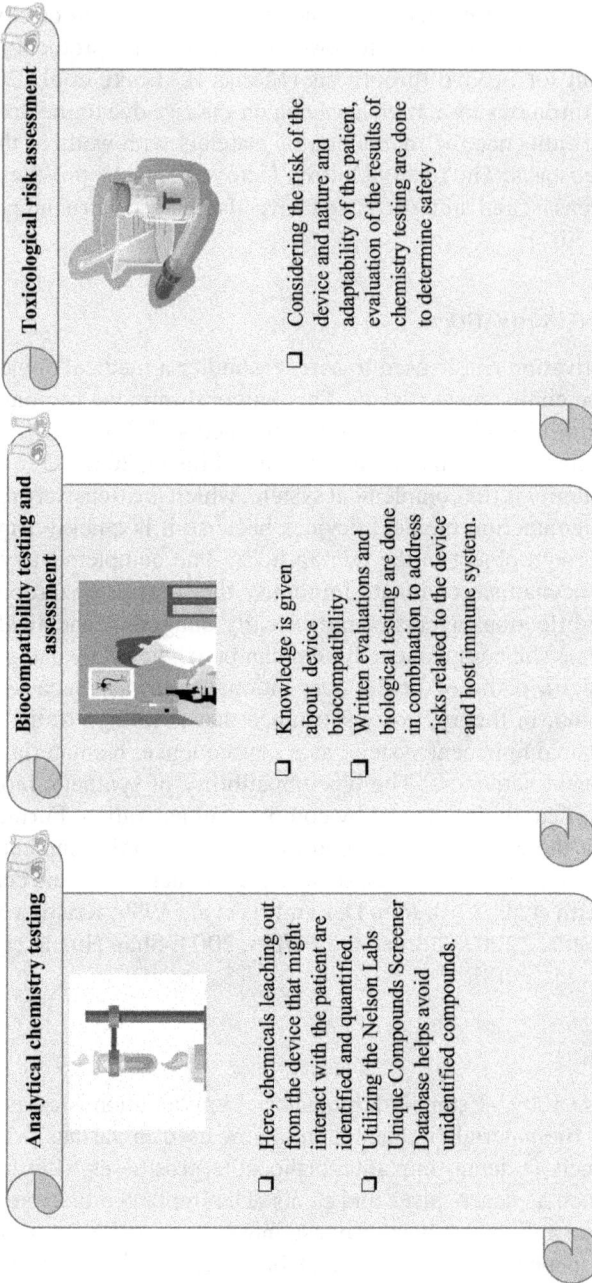

Analytical chemistry testing

❑ Here, chemicals leaching out from the device that might interact with the patient are identified and quantified.

❑ Utilizing the Nelson Labs Unique Compounds Screener Database helps avoid unidentified compounds.

Biocompatibility testing and assessment

❑ Knowledge is given about device biocompatibility

❑ Written evaluations and biological testing are done in combination to address risks related to the device and host immune system.

Toxicological risk assessment

❑ Considering the risk of the device and nature and adaptability of the patient, evaluation of the results of chemistry testing are done to determine safety.

FIGURE 7.3 Biological evaluation and risk assessment of medical devices. The figure describes the different methods for the evaluation of risks involved with techniques like analytical chemistry testing, where leak-outs of devices are tested. The test for biocompatibility is done pre-implantation. Also, to ensure the device is not toxic, a toxicological analysis is done to check its safety.

7.4.8.1   Influence of Shape and Characteristics

The parameters, like size, shape, and surface chemistry, are some of the most essential characteristics that play a major role in mitigating cellular responses and other biotechnological applications. The shapes that can be used are spheres, rods, and tubes (Zhengwei Mao et al., 2013). The shape of the implant should be simple in nature so as to avoid any complex problems. A biomaterial can have more than one form to change depending on the tissue. Size and shape are distinct from each other and have very different influences on biomedical applications. The biomaterial should be sustainable, bioinert, and biocompatible to surpass all adverse tissue reactions. Biocompatibility verifies whether a biomaterial is compatible with the living tissue (Meisam Omidi, 2017). Various quality tests and risk management processes are carried out to check the compatibility of the biomaterials (Davis, 2003). Other characteristics that should be carefully studied in biomaterials are the shape and size of the particles, tensile strength, host response, non-toxicity, corrosion, coatings, and so on (De Jong et al., 2002). The many types of materials that can be used are metals, polymers, ceramics, composites, and so on (Buddy Ratner et al., 2013). Sometimes, the biomaterials will be incompatible with the body even with all the characteristics mentioned earlier. This might be due to poor bio function, where the materials can shed contaminants on the body's surface. This release of contaminants can be avoided by coating the surface of the material either with the same component or bioactive materials, like zirconia or calcium phosphate, which gives a porous surface.

7.4.8.2   Rabbit Muscle Implantation Study

According to an experiment conducted in 2015, the intramuscular implantation of biomaterials explains to us the levels of evaluation of the reactions of the materials (Zhenyu Dai et al., 2015). The corrosion rate of the biomaterials depended majorly on the environment of the tissue. Apparently, complex environments had a lower corrosion rate, as they are more similar to the living environment when compared to simpler environments (Iulian Antoniac et al., 2020). Good results were observed with the biomaterials prepared with 3D bioprinting technology. The advantage of bioprinting is that the image and data can be used again to create similar organs (Kaile Zhang et al., 2017). The weight of the biomaterial also had a significant impact on the living tissue. In a few cases, the surrounding tissue acclimated to the surface of the implanted biomaterial and induced tissue healing. The substances of the materials also influenced the enzyme activity of the tissues (Wennberg et al., 1978). Magnesium alloys were found to have better biocompatibility and higher corrosion resistance than pure magnesium. Regardless, their low bioactivity can lead the implant to lose mechanical integrity. To overcome this problem, plasma electrolytic oxidation (PEO) is done to help provide a thick coating on the implant surface. The PEO-treated alloys had an overall positive outcome on the healing and recovery of the tissues (Seong Ryoung Kim et al., 2022).

7.4.8.3   Implant Studies as Part of Other Studies

The data from the earlier studies may not always be sufficient to evaluate the biomaterials, with the results being limited to local effects and sometimes extending to systemic effects. In general, simple in vitro tests are performed to assess biocompatibility and activity. If these studies show promising results, then additional functional and efficiency studies may be conducted to test the biomaterials.

7.4.9 IRRITATION

The selection of the biomaterials should be appropriate to minimize adverse body reactions while maintaining the functionality and longevity of the implantable device. The types of in vitro irritation assays used to assess biomedical devices are skin, ocular, mucosal, and intracutaneous reactivity. Irritation tests provide information on tissue response in a particular area (W.H. De Jong, 2020). Host reactions following implantation of biomaterials can be local, such as blood-material interactions (coagulation, fibrinolysis, platelet adhesion, complement activation, etc.), toxicity, infection, and tumorigenesis; or systemic, including embolization, hypersensitivity, injury, phagocytosis, acute inflammation, and chronic inflammation.

7.4.9.1 Skin Irritation

Biomaterial hypersensitivity is one of the most common issues after implantation. Hypersensitivity might occur because of the type of metal used for the manufacture of the material. Transdermal delivery of biomaterials has been one of the emerging technologies and has a comprehensive prospect for enhancing the penetration of a broad range of therapeutic agents through the skin barrier (Yang Chen et al., 2013). Transdermal delivery has numerous advantages over traditional routes, like oral or injectable. This delivery reduces toxicity and local irritation due to multiple sites for absorption. Polymeric hydrogels showed no toxicity or skin irritation. Sometimes, prostheses result in a blockage of airflow around the limb, causing sweat to become trapped where bacteria and fungi can thrive. This leads to skin irritation, abrasions, and damage. Designing better biomaterials with new cutting-edge technologies will reduce these side effects and help prevent skin diseases. Using chitosan as a biomaterial seems to be an ideal biopolymer because of its cell-binding and cell-activating properties (Bhaskara Rao and Sharma, 1997). Silk fibroin is another such material that has high biocompatibility and excellent mechanical strength with fewer after-effects. The advantages of silk fibroin include maintaining a moist environment for wound healing, preventing bacterial infection, and being easily applied and removed (Wei Zhang et al., 2017).

7.4.9.2 Ocular Irritation

When corresponding with other ways of drug delivery, the development of an ocular drug delivery system is one of the most technically demanding tasks, but due to the advanced technology, the sophisticated devices have been increasing rapidly in the last decade. Naturally derived monomers-based biopolymers were shown to possess low ocular irritation. Combinations of biopolymers also improved drug delivery by improving solubility and extending release. Ocular delivery systems are used to treat ocular diseases because of their properties (Allyn et al., 2022). Cases of ocular irritation were shallow after administering nanomaterials into the tissues. The nanomaterials did not cause any harm to the cell membrane and nucleus, and also no significant irritation of the cornea, iris, and conjunctiva was observed (Shen et al., 2015). Albumin nanocarriers have multiple effects, and albumin-based ocular drug delivery systems have significant physiological effects. Albumin helps in improving the transportation of drugs to the action sites. Nanostructured lipid carriers also reduced ocular irritation to a great extent (Diebold et al., 2007).

7.4.9.3 Mucosal Irritation

Mucosal irritation is mostly common in the gums due to dental implants. Substances from the biomaterials generate a reaction in the adjacent tissues, like mucosa. For the biomaterials that come into contact with the mucosa, there are many types of assays distinct to the kind of tissue exposure. A microscopic assessment of the tissue is performed to identify contamination. During mucosal administration, possible concerns, such as tissue irritation and tissue damage, are caused by the carrier. Polyelectrolytes showed no irritation when administered unless complexed with an oppositely charged electrolyte, making them an inert species (De Cock et al., 2011). Multilayer polyelectrolyte capsules were discovered to reduce these problems and are now being used for drug delivery applications. Mucoadhesive materials (adhesion between the biomaterials and the mucosal layer) offer prolonged contact and low enzymatic activity (Rahamatullah Shaikh et al., 2011).

7.4.9.4 Intracutaneous Reactivity

Intracutaneous reactivity is an in vitro assay that is used to assess the compatibility of the biomaterials and determine the localized reaction of tissue to extracts of medical devices, biomaterials, and prostheses (Huzum et al., 2021). It is a standard clinical assay irrespective of their exposure time during clinical use. Determination of irritation by intracutaneous reactivity may be applicable where skin or mucosal irritation tests are not suitable. Irritation can be assessed using many different models, and the choice of assessment should be based on the end use of the medical device or biomaterial. Exposure to minute amounts of potential leachables present in medical devices or biomaterials can result in sensitization or allergic reactions. Intracutaneous reactivity tests focus on determining the biological response of leachable agents that may be present in biomaterials. Silk fibroin and chitosan-based materials have no intracutaneous reactivity.

7.4.10 SENSITIZATION TEST

This in vivo test is used to detect immunological response, which is caused due to penetration of sensitizer or allergens into the skin and binds with different proteins. It is due to repeated prolonged exposure of leachable biomaterials or their extract to the dermis (Gerberick, 2004). This test is done to determine if the patient has any sensitization or allergic reaction to any biomaterial extract or compound causing erythema/swelling/eschar/edema in skin cells (Ghazali et al., 2021). According to OECD guidelines, the concentration of the dose used for induction of allergic reaction should be of the highest non-irritating level but should be concentrated and potent enough to cause very mild to moderate skin bioreaction or allergic reaction but not cause marked pain or distress and is systematically well tolerated (Badylak and Gilbert, 2008; Test No. 402: Acute Dermal Toxicity, 2017). The allergic reaction or hypersensitivity reaction is observed through histocompatibility and recorded after the administration or implantation of biomaterial extracts intracutaneously, or the leachability of biomaterials through direct skin contact uses a scoring matrix by comparing the test animals to the control animals using the same dose of biomaterial on both. Clinical trials are then conducted on human subjects. Both the animal and human trials mandatorily require approval from the institutional ethics committee (Greeshma Thrivikraman et al., 2014) Currently, there are three test models—guinea pig maximization test, guinea pig closed patch test, and lymph node assay—to detect the immunological response.

7.4.10.1 Guinea Pig Maximization Test

The guinea pig maximization test (GPMT) is an in vivo test used to screen substances that cause human sensitization by administering the same substance/biomaterial to the guinea pigs, which are the model for the test (Magnusson and Kligman, 1970). The guinea pig used in this test can be male or nulliparous female (pregnancy can reduce sensitization and can hamper the result). The dose should be the lowest effective dose, which causes a mild to moderate reaction. Ten or more guinea pigs are used to guarantee against counterfeit outcomes, and guinea pigs are divided into five distinct control groups (M. Kitano, 1992). They are given an intradermal administration of biomaterial extract, usually with a Freud adjuvant or physiological saline, which creates a stronger immune response in the guinea pig, followed by a topical epidermal induction for 48 hours of the same after 7 days of intradermal induction. After this weaker dose of biomaterial, the extract is administered to the test animals, and their immune response or allergic reaction is observed and recorded (Magnusson and Kligman, 1970). The response rate is expressed in terms of EC50. An EC50 is a statistical estimate of the concentration of a toxicant in the ambient medium necessary to produce a particular effect in 50% of a very large population under specified conditions (Rozman et al., 2010).

7.4.10.2 Guinea Pig Closed Patch Test

This is another type of skin sensitization test that provides information about the sensitization ability of a biomaterial and is almost akin to a closed patch test; the number of animals required and their sex and types are the same as in the guinea pig maximization test (E. V. Buehler, 1965). The guinea pig, taken as the test model, was consecutively exposed to the biomaterial extract or chemicals for six hours for three consecutive weeks. Then on days 27–28, which is 3 weeks after the last dermal exposure, a topical challenge of the untreated flank is given for 6 hours. The intensity of the allergic or hypersensitive reaction is then assessed at 21, 24, and 48 hours after the patch has been removed by comparing the affected animals with the control animals that had their skin exposed to non-irritating, non-sensitizing biomaterial, such as an organic cotton gauze (E. V. Buehler, 1965). To obtain a positive result, nearly 15% of the total guinea pig population should show mild to moderate allergic reactions.

7.4.10.3 Lymph Node Assay

This is another type of skin sensitization test, but this is considered to be less cruel than the previous two, so this is preferred and is used to measure the extent of allergic reaction of biomaterial in the host. Rodents, such as mice and guinea pigs, are used as model organisms for this assay (Leigh Ann Burns-Naas, 2005). The dose of biomaterial or its extract is administered by epicutaneous induction through the ears. The concentration of the dose should be of the highest non-irritant dosage and should cause mild to moderate hypersensitive or allergic reactions. Twenty guinea pigs are taken and divided into a test model and a negative control group. The first dose is given for three consecutive days and then left for the next three days undisturbed, and then on the sixth day, tracer substance 3-H methyl thymidine is injected intraperitoneally via the tail vein so that it incorporates into lymphocytes, and later, these lymphocytes are traced using bioluminescence, radiolabeling, and immunoassay, such as ELISA (Sharon Gwaltney-Brant, 2014). If the biomaterial is a potential allergen or irritant, then the proliferation will be high in lymph nodes present near the ears. After the administration, five hours later, the test animals are euthanized, and radioactive lymphocytes are collected from auricular lymph nodes, and a cell suspension is prepared. From this cell suspension, the tracer H2-thymidine is detected through scintillation. The endpoint considered for the local lymph node assay is an SI index of greater or equal to three cells. When the stimulation index is greater (SI > 3), a relevant sensitizing potential is assumed. In contrast to the classical guinea pig tests, the LLNA provides a quantitative measurement of the sensitizing potency of a tested chemical (Thomas Clausen et al., 2006; Stacey E. Anderson et al., 2011). The limitation of these three assays mentioned earlier is that although rodents (guinea pig) are considered the closest model for various toxicity tests and trials, their penetration rate to the chemical or biomaterial extract in different hosts and model organisms is different, and they can't distinguish between the hypersensitivity types (A. Garnett et al., 1994). Sensitizer, as well as a non-sensitizing skin irritant, causes lymphocyte proliferation with the sensitizer causing specific lymphocyte differentiation, and the non-sensitizing skin irritant causing non-specific lymphocyte differentiation. This sometimes gives a false positive result and hampers the actual result (Kligman and Basketter, 1995).

7.4.11 SYSTEMIC TOXICITY

This refers to the short-term toxic effects caused after oral administration, implantation, percutaneous absorption, or intradermal injection of a biomaterial or its extract. It should be noted that some chemicals are more readily absorbed than others due to their difference in hydrophobicity, and their effect on the vital organ may differ (Pan et al., 2020). The absorption rate is measured using the water uptake ratio (WUR) (Robinson, 2022). The extent of the effects seen after the exposure depends upon several other factors, apart from the duration of the exposure, such as the physical properties (such as the porosity and density of the biomaterial, solubility, hardness, and boiling and melting temperature), chemical properties (such as bioreactivity, electronegativity, corrosive property, biodegradability, acidity, and basicity of the cells and tissues in contact), duration and nature of exposure, as well as administration route (whether it is given orally, through the intraperitoneal route, or through tail veins) (Sylwia Grabska-Zielińska et al., 2020; Matthias Schnabelrauch, 2017; Zhang, 2010). Some biomaterial extracts induce more allergic reactions or hypersensitivity when administered through percutaneous absorption than oral administration (Villa-Ruano et al., 2016).

7.4.11.1 Acute Systemic Toxicity

Acute system toxicity test refers to the short-term effects observed after the acute exposure of biomaterials to the testing subject. Acute systemic toxicity can be studied either in rodent or non-rodent animals for testing. After the implantation of the biomaterial extract or intraperitoneal or intravenous administration of liquid chemicals, the bioactivity of the same is observed at predictable intervals of 4, 16, 24, 48, and 72 hours, and detrimental effects (if any) can be analyzed by its biochemical, histological, morphological, and pathological changes, and noted precisely, and an appropriate conclusion is drawn from the findings. It is important to note that this implantation is only carried out in animals after the defect is created for a particular biomaterial, biodevice, or prosthetic (Anderson and Jiang, 2019). A different model of animals, including rodents as well as primates, is used for testing the same biomaterial, and the model animal that most accurately mimics the actual host (human) for that defect is chosen. For a model to be scientifically valid, it is necessary to show that the knowledge gained from the model can be extrapolated to the condition in the original species, mainly humans (M Egermann et al., 2008). From these findings, the short-term effect of the biomaterials and chemicals/pyrogens used can be analyzed and checked for any health hazard posed by it. Acute toxicity is measured in terms of LD, a non-lethal, non-toxic median dose that causes the death of 50% of the total population. It is used as an index to classify the toxicity of biomaterials used in industries and the environment. Although, it does not provide the toxicity data of the pharmaceuticals products (Ricardo Ochoa, 2002).

7.4.11.2 Subacute/Subchronic Toxicity

Subacute toxicity is defined as a negative effect observed after the repeated exposure of biomaterials or pyrogens, their extract, or chemicals for 24 hours and 28 days, not greater than 10% of the life span of the animal or rodent model (Jeffrey A. Handler, 2013; De Jong et al., 2002). Its testing time is greater than that of acute systemic toxicity testing but less than that of chronic systemic testing. It is akin to acute toxicity except for the period when the dose of the test sample is given. The route of administration and baseline parameters of changes are the same as those of acute systemic toxicity. It generally doesn't have a defined protocol, as dictated by ISO 10993-11. As biomaterial extract is being used, the relationship between the dosage level or the exposure time and safety factor cannot be estimated (Jean Boutrand, 2019).

7.4.11.3 Chronic Toxicity

Chronic toxicity refers to the continuous and repeated exposure of biomaterial and its extract after implantation for 12 months to the testing animal to determine its prolonged effect (much longer than acute toxicity) (Figure 7.4). It is carried out to determine and analyze the very long-term effects on the host, and it is extrapolated to the human safety of the test substance (Badylak and Gilbert, 2008). The effects can be studied by comparing the same parameter of changes observed in the control test group and negative test group model animals. Chronic toxicity is a type of acute toxicity but with longer exposure to a biomaterial or its extract and delayed effect.

In vivo testing of biomaterials		
Implantation	**Sensitization**	**Immune Responses**
- Depends on shape and characteristics of the device - Tested on animal models to check for the biocompatibility of the materials - Synthetic and biological materials are used as biomaterials for implantation purposes	- Immune system response to chemicals - Tests estimate the sensitizing capacity to the prolonged exposure of a test material - These tests help in improving the function of the biomaterials - Example: Buehler test, h-CLAT test.	- Host response as first step of tissue repair - Steps: 1. Provisional matrix deposition 2. Neutrophil and monocyte recruitment 3. Macrophage adhesion and fusion 4. Giant cell formation 5. Encapsulation

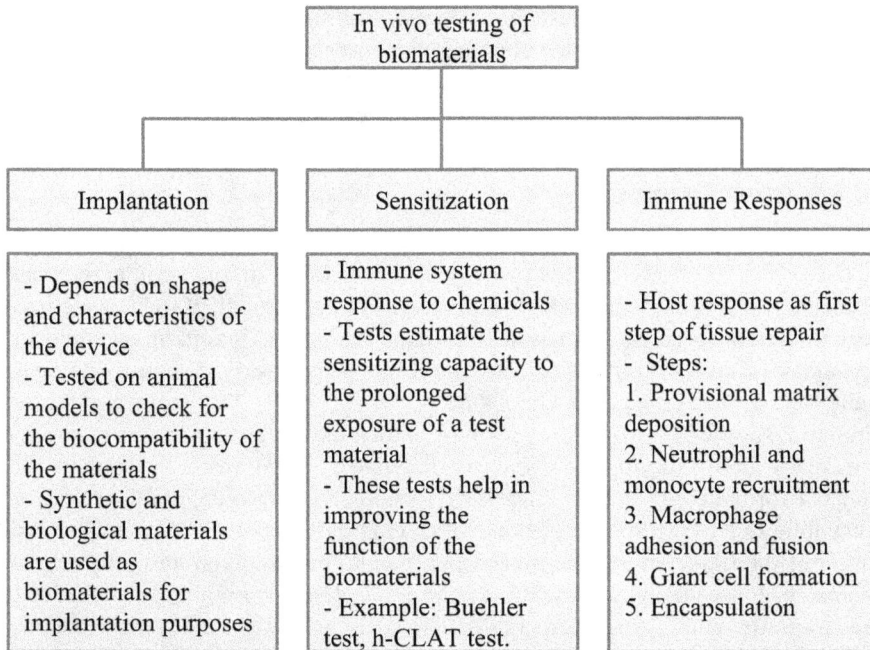

FIGURE 7.4   Considerations for the testing of biomaterials: The figure explains the important factors that need to be considered when testing biomaterials in vivo. The main factors are implantation, sensitization, and immune responses. Other factors include carcinogenicity, irritation, genotoxicity, and systemic toxicity.

Some drugs, biomaterial extracts, or chemicals don't show any effect in acute systemic toxicity but show significant bioreaction in chronic systemic toxicity (Medinat Y. Abbas et al., 2018).

7.5   IMMUNE RESPONSES TO MEDICAL DEVICES

The field of regenerative medicine is enormously progressing toward clinical translation (Ribitsch et al., 2020). Host immune responses to the implanted devices are dependent not only on the material and design of the device but also on the host's environment (Barré-Sinoussi and Montagutelli, 2015). Soon after the implantation of the medical device, the host tends to generate an immune response. The immune responses that are generated may include tissue remodeling, tissue injury, inflammation, proliferation, foreign body reactions, and changes in the vascular system (James M. Anderson, 2001). The medical devices are designed and manufactured in such a way that they meet the conditions of biocompatibility, which is the potential of a medical device or prosthesis to regulate and perform with a particular host response. The time and measure of ill effects in homeostatic mechanisms have to be considered while testing the biocompatibility of the device (Anderson and Jiang, 2016).

Following an injury, homeostasis gets altered, leading to a resolution that includes restitution and reorganization. Immune responses post-implantation could also include various types of irritation reactions (W.H. De Jong et al., 2012). Implantation may have both positive and negative effects (James M Anderson, 2001).

7.5.1 TISSUE RESPONSES

After the implant of a device, the initiation for a response begins from an injury to the tissue and is followed by the other parts of the body, and in turn, activation of the mechanisms to maintain homeostasis (James M Anderson, 2001). Tissue injury leads to cellular cascade formation for wound healing to maintain a homeostatic mechanism. Based on various factors, the response may vary, affecting the degree of the inflammatory response (James M Anderson, 2001). Depending on the host immune response following tissue injury, either tissue resolution or organization takes place within the injured tissue. Following the inflammatory response, there occurs a formation of scar tissue (Barré-Sinoussi and Montagutelli, 2015). The injury follows a host response of innate and adaptive immune responses. In consideration of the tissue responses, macrophages can be considered an orchestrator of the host response (Badylak and Gilbert, 2008). Protein adsorption is also one of the steps in tissue injury (Anderson, 1988). The tissue injury is followed by responses leading to wound healing, which involve a series of steps, like injury, coagulation, inflammation, granulation tissue, and healed wound (James M. Anderson et al., 2008).

7.5.2 BLOOD RESPONSES

Immediately after implantation, an injury occurs, following which modulations in vascular flow are generated. The responses to blood-device interactions and inflammation are closely linked, and usually, the initial responses to injury involve the blood and vascular system. In the blood response, the fluid, protein, and blood cells move from the vascular system into the injured tissue, and this action is known as exudation (James M. Anderson, 2001). The prior events in blood responses involve the adsorption of plasma proteins at the blood-device interface. The responses and reaction of the implanted material to the blood would depend on the components of the implant and the composition of the material (Tomaz Velnar, 2016). Also, during blood responses, damage is observed to the local lymphatics (Doke and Dhawale, 2015). To understand the degree of interaction between the blood and the device, the properties of the materials should be identified and studied (James M. Anderson, 2001).

7.5.3 LONG-TERM RESPONSES

In the long run, the implants may cause severe injuries and problems in response to the implantation. Many times, there are chances for a rejection of the implant that has been placed inside the body after the surgical site has healed (Barré-Sinoussi and Montagutelli, 2015). There may be a potential for excruciating discomfort and anguish in the case of implants in the future, which shows the body is trying to reject the implant, and thus, it has failed. Through stimulation of electrical signals, the medical devices also start reacting with nerve impulses, which may cause aggressive responses (Outman Akouissi et al., 2022). After implantation, there is a probability that dangers from biofilm infection could develop in the future (Stewart and Bjarnsholt, 2020). The positive effects of the implants occur when materials used in device design help in tissue growth and remodeling mechanisms. Improper functioning of the implant due to altered physiology is an example of a negative effect of the implant (James M. Anderson, 2001). Neointima growth on artery prostheses, hard tissue remodeling in the presence of implants, tendon prosthesis attached to soft tissue, and other favorable consequences are a few instances (James M. Anderson, 2001).

7.6   DISCUSSION AND FUTURE PERSPECTIVES

There has been a long-standing practice in biological research for the use of animal models for testing medical practices. The mouse models are especially used because of their 99% gene similarity with human beings (Barré-Sinoussi and Montagutelli, 2015). But with animal ethics and future prospects in mind, all focus on navigating high-tech products. The growing era of interconnected fields and interdisciplinary approaches to modern problems help to find modern solutions (Barré-Sinoussi and Montagutelli, 2015). This would basically involve an interaction between the doctors, engineers, scientists, and technicians who would all work together hand in hand to implement new strategies and devices that would be more effective and beneficial. Devices like microelectronic implants are emerging, which would work as a single system for diagnosis and treatment. In terms of the safety of medical devices, the probability of species differences in homeostatic mechanisms may be considered (James M Anderson, 2001). Treatments are coming up with lesser surgical pains and recovery. Disease treatment with electrical stimulation is increasingly becoming the focus of medicine (Barré-Sinoussi and Montagutelli, 2015). Risk assessment can also be carried out to analyze the level of risk of a medical device and its danger to the patient. This can be done by a combination of in vitro and in vivo testing on the toxicity of a medical device (James M. Anderson, 2001).

7.6.1   EXPLORING THE USE OF HUMAN CELLS AND TISSUES TO REPLACE ANIMAL MODELS

In order to replace animal models for testing, the implication of biotechnology can be brought into use. With the help of this application, we can make use of embryonic stem cells onto which the experiments can be done (Doke and Dhawale, 2015). The use of bioresorbable material is encouraged for device implants, as it makes use of transition metals that are present in the body and can be biocompatible with the host (Yingchao Su et al., 2022) Also, cells, tissues, and organs can be grown in labs so as to reduce the use of animals and use the parts grown in the lab. The use of 3Rs, viz. reduction, refinement, and replacement, is put into practice to find alternatives to animal models. Mouse embryonic stem cells are studied and manipulated in such a way that can be used as an alternative for mouse models (Nadia Rosenthal and Steve

Brown, 2007). Computer models are discovered and have been used where software is developed to test drugs instead of animals. The use of lower vertebrates that have a similarity with higher vertebrates is also an option (Doke and Dhawale, 2015). Different formulations of chemicals, like nitric oxide and its derivative compounds, can be used for designing a medical device, as it has cell messenger abilities and antimicrobial properties (Mitchell Lawrence Jones et al., 2010).

7.6.2 ORGAN-ON-A-CHIP MODEL

With recent advancements, the use and development of the organ-on-a-chip model are prevalent today. Engineering of various human tissues in micro physiologically relevant platforms is known as organs-on-chips (OOCs). Two or more tissue types that are organized in an orderly manner in a unique 3D structure form an OOC (Sushila Maharjan et al., 2020). There are various on-a-chip models, like the lymph-node-on-a-chip model, bone-marrow-on-a-chip model, and lymphatic-vessel-on-a-chip model. All these have widespread applications in medicine and healthcare (Sushila Maharjan et al., 2020). In a research study, it is found that OOC models can be inserted into various tissue injuries and can be modulated accordingly. But the most relevant OOC that has been studied today includes a stem cell OOC model that will create a whole new set of regenerative medicinal worlds. To complement the present-day preclinical model and to ease patient use, these OOC models are being designed with host specificity for drug screening and treatment of diseases (Wnorowski et al., 2019). Recent advancements have been able to structure a design of a 3D-organ-on-a-chip model in order to improve the reproducibility of in vitro organs. In this model, the source for 3D in vitro culture models has majorly been human pluripotent embryonic stem cells (D'Costa et al., 2020). The techniques of cell biology, tissue engineering, and technology have been combined to make an organ-on-a-chip model. It is designed in a way to depict and mimic human tissue and organ models (Qirui Wu et al., 2020). Studies also reveal that OOC has been showing consistency in its functioning ability and is being used at a large scale for healthcare and medicine (Gordana Vunjak-Novakovic et al., 2021). There is a clear difference between the terms "OOC" and "organoids". Organoids develop into multicellular forms and provide models for studying early development and a few diseases, whereas OOCs make use of bioengineering tools to combine matured tissue constructs to develop organs and their functions (James M. Anderson, 2001). Systemic diseases and various other drug formulation–like studies can be studied by coupling multiple OOCs together. OOC is designed in a way to provide human organ-specific readouts. OOCs can be divided into barrier function devices and parenchymal function devices (Gordana Vunjak-Novakovic et al., 2021). Among the wide study of OOCs being carried out, the human heart muscle has been studied as an OOC device, and most of the deaths occur due to cardiovascular diseases rather than cancers (Gordana Vunjak-Novakovic et al., 2021). The multi-OOC model gives clarity for therapeutic screening prior to clinical trials (Gordana Vunjak-Novakovic et al., 2021).

7.6.3   A NOVEL DEVELOPMENT IN TOXICOLOGY—NANOPARTICLES

A famous American physicist quoted that "there is plenty of room in the bottom," which is considered the inspirational beginning of the nanotechnology field (Richard P. Feynman, 2011). The nanoparticle is a revolutionary discovery in the field of modern biomedical science, extensively used for drug delivery into individual cells. As the name suggests, its overall dimension is in the nanoscale (i.e., 1–100 nm) (Zhang, 2010). The nanoparticle can be made up of gold, silver, platinum, and palladium, among which the gold nanoparticle is used commonly due to its unreactive and inert chemical properties, and its discovery is considered the new golden age of biomedical technology. They can be of different sizes, colors, and shapes, and the material from which it is made can be organic as well as inorganic and metals as well as non-metals (Erik C. Dreaden et al., 2012). Due to the very small size of nanoparticles, they can reach tumors and target tissue and cells more easily than other small molecules and with a mechanism and pathway different from others. They can be carbon-based nanoparticles, metal nanoparticles, ceramic nanoparticles, semiconductor nanoparticles, polymeric nanoparticles, and lipid-based nanoparticles (Ibrahim Khan et al., 2019). Their optical properties are an important deciding factor for their physicochemical properties. Altering the size of the nanoparticles can alter the surface area of the nanoparticles, and hence, their absorption peak is shifted to red in the visible spectra (Tali Dadosh, 2009). Nanoparticles are used in protein detection, tissue engineering, multicolor optical coding for biological assays, manipulation of cells and biomolecules, cancer therapy, environmental remediation, food processing, packaging, and agriculture (Wang et al., 2002; Cao et al., 2003; D.H. Reich et al., 2003; Mingyong Han et al., 2001; O.V. Salata, 2004; Ray and Iroegbu, 2021; Nandita Dasgupta et al., 2015).

7.6.4   THRESHOLD OF TOXICOLOGICAL CONCERN INITIATIVES FOR MEDICAL DEVICES

The threshold of toxicological concern refers to the non-lethal, non-irritant, non-toxic acceptable dose that does not cause any hypersensitive reaction or allergic reaction or, in other words, protective index of dose of biomaterial that does not pose any risk of endpoint bioreaction in the host. TTC is based on general endpoint toxicity as well as specific end toxicity, which includes carcinogenicity, immunotoxicity, as well as reproductive toxicity. It can identify the toxicity of many chemicals whose toxicity is not known, just by their chemical structure as well as the toxicity of those chemicals that have minimal to no toxicity effect on the host (Kroes, 2006). Almost all chemicals are placed under one class among three classes, which are classified based on their toxicity level expanding from low to moderate to high to serious toxicity (G.M. Cramer et al., 1976).

Understanding the toxicological data for a chemical or biomaterial extract is very important to calculate its biocompatibility and bioreaction risks in the host. And if the full toxicity data from all the published or non-published pieces of literature, from the supplier or any other trusted source about composition, polarity, molecular weights, and other chemical properties are known about leachable chemicals, then an appropriate toxicological conclusion can be drawn from the data experimentally, but if there is limited chemical-specific toxicity data, the TTC concept is used to draw appropriate conclusion and results (Simon J. More et al., 2019). According to ISO 10993-1, TTC is based on the compilation of data from the host exposure to the device leachable or biomaterial extract or device component concerning the number of high toxicities that probably exist. No further data is needed if there is no sign of the toxicity concern even after all the chemicals are released from the biomaterial source, but if toxicity concern exists after the release of all the chemicals, then further information about its target site and the amount released in the host body is required. If human exposure to a substance is below that threshold, the substance can be judged, with reasonable confidence, to present a low probability of risk regardless of structure, even if there is no toxicological data available (I.C. Munro et al., 1996).

7.7 CONCLUSION

With all the previously stated procedures/requirements/evaluations, it can be concluded that to carry out any risk assessment of the medical device biomaterial in vivo, animal models that closely mimic humans are being used. With these animals, after administration with the biomaterial either orally, intracutaneously injected, or implanted, various tests, such as in vivo genotoxicity, in vivo mouse micronucleus assays, in vivo chromosomal aberration assay, carcinogenicity, hemocompatibility tests, and skin sensitization tests, are conducted. These tests provide a basis for the analysis of hypersensitivity reactions, which include skin irritation, mucosal irritation, and ocular irritation, as well as tissue and blood response. The tissue, blood, and cellular response also depend on the duration for which the tests are conducted; the shape, size, and weight of the implants; the route of exposure; the temperature of the host and the environment; and the chemical and physical properties of the biomaterials. Time of exposure to biomaterial plays a huge role in the immunogenic response of the host. Some biomaterials do not cause any bioreaction or immunogenic response when exposed for a short period but are able to show an immunogenic response when given for a longer period. Though in vivo testing of biomaterial is realistic, efficient, and reliable in providing sufficient data for toxicity analysis, it requires the death of a number of animal models for testing and, hence, raises ethical issues. With recent advancements, the use of the 3D organ-on-a-chip model, bioresorbable material, computer model for testing drugs, nitric oxide for designing biomaterial, and human cells and tissues to replace animal models are very much prevalent nowadays. This not only eliminates the use of animal models for tests but also is a more reliable and efficient strategy/method of testing.

7.8 ABBREVIATIONS

ISO—International Organization for Standardization
OECD—Organization for Economic Co-operation and Development
CAb—Chromosomal aberration assay

GPMT—Guinea pig maximization test
PEO—Plasma electrolytic oxidation
DAMP—Damage-associated molecular patterns
ELISA—Enzyme-linked immunosorbent assay
LLNA—Local lymph node assay
SI—Stimulation index
OOC—Organ-on-chip
TTC—Threshold of toxicological concern

Authors' Contributions
All authors contributed to writing the manuscript and reviewing.

Conflict of Interest
The authors declare that they have no competing interests.

Consent for Publication
Not applicable.

Acknowledgments
Not applicable.

Funding Information
Not received.

Compliance with Ethical Standards
Not applicable.

REFERENCES

Abbas, M. Y., Ejiofor, J. I., & Yakubu, M. I. (2018). Acute and chronic toxicity profiles of the methanol leaf extract of Acacia ataxacantha D.C. (Leguminosae) in Wistar rats. *Bulletin of Faculty of Pharmacy, Cairo University*, *56*(2), 185–189. https://doi.org/10.1016/j.bfopcu.2018.09.001.

Akouissi, O. et al. (2022). A finite element model of the mechanical interactions between peripheral nerves and intrafascicular implants. *Journal of Neural Engineering*, *19*(4), 046017. IOP Publishing. Retrieved August 7, 2022, from https://doi.org/10.1088/1741-2552/ac7d0e.

Albert, D. (2012). Material and chemical characterization for the biological evaluation of medical device biocompatibility. *Biocompatibility and Performance of Medical Devices*, 65–94. https://doi.org/10.1533/9780857096456.2.63.

Allyn, M. M., Luo, R. H., Hellwarth, E. B., & Swindle-Reilly, K. E. (2022). Considerations for polymers used in ocular drug delivery. *Frontiers in Medicine*, *8*, 787644. https://doi.org/10.3389/fmed.2021.787644.

Anderson, J. M. (1988). Inflammatory response to implants. *ASAIO Journal*, *34*(2), 101–107. Ovid Technologies (Wolters Kluwer Health). https://doi.org/10.1097/00002480-198804000-00005.

Anderson, J. M. (2001). Biological responses to materials. *Annual Review of Materials Research*, *31*(1), 81–110. Annual Reviews. https://doi.org/10.1146/annurev.matsci.31.1.81.

Anderson, J. M. (2012). *Polymer science: A comprehensive reference*. Retrieved August 9, 2022, from www.sciencedirect.com/referencework/9780080878621/polymer-science-a-comprehensive-reference.

Anderson, J. M. (2020). *Perspectives on in vivo testing of biomaterials, prostheses, and artificial organs*. Retrieved August 10, 2022, from https://journals.sagepub.com https://doi.org/10.3109/10915818809019520.

Anderson, J. M., & Jiang, S. (2016). Implications of the acute and chronic inflammatory response and the foreign body reaction to the immune response of implanted biomaterials. In *The immune response to implanted materials and devices*, 15–36. Springer International Publishing. Retrieved August 7, 2022, from https://doi.org/10.1007/978-3-319-45433-7_2.

Anderson, J. M., & Jiang, S. (2019). Animal models in biomaterial development. *Encyclopedia of Biomedical Engineering*, 237–241. https://doi.org/10.1016/b978-0-12-801238-3.99882-9.

Anderson, J. M., Rodriguez, A., & Chang, D. T. (2008). Foreign body reaction to biomaterials. *Seminars in Immunology*, *20*(2), 86–100. Elsevier BV. Retrieved August 7, 2022, from https://doi.org/10.1016/j.smim.2007.11.004.

Anderson, S. E., Siegel, P. D., & Meade, B. J. (2011). The LLNA: A brief review of recent advances and limitations. *Journal of Allergy*, 1–10. https://doi.org/10.1155/2011/424203.

Antoniac, I., Adam, R., Biţă, A., Miculescu, M., Trante, O., Petrescu, I. M., & Pogărăşteanu, M. (2020). Comparative assessment of in vitro and in vivo biodegradation of Mg-1Ca magnesium alloys for orthopedic applications. *Materials*. https://doi.org/10.3390/ma14010084.

Arnold, B. (2019, April 19). Shape memory alloys for biomedical applications. *AZoM*. Retrieved August 11, 2022 from www.azom.com/article.aspx?ArticleID=13303.

Badylak, S. F., & Gilbert, T. W. (2008). Immune response to biologic scaffold materials. *Seminars in Immunology*, *20*(2), 109–116. Elsevier BV. Retrieved August 7, 2022, from https://doi.org/10.1016/j.smim.2007.11.003.

Barré-Sinoussi, F., & Montagutelli, X. (2015). Animal models are essential to biological research: Issues and perspectives. *Future Science OA*, *1*(4). Future Science Ltd. https://doi.org/10.4155/fso.15.63.

Bhaskara Rao, S., & Sharma, C. P. (1997). Use of chitosan as a biomaterial: Studies on its safety and hemostatic potential. *34*(1), 21–28. https://doi.org/10.1002/(sici)1097-4636(199701)34:1<21::aid-jbm4>3.0.co;2-p.

Boutrand, J. (2019). *Biocompatibility and performance of medical devices*, 2nd ed. (Woodhead Publishing Series in Biomaterials). Woodhead Publishing.

Brake, M. A., Ivanciu, L., Maroney, S. A., Martinez, N. D., Mast, A. E., & Westrick, R. J. (2019). Assessing blood clotting and coagulation factors in mice. *Current Protocols in Mouse Biology*, *9*(2). https://doi.org/10.1002/cpmo.61.

Buehler, E. V. (1965). Delayed contact hypersensitivity in the Guinea pig. *Archives of Dermatology*, *91*(2), 171. https://doi.org/10.1001/archderm.1965.01600080079017.

Burns-Naas, L. A. (2005). Hypersensitivity, delayed type*. *Encyclopedia of Toxicology*, 559–561. https://doi.org/10.1016/b0-12-369400-0/00510-x.

Cao, Y. C., Jin, R., Nam, J. M., Thaxton, C. S., & Mirkin, C. A. (2003). Raman dye-labeled nanoparticle probes for proteins. *Journal of the American Chemical Society*, *125*(48), 14676–14677. https://doi.org/10.1021/ja0366235.

Chen, F. M., & Liu, X. (2016). Advancing biomaterials of human origin for tissue engineering. *Progress in Polymer Science*, *53*, 86–168. https://doi.org/10.1016/j.progpolymsci.2015.02.004.

Chen, Y., Wang, M., & Fang, L. (2013). Biomaterials as novel penetration enhancers for transdermal and dermal drug delivery systems. *Drug Delivery*, *20*(5), 199–209. https://doi.org/10.3109/10717544.2013.801533.

Cheung, V. V., Jha, A., Owen, R., Depledge, M. H., & Galloway, T. S. (2006). Development of the in vivo chromosome aberration assay in oyster (*Crassostrea gigas*) embryo–larvae for genotoxicity assessment. *Marine Environmental Research, 62*. https://doi.org/10.1016/j.marenvres.2006.04.018.

Clausen, T., Schwan-Jonczyk, A., Lang, G., Schuh, W., Liebscher, K. D., Springob, C., Franzke, M., Balzer, W., Imhoff, S., Maresch, G., & Bimczok, R. (2006). Hair preparations. In *Ullmann's Encyclopedia of Industrial Chemistry*. https://doi.org/10.1002/14356007.a12_571.pub2.

Cramer, G., Ford, R., & Hall, R. (1976). Estimation of toxic hazard—A decision tree approach. *Food and Cosmetics Toxicology, 16*(3), 255–276. https://doi.org/10.1016/s0015-6264(76)80522-6.

Dadosh, T. (2009). Synthesis of uniform silver nanoparticles with controllable size. *Materials Letters, 63*(26), 2236–2238. https://doi.org/10.1016/j.matlet.2009.07.042.

Dai, Z., Li, Y., Lu, W., Jiang, D.-M., Hong, H., Yan, Y., Lv, G., & Yang, A. (2015). In vivo biocompatibility of new nano-calcium-deficient hydroxyapatite/poly-amino acid complex biomaterials. *International Journal of Nanomedicine*, 6303. https://doi.org/10.2147/IJN.S90273.

Dasgupta, N., Ranjan, S., Mundekkad, D., Ramalingam, C., Shanker, R., & Kumar, A. (2015). Nanotechnology in agro-food: From field to plate. *Food Research International, 69*, 381–400. https://doi.org/10.1016/j.foodres.2015.01.005.

Davis, J. R. (2003). *Handbook of materials for medical devices*. ASM International.

D'Costa, K. et al. (2020). Biomaterials and culture systems for development of organoid and organ-on-a-chip models. *Annals of Biomedical Engineering, 48*(7), 2002–2027. Springer Science and Business Media LLC. Retrieved August 7, 2022, from https://doi.org/10.1007/s10439-020-02498-w.

De Cock, L. J., Lenoir, J., De Koker, S., Vermeersch, V., Skirtach, A. G., Dubruel, P., Adriaens, E., Vervaet, C., Remon, J. P., & De Geest, B. G. (2011). Mucosal irritation potential of polyelectrolyte multilayer capsules. *32*(7), 1967–1977. https://doi.org/10.1016/j.biomaterials.2010.11.012.

De Jong, W. H. (2020). *Biocompatibility and performance of medical devices || in vivo and in vitro testing for the biological safety evaluation of biomaterials and medical devices*, 123–166. https://doi.org/10.1016/B978-0-08-102643-4.00007-0.

De Jong, W. H., Carraway, J., & Geertsma, R. et al. (2012). In vivo and in vitro testing for the biological safety evaluation of biomaterials and medical devices. *Biocompatibility and Performance of Medical Devices*, 120–158. Elsevier. Retrieved August 12, 2022 from https://doi.org/10.1533/9780857096456.2.120.

De Jong, W. H., Geertsma, R., & Tinkler, J. (2002). Medical devices manufactured from latex: European regulatory initiatives. *Methods, 27*(1), 93–98. https://doi.org/10.1016/s1046-2023(02)00057-9.

Dewanjee, M. (2017, April 6). *Methods of assessment of thrombosis in vivo*. Retrieved August 5, 2022, from www.academia.edu/32303070/Methods_of_Assessment_of_Thrombosis_in_Vivo?from=cover_page

Diebold, Y., Jarrín, M., Sáez, V., Carvalho, E. L. S., Orea, M., Calonge, M., Seijo, B., & Alonso, M. J. (2007). Ocular drug delivery by liposome–chitosan nanoparticle complexes (LCS-NP). *Biomaterials, 28*(8), 1553–1564. https://doi.org/10.1016/j.biomaterials.2006.11.028.

Doke, S. K., & Dhawale, S. C. (2015). Alternatives to animal testing: A review. *Saudi Pharmaceutical Journal, 23*(3), 223–229. doi: 10.1016/j.jsps.2013.11.002. Epub 2013 Nov 18. PMID: 26106269; PMCID: PMC4475840.

Dornell, J. (2022, March 14). *In vivo vs in vitro: Definition, pros and cons*. Drug Discovery from Technology Networks. www.technologynetworks.com/drug-discovery/articles/in-vivo-vs-in-vitro-definition-pros-and-cons-350415.

Dreaden, E. C., Alkilany, A. M., Huang, X., Murphy, C. J., & El-Sayed, M. A. (2012). Chem-Inform abstract: The golden age: Gold nanoparticles for biomedicine. *ChemInform*, *43*(27). https://doi.org/10.1002/chin.201227268.

Egermann, M., Goldhahn, J., Holz, R., Schneider, E., & Lill, C. A. (2008). A sheep model for fracture treatment in osteoporosis: Benefits of the model versus animal welfare. *Laboratory Animals*, *42*(4), 453–464. https://doi.org/10.1258/la.2007.007001.

Ekdahl, K. N., Lambris, J. D., Elwing, H., Ricklin, D., Nilsson, P. H., Teramura, Y., Nicholls, I. A., & Nilsson, B. (2011). Innate immunity activation on biomaterial surfaces: A mechanistic model and coping strategies. *Advanced Drug Delivery Reviews*, *63*, 1042–1050.

Eske, J. (2020, August 31). *What is the difference between in vivo and in vitro?* www.medical-newstoday.com/articles/in-vivo-vs-in-vitro.

Feynman, R. P. (2011). There's plenty of room at the bottom. *Resonance*, *16*(9), 890–905. https://doi.org/10.1007/s12045-011-0109-x.

Furie, B. (2005). Thrombus formation in vivo. *Journal of Clinical Investigation*, *115*(12), 3355–3362. https://doi.org/10.1172/jci26987.

Gad, S. (2013). Standards and methods for assessing the safety and biocompatibility of biomaterials. *Characterization of Biomaterials*, 285–306. https://doi.org/10.1533/9780857093684.285.

Garnett, A., Hotchkiss, S., & Caldwell, J. (1994). Percutaneous absorption of benzyl acetate through rat skin in vitro. 3. A comparison with human skin. *Food and Chemical Toxicology*, *32*(11), 1061–1065. https://doi.org/10.1016/0278-6915(94)90147-3.

Gerberick, G. F. (2004). Development of a peptide reactivity assay for screening contact allergens. *Toxicological Sciences*, *81*(2), 332–343. https://doi.org/10.1093/toxsci/kfh213.

Ghazali, A. R., Rajab, N. F., Zainuddin, M. F., & Ahmat, N. (2021). Assessment of skin irritation and sensitisation effects by topical pterostilbene. *Biomedical and Pharmacology Journal*, *14*(4), 1917–1927. https://doi.org/10.13005/bpj/2290.

Goldberg, A. M. (2010). The principles of humane experimental technique: Is it relevant today? *ALTEX—Alternatives to Animal Experimentation*, *27*(2), 149–151. https://doi.org/10.14573/altex.2010.2.149.

Gorbet, M. B., & Sefton, M. V. (2004). Biomaterial-associated thrombosis: Roles of coagulation factors, complement, platelets and leukocytes. *Biomaterials*, *25*, 5681–5703.

Grabska-Zielińska, S., Sionkowska, A., Reczyńska, K., & Pamuła, E. (2020). Physico-chemical characterization and biological tests of collagen/silk fibroin/chitosan scaffolds cross-linked by dialdehyde starch. *Polymers*, *12*(2), 372. https://doi.org/10.3390/polym12020372.

Han, M., Gao, X., Su, J. Z., & Nie, S. (2001). Quantum-dot-tagged microbeads for multiplexed optical coding of biomolecules. *Nature Biotechnology*, *19*(7), 631–635. https://doi.org/10.1038/90228.

Handler, J. A. (2013). Book review: Biocompatibility and performance of medical devices. *International Journal of Toxicology*, *32*(5), 396–397. https://doi.org/10.1177/1091581813493612.

Hayashi, M., Tice, R. R., MacGregor, J. T., Anderson, D., Blakey, D. H., Kirsch-Volders, M., . . . Vannier, B. (1994). In vivo rodent erythrocyte micronucleus assay. *Mutation Research/Environmental Mutagenesis and Related Subjects*, *312*(3), 293–304. https://doi.org/10.1016/0165-1161(94)90039-6.

Hu, L. X., Hu, S. F., Rao, M., Yang, J., Lei, H., Duan, Z., Xia, W., & Zhu, C. H. (2018). Studies of acute and subchronic systemic toxicity associated with a copper/low-density polyethylene nanocomposite intrauterine device. *International Journal of Nanomedicine*, *13*, 4913–4926. https://doi.org/10.2147/ijn.s169114.

Huang, S., Engberg, A. E., Jonsson, N., Sandholm, K., Nicholls, I. A., Mollnes, T. E., Fromell, K., Nilsson, B., & Ekdahl, K. N. (2016). Reciprocal relationship between contact and complement system activation on artificial polymers exposed to whole human blood. *Biomaterials*, *77*, 111–119.

Huzum, B., Puha, B., Necoara, R. M., Gheorghevici, S., Puha, G., Filip, A., Sirbu, P. D., & Alexa, O. (2021, November). Biocompatibility assessment of biomaterials used in orthopedic devices: An overview (review). *Experimental and Therapeutic Medicine, 22*(5), 1315. https://doi.org/10.3892/etm.2021.10750. Epub 2021 Sep 17. PMID: 34630669; PMCID: PMC8461597.

Jamiolkowski, M. A., Snyder, T. A., Perkins, I. L., Malinauskas, R. A., & Lu, Q. (2020). Preclinical device thrombogenicity assessments: Key messages from the 2018 FDA, industry, and Academia Forum. *ASAIO Journal, 67*(2), 214–219. https://doi.org/10.1097/mat.0000000000001226.

Johannes, C., & Obe, G. (2019). Chromosomal aberration test in human lymphocytes. *Methods in Molecular Biology*, 121–134. https://doi.org/10.1007/978-1-4939-9646-9_6.

Jones, M. L. et al. (2010). Antimicrobial properties of nitric oxide and its application in antimicrobial formulations and medical devices. *Applied Microbiology and Biotechnology, 88*(2), 401–407. Springer Science and Business Media LLC. https://doi.org/10.1007/s00253-010-2733-x.

Jung, F., Braune, S., & Lendlein, A. (2013). Hemocompatibility testing of biomaterials using human platelets. *Clinical Hemorheology and Microcirculation, 53*(1–2), 97–115. https://doi.org/10.3233/ch-2012-1579.

Kang, S. H., Kwon, J. Y., Lee, J. K., & Seo, Y. R. (2013). Recent advances in in vivo genotoxicity testing: Prediction of carcinogenic potential using comet and micronucleus assay in animal models. *Journal of Cancer Prevention, 18*(4), 277–288. https://doi.org/10.15430/jcp.2013.18.4.277.

Khamar, K., & Richmond, F. (2018). Testing of tissue engineered products in the US. *Reference Module in Biomedical Sciences*. https://doi.org/10.1016/b978-0-12-801238-3.65573-3.

Khan, I., Saeed, K., & Khan, I. (2019). Nanoparticles: Properties, applications, and toxicities. *Arabian Journal of Chemistry, 12*(7), 908–931. https://doi.org/10.1016/j.arabjc.2017.05.011.

Kim, S. R., Lee, K. M., Kim, J. H. et al. (2022). Biocompatibility evaluation of peotreated magnesium alloy implants placed in rabbit femur condyle notches and paravertebral muscles. *Biomaterials Research, 26*, 29 (2022). https://doi.org/10.1186/s40824-022-00279-1.

Kitano, M. (1992). Updating OECD guidelines for the testing of chemicals. *Water Science and Technology, 25*(11), 465–472. https://doi.org/10.2166/wst.1992.0327.

Klien, K., & Godnić-Cvar, J. (2012). Genotoxicity of metal nanoparticles: Focus on in vivo studies. *Archives of Industrial Hygiene and Toxicology, 63*(2), 133–145. https://doi.org/10.2478/10004-1254-63-2012-2213.

Kligman, A. M., & Basketter, D. A. (1995). A critical commentary and updating of the guinea pig maximization test. *Contact Dermatitis, 32*(3), 129–134. https://doi.org/10.1111/j.1600-0536.1995.tb00801.x.

Krishna, G., & Hayashi, M. (2000). In vivo rodent micronucleus assay: Protocol, conduct and data interpretation. *Mutation Research/Fundamental and Molecular Mechanisms of Mutagenesis, 455*(1–2), 155–166. https://doi.org/10.1016/s0027-5107(00)00117-2.

Kroes, R. (2006). The threshold of toxicological concern concept in risk assessment. *Toxicology Letters, 164*, S48. https://doi.org/10.1016/j.toxlet.2006.06.102.

Lambris, J. D., Reid, K. B., & Volanakis, J. E. (1999). The evolution, structure, biology and pathophysiology of complement. *Immunology Today, 20*, 207–211.

Liu, X., Yuan, L., Li, D., Tang, Z., Wang, Y., Chen, G., . . . Brash, J. L. (2014). Blood compatible materials: State of the art. *Journal of Materials Chemistry B. Materials, 2*(35), 5718–5738. https://doi.org/10.1039/c4tb00881b.

Magnusson, B., & Kligman, A. M. (1970). The identification of contact allergens by animal assay. The guinea pig maximization test. *Journal of Occupational and Environmental Medicine*, *12*(2), 59. https://doi.org/10.1097/00043764-197002000-00023.

Maharjan, S. et al. (2020). 3D immunocompetent organ-on-a-chip models. *Small Methods*, *4*(9), 2000235. Wiley. https://doi.org/10.1002/smtd.202000235.

Mao, Z., Zhou, X., & Gao, C. (2013). *Influence of structure and properties of colloidal biomaterials on cellular uptake and cell functions*, 896–911. Royal Society of Chemistry. https://doi.org/10.1039/C3BM00137G.

Mödinger, Y., Teixeira, G., Neidlinger-Wilke, C., & Ignatius, A. (2018). Role of the complement system in the response to orthopedic biomaterials. *International Journal of Molecular Sciences*, *19*(11), 3367. https://doi.org/10.3390/ijms19113367.

Moeller, M., & Matyjaszewski, K. (2012). *Polymer science: A comprehensive reference*, 1st ed. Elsevier Science.

Mohan, V. (2007). Chromosome 11 aneusomy in esophageal cancers and precancerous lesions—an early event in neoplastic transformation: An interphase fluorescence in *situ hybridization* study from South India. *World Journal of Gastroenterology*, *13*(4), 503. https://doi.org/10.3748/wjg.v13.i4.503.

Morais, J. M., Papadimitrakopoulos, F., & Burgess, D. J. (2010). Biomaterials/tissue interactions: Possible solutions to overcome foreign body response. *The AAPS Journal*, *12*(2), 188–196. https://doi.org/10.1208/s12248-010-9175-3.

More, S. J., Bampidis, V., Benford, D., Bragard, C., Halldorsson, T. I., Hernández-Jerez, A. F., Hougaard Bennekou, S., Koutsoumanis, K. P., Machera, K., Naegeli, H., Nielsen, S. S., Schlatter, J. R., Schrenk, D., Silano, V., Turck, D., Younes, M., Gundert-Remy, U., Kass, G. E. N., Kleiner, J., . . . Wallace, H. M. (2019). Guidance on the use of the threshold of toxicological concern approach in food safety assessment. *EFSA Journal*, *17*(6). https://doi.org/10.2903/j.efsa.2019.5708.

Munro, I., Ford, R., Kennepohl, E., & Sprenger, J. (1996). Correlation of structural class with no-observed-effect levels: A proposal for establishing a threshold of concern. *Food and Chemical Toxicology*, *34*(9), 829–867. https://doi.org/10.1016/s0278-6915(96)00049-x.

Nilsson, B., Ekdahl, K. N., Mollnes, T. E., & Lambris, J. D. (2007). The role of complement in biomaterial-induced inflammation. *Molecular Immunology*, *44*, 82–94.

Ochoa, R. (2002). Pathology issues in the design of toxicology studies. In *Handbook of toxicologic pathology*, 307–326. https://doi.org/10.1016/b978-012330215-1/50015-6.

OECD Guidelines for the testing of chemicals, Section 4. (2016). https://doi.org/10.1787/20745788.

Omidi, M. (2017). *Biomaterials for oral and dental tissue engineering || characterization of biomaterials*, 97–115. https://doi.org/10.1016/B978-0-08-100961-1.00007-4.

Pan, Y., Lin, Y., Jiang, L., Lin, H., Xu, C., Lin, D., & Cheng, H. (2020). Removal of dental alloys and titanium attenuates trace metals and biological effects on the liver and kidney. *Chemosphere*, *243*, 125205. https://doi.org/10.1016/j.chemosphere.2019.125205.

Ratner, B. D., Hoffman, A. S., Schoen, F. J., & Lemons, J. E. (2013). *Biomaterials science*. Elsevier Gezondheidszorg.

Ray, S. S., & Iroegbu, A. O. C. (2021). Nanocelluloses: Benign, sustainable, and ubiquitous biomaterials for water remediation. *ACS Omega*, *6*(7), 4511–4526. https://doi.org/10.1021/acsomega.0c06070.

Reich, D. H., Tanase, M., Hultgren, A., Bauer, L. A., Chen, C. S., & Meyer, G. J. (2003). Biological applications of multifunctional magnetic nanowires (invited). *Journal of Applied Physics*, *93*(10), 7275–7280. https://doi.org/10.1063/1.1558672.

Remes, A., & Williams, D. (1992). Immune response in biocompatibility. *Biomaterials*, *13*(11), 731–743. https://doi.org/10.1016/0142-9612(92)90010-1/.

Ribitsch, I. et al. (2020). Large animal models in regenerative medicine and tissue engineering: To do or not to do. *Frontiers in Bioengineering and Biotechnology, 8.* Frontiers Media SA. Retrieved August 7, 2022, from https://doi.org/10.3389/fbioe.2020.00972.

Richard, F. Wallin | January 1. (2017, August 7). *A practical guide to ISO 10993–3: Carcinogenicity.* Retrieved August 10, 2022, from www.mddionline.com/news/practical-guide-iso-10993-3-carcinogenicity.

Ricklin, D., Hajishengallis, G., Yang, K., & Lambris, J. D. (2010). Complement: A key system for immune surveillance and homeostasis. *Nature Immunology, 11,* 785–797.

Robinson, A. (2022). Ann Robinson's research reviews—21 July 2022. *BMJ,* o1789. https://doi.org/10.1136/bmj.o1789.

Rogers, W. (2012). Sterilization techniques for polymers. *Sterilization of Biomaterials and Medical Devices,* 151–211. https://doi.org/10.1533/9780857096265.151.

Rosenthal, N., & Brown, S. (2007). The mouse ascending: Perspectives for human-disease models. *Nature Cell Biology, 9*(9), 993–999. Springer Science and Business Media LLC. https://doi.org/10.1038/ncb437.

Rozman, K. K., Doull, J., & Hayes, W. J. (2010). Chapter 1—Dose and time determining, and other factors influencing toxicity. In *Hayes' handbook of pesticide toxicology,* 3rd ed., Academic Press, New York, vol. 24, 3–101. https://www.sciencedirect.com/science/article/pii/B978012374367100001X.

Saeidnia, S., Manayi, A., & Abdollahi, M. (2016). From in vitro experiments to in vivo and clinical studies: Pros and Cons. *Current Drug Discovery Technologies, 12*(4), 218–224. https://doi.org/10.2174/1570163813666160114093140.

Salata, O. (2004). Applications of nanoparticles in biology and medicine. *Journal of Nanobiotechnology, 2*(1), 3. https://doi.org/10.1186/1477-3155-2-3.

Santella, R. M. (1997). DNA damage as an intermediate biomarker in intervention studies. *Experimental Biology and Medicine, 216*(2), 166–171. https://doi.org/10.3181/00379727-216-44166.

Schnabelrauch, M. (2017). Chemical bulk properties of biomaterials. *Biomaterials in Clinical Practice,* 431–459. https://doi.org/10.1007/978-3-319-68025-5_15.

Shaikh, R., Raj Singh, T. R., Garland, M. J., Woolfson, A. D., & Donnelly, R. F. (2011). Mucoadhesive drug delivery systems. *Journal of Pharmacy & Bioallied Sciences, 3*(1), 89–100. https://doi.org/10.4103/0975-7406.76478.

Shen, C., Han, Y., Wang, B., Tang, J., Chen, H., & Lin, Q. (2015). Ocular biocompatibility evaluation of POSS nanomaterials for biomedical material applications. *RSC Advances, 5*(66), 53782–53788. https://doi.org/10.1039/c5ra08668j.

Stewart, P. S., & Bjarnsholt, T. (2020). Risk factors for chronic biofilm-related infection associated with implanted medical devices. *Clinical Microbiology and Infection, 26*(8), 1034–1038. Elsevier BV. https://doi.org/10.1016/j.cmi.2020.02.027.

Su, Y. et al. (2022). Blending with transition metals improves bioresorbable zinc as better medical implants. *Bioactive Materials, 20,* 243–258. Elsevier BV. Retrieved August 7, 2022, from https://doi.org/10.1016/j.bioactmat.2022.05.033.

Tang, C. (n.d.). *In vitro vs. in vivo: Is one better?* Retrieved August 12, 2022, from www.uhn-research.ca/news/vitro-vs-vivo-one-better.

Tang, L., & Eaton, J. W. (1995). Inflammatory responses to biomaterials. *American Journal of Clinical Pathology, 103*(4), 466–471. https://doi.org/10.1093/ajcp/103.4.466.

Test No. 402: Acute Dermal Toxicity. (2017). *OECD guidelines for the testing of chemicals, section 4.* https://doi.org/10.1787/9789264070585-en.

Thomas, S., Grohens, Y., & Ninan, N. (Eds.). (2015). *Nanotechnology applications for tissue engineering.* William Andrew Publishing. https://doi.org/10.1016/c2014-0-00006-8).

Thrivikraman, G., Madras, G., & Basu, B. (2014). In vitro/In vivo assessment and mechanisms of toxicity of bioceramic materials and their wear particulates. *RSC Advances, 4*(25), 12763. https://doi.org/10.1039/c3ra44483j.

Velnar, T. et al. (2016). Biomaterials and host versus graft response: A short review. *Bosnian Journal of Basic Medical Sciences*. Association of Basic Medical Sciences of FBIH. https://doi.org/10.17305/bjbms.2016.525.

Villa-Ruano, N., Lozoya-Gloria, E., & Pacheco-Hernández, Y. (2016). Kaurenoic acid. *Studies in Natural Products Chemistry*, 151–174. https://doi.org/10.1016/b978-0-444-63932-5.00003-6.

Vunjak-Novakovic, G. et al. (2021). Organs-on-a-chip models for biological research. *Cell*, *184*(18), 4597–4611. Elsevier BV. Retrieved August 7, 2022 from https://doi.org/10.1016/j.cell.2021.08.005.

Wang, S., Mamedova, N., Kotov, N. A., Chen, W., & Studer, J. (2002). Antigen/antibody immunocomplex from CdTe nanoparticle bioconjugates. *Nano Letters*, *2*(8), 817–822. https://doi.org/10.1021/nl0255193.

Weber, M., Steinle, H., Golombek, S., Hann, L., Schlensak, C., Wendel, H. P., & Avci-Adali, M. (2018). Blood-contacting biomaterials: In vitro evaluation of hemocompatibility. *Frontiers in Bioengineering and Biotechnology*, *6*. https://doi.org/10.3389/fbioe.2018.00099.

Wennberg, A., Hasselgren, G., & Tronstad, L. (1978). A method for evaluation of initial tissue response to biomaterials. *Acta Odontologica Scandinavica*, *36*(2), 67–73. https://doi.org/10.3109/00016357809027568.

Wnorowski, A. et al. (2019). Progress, obstacles, and limitations in the use of stem cells in organ-on-a-chip models. *Advanced Drug Delivery Reviews*, *140*, 3–11. Elsevier BV. https://doi.org/10.1016/j.addr.2018.06.001.

Wu, Q. et al. (2020). Organ-on-a-chip: Recent breakthroughs and future prospects. *Biomedical Engineering Online*, *19*(1). Springer Science and Business Media LLC. https://doi.org/10.1186/s12938-020-0752-0.

Zhang, K., Fu, Q., Yoo, J., Chen, X., Chandra, P., Mo, X., Song, L., Atala, A., & Zhao, W. (2017). 3D bioprinting of urethra with PCL/PLCL blend and dual autologous cells in fibrin hydrogel: An in vitro evaluation of biomimetic mechanical property and cell growth environment. *Acta Biomaterialia*, *50*, 154–164. https://doi.org/10.1016/j.actbio.2016.12.008.

Zhang, W., Chen, L., Chen, J., Wang, L., Gui, X., Ran, J., Xu, G., Zhao, H., Zeng, M., Ji, J., Qian, L., Zhou, J., Ouyang, H., & Zou, X. (2017). Silk fibroin biomaterial shows safe and effective wound healing in animal models and a randomized controlled clinical trial. *Advanced Healthcare Materials*, 1700121. https://doi.org/10.1002/adhm.201700121.

Zhang, X. (2010). Toxicologic effects of gold nanoparticles in vivo by different administration routes. *International Journal of Nanomedicine*, 771. https://doi.org/10.2147/ijn.s8428.

8 Clinical Trials of Materials for Medical Applications—Materials Testing for Toxicity, Efficacy, Disease Treatment, and Diagnosis in Humans (Clinical Trial Phase I, Phase II, Phase III, and Phase IV)

Sundus Iftikhar, Hina Ashraf, Muhammad Ali Faridi, Maria Khan, and Abdul Samad Khan

8.1 INTRODUCTION

Recently, biomedicine has been hugely interested in biomaterials because of the diversity they have to offer in applications. Biomaterials (natural or synthetic materials) are used to synthesize medical prostheses, devices, drug delivery systems, and implants (Aguilera-Márquez et al., 2022). When performing clinical trials for materials, a few considerations must be kept in mind: first, the device in which this material would be used; second, the objective and purpose of that device depending upon its location; and third, the regulatory body considerations (Hench, 1998). Biomaterials are also being increasingly studied for their ability to diagnose certain diseases (Huebsch & Mooney, 2009). Drug development is a tiresome and extensive process lasting for years. A drug undergoes different testing regimes before coming into the market. It is tested on humans after it has cleared laboratory testing. In order to utilize them to their maximum potential, researchers need to conduct rigorous clinical trials. This testing in humans is termed a clinical trial. Clinical trials are a trial or a study based on research carried out on human beings in order to reach a definite conclusion for health-related questions. It includes identifying, considering, and evaluating distinctive medical and dental devices or drugs and ultimately labeling them as non-toxic and effective products. Strict ethical and scientific protocols are followed for clinical trials (Abi Jaoude et al., 2021).

Clinical trials are the fundamental way of evaluating new interventions and provide reliable sources of evidence on the efficacy of interventions. They are a means of improving basic life quality with the help of monitoring and evaluation of new drugs, devices, or medical procedures. Any new device, drug, or medical tool must pass through all phases of clinical trials to be able to proceed from laboratory to marketplace (Clinical Trial Startup Material, 2020). Clinical trial studies are prospective and are formulated in such a way as to answer specific questions related to behavioral or biomedical intrusions and must stick to the codes of good clinical practice (GCP) (Rock et al., 2010).

The principles of GCP (Figure 8.1) were approved by the International Conference on Harmonization (ICH) steering committee in May 1996. It demonstrates a globally accepted standard of moral and scientific value for the conduct, scheme, reporting, and recording of clinical trials. Compliance with GCP is a declaration that participant security is safeguarded and clinical trial results are plausible (Lattermann et al., 2014). Clinical results obtained from different experiments are evaluated by researchers/clinicians to identify appropriate doses and efficiency of evolving, instead of; identify innovative preparations or tools; and govern the safety, efficacy, trustworthiness, and benefits of newly emerging medical gear. The test results are compared with their desired expectations, which leads to the development or redesigning of new preparations and medical devices, optimizing the risk/benefit ratios. The selection of participants or volunteers in each clinical research is based on a criterion that includes age, gender, and specific health-related issues, which govern their inclusion or exclusion in the study (Faris, 2013).

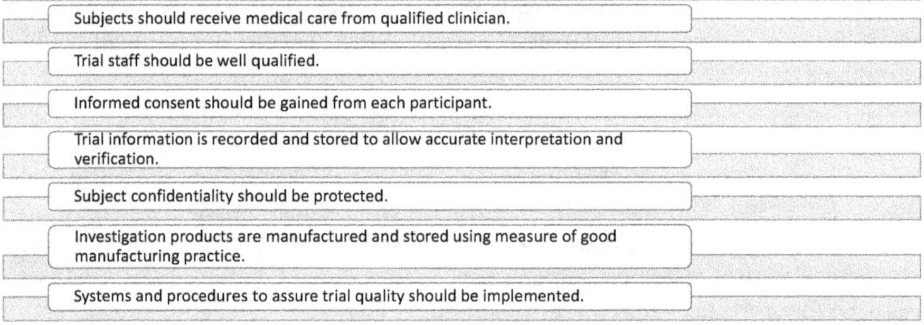

A trial should proceed only if the proposed benefits outlie the possible risks.

Rights, well-being, and safety of trial participants is of utmost interest.

Available clinical and non-clinical data should be adequate to support the trial.

Trials should be explained in clear, detailed, and scientifically sound protocol.

Clinical trial protocols should undergo local, independent, and ethical review.

Subjects should receive medical care from qualified clinician.

Trial staff should be well qualified.

Informed consent should be gained from each participant.

Trial information is recorded and stored to allow accurate interpretation and verification.

Subject confidentiality should be protected.

Investigation products are manufactured and stored using measure of good manufacturing practice.

Systems and procedures to assure trial quality should be implemented.

FIGURE 8.1 The principles of good clinical practice per the International Conference on Harmonization Committee.

## 8.2	PHASES OF CLINICAL TRIALS

No matter how promising the preclinical data seems, it still cannot confirm how a material or a drug would behave in the human body; that is, its toxicity and efficacy. Clinical trials are classified into different phases, marked as 0, 1, 2, 3, and 4, as shown in Figure 8.2. There is one prephase and four main phases. Phase 0 (1–20 people) is known as the prephase. Phases I, II, III, and IV are the main phases of clinical trials. Phases I (small group: 20–50 people) and II (medium group: over 100) are aimed at identifying the safety and effectiveness of a drug, respectively. These phases are performed on a small number of participants as compared to subsequent phases. After getting cleared from phases I and II, the drug proceeds to phase III (large group: 100–1,000 people) of the clinical trial (Nikkho et al., 2020). Rigorous four-phase clinical trials are required to satisfy legal and ethical considerations. The clinical trials are regulated according to the United States Public Health Service (USPHS) or Ryge criteria before they are allowed to enter commercial markets (Murray et al., 2007).

### 8.2.1	PHASE I

Generally, phase I trials are carried out to determine the maximum tolerated dose (MTD) that can be safely given to humans. This phase is crucial for the subsequent phases, as it identifies a safe starting point by determining the biomaterial's toxicity. This is why they are commonly referred to as "toxicity trials" (van Norman, 2021). However, the objectives of Phase I trials are expanding to include endpoints like molecular targeted effects, which is making the distinction between Phase I and II progressively obscure.

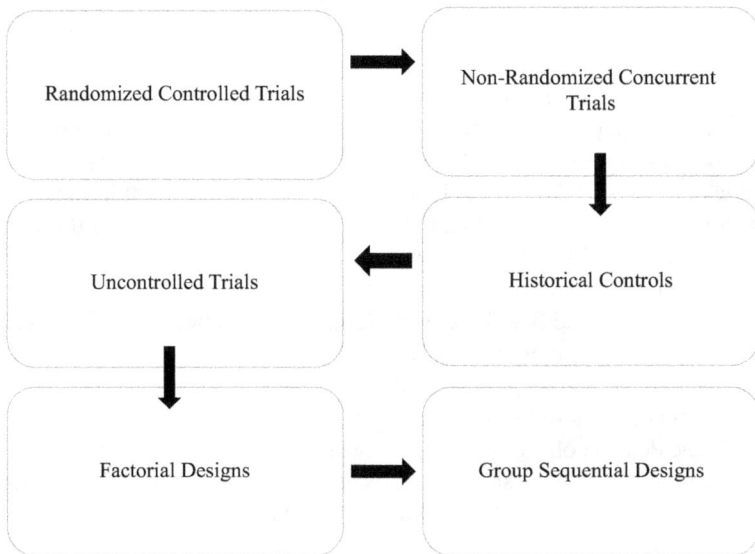

FIGURE 8.2	The preclinical and clinical trial phases.

Phase I trials are an essential part of any clinical trial because of the unpredictable nature of the newly synthesized material being introduced into the human body. Ideally, a meticulously designed Phase I trial should be able to determine the maximum tolerated dose accurately while at the same time attempting to keep the number of subjects to the minimum. It is important to keep the number of subjects as few as possible to reduce the number of participants being exposed to inefficient or overly toxic doses (Li & Bergan, 2020).

8.2.1.1 Types of Phase I Study Designs

The main purpose of the Phase I trial is to determine the safe dose of the drug or material by keeping the number of participants being exposed to the minimum. Therefore, most Phase I trials are based on dose-escalation designs where the major decision of the researcher lies in whether to escalate the dose rapidly or slowly. On the whole, Phase I designs are divided into rule-based or model-based designs.

8.2.1.1.1 Rule-Based Design

As the name suggests, this design is based on predefined rules. It relies on previously available data to use the doses based on actual observations rather than assuming the dose toxicity. It typically uses the 3 + 3 design or its variations (Siu et al., 2009).

8.2.1.1.2 3+3 Design and Modifications

The 3 + 3 design follows the protocol in which cohorts of three participants (patients) are used. For the first cohort, the researcher uses the starting dose that is observed to be safe based on preclinical or animal trials. The subsequent cohorts are treated with increasing dose levels that have been decided before starting the trial. The principle for increasing the dose is based on a modified Fibonacci sequence; this means that the dose increments become less as the dose increases. That is, the first dose is increased by 100%; the second is increased by 67%, then 50%, 40%, and so on and so forth (Rogatko et al., 2007). After beginning the trial, all three patients in the first cohort are carefully observed for adverse effects. If none of the three patients experience any toxicity, the dose is increased for the next cohort. If any one of the patients experiences toxicity, then the next cohort of three participants is treated with the same level of dose. The dose is increased or escalated until at least two patients in a cohort experience toxicity from the dose. The dose level just a little below this dose is then considered for the subsequent phases of clinical trials; that is, Phase II and onwards (Siu et al., 2009).

Alternatively, modified 3 + 3 study designs have also been used by researchers. A few of these modifications include 2 + 4, 3 + 3 + 3, and 3 + 1 + 1 (best of five). The 2 + 4 design includes two patients in the first cohort, and four patients are included in the next cohort if toxicity is observed in one of the two patients of the first cohort. In 3 + 3 + 3, the design cohort of three patients is used; however, a third cohort is also added if two patients in the first two cohorts experience toxicity. If three patients out of these nine experience toxicities at some level, the trial is terminated. In the best of five (3 + 1 + 1) design, stricter measures are employed, and one patient is added if toxicity is observed in the first cohort, and another patient is added if two patients have toxic symptoms among the first four being treated (Hansen et al., 2014).

8.2.1.1.3 Accelerated Titration Design

This design is a combination of the 3 + 3 and the model-based design. However, it is classified under the rule-based design because the doses are decided beforehand based on prespecified rules. The main reason for its existence is to reduce the number of patients who are being treated on sub-therapeutic levels and speed up Phase I of the trial. In this type of design, only one patient is included per dose level and intra-patient escalation of the dose is also allowed. It provides the patient with the possibility of being treated at a higher dose level, which could be more effective (Simon et al., 1997).

8.2.1.1.4 Pharmacologically Guided Dose Escalation

This is also a variation of the traditional 3 + 3 design but is used infrequently. It is largely based on the assumption that dose-limiting toxicities depend on plasma drug concentrations and that results obtained from animal studies can be generalized for humans as well. This study is carried out by using one patient whose pharmacokinetic data is taken in real time. The dose is increased at 100% until the prespecified plasma concentration is reached. If toxicity is observed, then the design is changed to the traditional 3 + 3 design (Siu et al., 2009).

Several other rule-based designs have been employed by researchers over time, like the isotonic regression model, biased coin design, and rolling six (Leung and Wang, 2002; Ivanova et al., 2003).

8.2.1.1.5 Model-Based Designs

These methods utilize statistical models, implemented through software, to determine a dose level that predicts the probability of dose-limiting toxicity by using patient data. The data is used to plot a graph. This whole process is carried out using the Bayesian model. The continual reassessment method was the first method based on the Bayesian model that was accepted for the running phase clinical trial.

The initial dose is based on the preclinical data by predicting the maximum tolerated dose (MTD). All the patients are treated at this predicted MTD. Unlike rule-based designs where only prespecified dose levels are used, model-based designs allow the researchers to skip a dose or determine new dose levels during the based trial run. It results in a fewer number of patients being exposed to the drug at sub-therapeutic levels. It also makes use of all the data acquired from all the patients. Despite visible advantages, model-based designs are seldom preferred. The major reason is the logistics required to carry out statistical analysis for every patient in each cohort. In addition, some clinical researchers are apprehensive because Phase I trials are the first time humans are being exposed to a new material or drug; consequently, the uncertainty is high. The significant amount of data required for model-based designs can only be acquired after the trial starts, which makes it risky (Love et al., 2017). Therefore, the researchers usually side with rule-based designs over model-based designs despite the latter being less time-consuming. One of the reasons for not selecting the model-based design could be the lack of statistical expertise of the researchers (van Brummelen et al., 2016).

8.2.1.2 Selection of Humans for Clinical Trials

The main and single most grave adverse effect of novel materials or drugs being investigated at the Phase I stage is death. Other adverse effects include certain conditions or disabilities that may be irreversible. Therefore, the question arises, how do we select humans for testing the material in the Phase I clinical trial? Phase I oncology treatments are usually offered to patients with progressive or last-stage malignancies as the last resort.

For drugs or materials not involving oncological treatment, healthy individuals have also been accrued as participants. Recruitment of healthy individuals raises ethical concerns, but a systematic review of 475 studies revealed that severe harms to the participants were rare (Johnson et al., 2016).

Phase I trials usually have a broad eligibility criterion so that the patients can be recruited for the trial in a short period. This reduces the cost of the study and also makes it easier to generalize the findings (Malik & Lu, 2019). Historically, the therapeutic intent of Phase I trials has been questioned for ethical reasons, as patients enroll with positive expectations to receive clinical benefits. Currently, Phase I trials have been seen to identify specific target populations with therapeutic intent. However, this needs further investigation because the researchers have conflicting opinions on whether Phase I trials should be expanded beyond the toxicity trial (Ivy et al., 2010).

8.2.2 PHASE II

8.2.2.1 Selection of Humans for Clinical Trials

Phase I ensures that before enrolling any human subjects in this phase of the study, it is essential to have preclinical data that is acceptable to be used in humans for the first time. Affirmative results from the first phase allow the researchers to move ahead with Phase II trials that are conducted to determine the preliminary efficacy and toxicity of the intervention limited to a smaller sample size. The dose that has been categorized as the maximum tolerated dose (MTD) in the Phase I trial is then used to investigate the efficacy and toxicity of the drug in Phase II. This in turn will decide whether the material tested should move on to the confirmatory Phase III trial on a larger scale. The key aspects identified in the Phase II trial are as follows:

- Therapeutic considerations (e.g., toxicity)
- Aim of the trial (treatment selection)
- Outcome of interest
- Features of study design

The previously mentioned reasons, along with other things like the availability and usefulness of previous data and other practical considerations, form the basis for discontinuing the trial at Phase II or proceeding toward Phase III (Torres-Saavedra & Winter, 2022).

Since the results are obtained from Phase II studies, it is essential to have strict inclusion and exclusion criteria for Phase II studies. The strict criteria ensure that there are minimum chances of getting a false positive or false negative result. Generally, Phase II studies involve 100–300 participants and can continue for up to two to three years (Blass, 2015).

8.2.2.2   Types of Phase II Study Designs

The endpoint of a clinical trial is explained as quantifiable data that can be used to evaluate the probable effects of the intervention being studied. It bridges the gap between what the theory states about the intervention and how it responds to human subjects. Therefore, it largely depends on the patient-reported outcomes and quality of life. The primary endpoints of Phase II and phase III trials are similar except for one notable difference: Phase II endpoints can be assessed in a shorter period (Gottlieb et al., 2015). Phase II studies are designed keeping in mind the expected endpoints.

8.2.2.2.1   Single-Arm

One-stage single-arm: Human subjects are selected as the ones having the disease for which the intervention is being done. The subjects are exposed to the intervention, and the endpoint is only assessed at the end of the trial. However, in such designs, it is necessary that a smaller sample size is considered so that the minimum number of patients are exposed to ineffective or toxic interventions (Torres-Saavedra & Winter, 2022). This type of study usually has a short-term endpoint because it ensures minimum selection bias (patients showing promising results are more favorably chosen for further trials) (Rubinstein et al., 2014).

Two-stage single-arm: This type of design is used in multi-institutional studies. The main objective of the design is to recruit a minimum number of participants in the first stage. Usually, fewer than 30 participants are recruited in the first stage, and the intervention is carried out. An analysis of the outcome is determined at the end of this stage, known as the interim analysis. The analysis of the outcome determines whether the intervention is ineffective and should be discontinued or has acceptable efficacy to continue. In the latter scenario, additional patients are enrolled, and a second stage is initiated (Simon, 1989).

8.2.2.2.2   Non-Comparative Randomized Trials (NCRTs)

In recent times, newer agents and drugs are being introduced rapidly, so the interest in randomized trials is growing at the same rate. There are times when no historical data is present or the new material has never been used before. At other times, recruiting patients is an arduous task due to the complexity or rarity of the condition. Randomized trials usually require at least four times the number of patients required by single-arm studies. In order to deal with these situations while maintaining some degree of randomization, researchers have attempted to modify randomized trials according to their needs. One such modification gave rise to non-comparative randomized trials (NCRTs). In this study design, the participants are randomized into two experimental groups. Each group acts as a one-stage single-arm study. At the end of the intervention, the endpoint of both groups is analyzed to decide which group shows better results or the highest observed response rate. The group depicting better results is then carried forward to the next step—Phase III (Rubinstein et al., 2014). It provides convenience to the researcher in deciding the treatment/dose regimen without prior data; however, it shares the same shortcomings of single-arm studies, as both the groups cannot be compared statistically (Torres-Saavedra & Winter, 2022).

8.2.2.2.3 Comparative Randomized Trials

Randomized trials have been considered the gold standard in clinical research studies. In Phase II studies, it is particularly employed to compare existing data or treatment protocol with the new regimen or intervention. A small randomized trial conducted at the Phase II level to vaguely compare intervention with the existing standard therapies is called the randomized Phase II screening trial. Although the results are inconclusive statistically, owing to a smaller sample size, it gives an idea of whether to discontinue or move on to the next phase. Evidently, this type of study involves two groups randomized into interventional and control groups (Torres-Saavedra & Winter, 2022).

As attractive as it may seem on the surface, the use of randomized control trials has been argued by clinical researchers. The researchers who deem it unnecessary at the Phase II stage claim that at this stage, it is harder to convince the patients to enroll in a study in which they will be randomly assigned to groups. This claim was supported by a result of a study that indicated that 27% of Phase II randomized trials failed due to major problems. The small scale of the Phase II trial is not adequate to give definite results about prognosis or treatment, and the results obtained might not coincide with the literature (Gan et al., 2010). Hence, there is always a risk of researchers interpreting the data incorrectly, as if it were obtained from a Phase III trial (Grayling et al., 2019). The cost and complexity of a randomized control trial are also high, with opponents arguing the futility of this type of trial at Phase II. However, the proponents of RCT Phase II trials are of the opinion that RCTs are absolutely necessary for improving the efficiency of Phase II trials, as a successful Phase II trial would be reliable to predict success in a Phase III trial (Mandrekar & Sargeant, 2009). Researchers have voiced their opinions vehemently in favor of any one type of study design in Phase II trials. Single-arm studies use data from historical controls; that is, data present already in literature, assuming that the controls would act in a similar way in the new study as well. This reduces the number of participants needed for the study for conditions that have been well-established through decades of research. However, this may not stand true for all interventions because comparing with historical controls may give unreliable results. The treatment protocols, facilities, and standards of care are rapidly improving; therefore, these variables cannot be accounted for in historical controls, resulting in an inaccurate comparison in single-arm studies. Single-arm studies are not considered the first choice when determining the closest accuracy of dose efficacy and dose toxicity (Ratain & Sargent, 2008). Hence, the selection of study design in Phase II largely depends on the discretion and intellectual judgment of the researcher. The selection is made by weighing the pros and cons of the study designs against each other, keeping in mind the expected endpoint of the trial (Figure 8.4).

8.2.2.3 Materials Testing for Toxicity in Phase II

"Toxicity" is defined as the extent to which a substance can be harmful to humans or animals (Longo et al., 2011). Clinical testing for toxicity is carried out to investigate the hemostatic imbalances in human organisms by monitoring the biochemical balance and metabolism (Madorran et al., 2020). Researchers face a big challenge when classifying material safety and toxicity because the protocol has to be meticulous. Researchers gather the data (toxicity, safety, physical, and chemical properties of the material) and submit an Investigational New Drug (IND) application to FDA for approval. The human trial cannot begin until approval is gained from FDA (Bobo et al., 2016).

Generally, Phase I and II recruit healthy participants for trials. However, in cases when the drug has known toxicity, healthy participants are not recruited; for example, while testing a new antiviral drug for HIV patients, only HIV-positive participants are recruited (Chan-Tack et al., 2008). In cases where the efficacy and toxicity of a drug are not known, Phase I and Phase II trials are often merged into one in order to reduce the number of participants being exposed to the potential side effects (Blass, 2015). It has been noted that this component of the Phase II trial is usually not well-reported in the literature. The issues noted with toxicity studies are as follows:

- There is a lack of uniformity among different protocols to investigate toxicity.
- Toxicity studies, in the case of therapeutic applications, need long-term study, whereby a long phase II trial can exhaust the funding.

8.2.2.4 Data Collection

The trials designed at the Phase II stage are intended to provide initial efficacy data to determine whether the intervening compound is safe and has the potential to improve the lives of humans. A study conducted in 2014 revealed that from 5,800 studies conducted by different institutes, only 60% of the studies that had positive results in Phase II also had positive results in Phase III trials (Hay et al., 2014). Since the data obtained in this phase of the trial determines future studies, it is important to analyze and scrutinize the data strictly within the given time. It should be strong enough to form the basis of the next phase. Failure to provide reliable data within the limited time available would affect the trial adversely. Since Phase II clinical trials depend largely on accruing patients in a timely manner, it faces numerous challenges owing to the slow accrual. The reasons identified for slow accrual are as follows (Massett et al., 2016):

- Safety and toxicity issues of the material that halts accrual
- Study design or protocol takes longer than expected; for example, the requirements and complexity of the trial and procedures involved in the treatment burden a lot of patients
- The strict eligibility criteria or involvement of a rare condition/disease
- Extended delays due to administrative reasons; for example, delayed IRB (institutional review board) approvals
- Lack of funding

Another challenge that researchers face during data collection is known as the excessive collection of adverse effects. It was reported that 50% of the adverse effects on the placebo arm of the clinical trial could be attributed to the treatment being tested. This makes adverse effect reporting unreliable. Therefore, to reduce the burden on the clinical trials, the researchers advise against the collection of low-grade adverse effects because, ultimately, the clinical trial needs to be fast, reliable, and cost-effective (Sargent & Oncol, 2010).

8.2.2.5   Data Storage and Presentation

Reporting and presenting the results of RCT are essential parts of the research because to understand randomized control trials, the reader must be fully aware of the study design, intervention, analysis, and interpretation of results. This requires the researchers to report their studies transparently and in-depth. The readers have the right to know why that particular study design was chosen, what the steps involved in the study are, and how the results were interpreted because the strengths and limitations of a study depend on these constructs. Inadequate reporting of RCT has been associated with bias in interpreting the results of the study (Moher et al., 1998). Unfortunately, nearly 50% of RCTs cannot be used due to inadequate reporting. To achieve maximum transparency in the process of reporting, a group of clinical scientists, statisticians, biomedical editors, and epidemiologists designed a protocol (Moher et al., 2001). It was first published as the Consolidated Standards of Reporting Trials (CONSORT) statement in 1996, and the latest revision was presented in 2010. The main objective of the CONSORT statement is to provide the researchers with a checklist in order to ensure clear, transparent, and concise reporting of the clinical trials (Moher et al., 2010).

Since the publication of the CONSORT statement, several recommendations have come forward from various researchers regarding the aspects that were missing from the initial statement. It was noted that although the CONSORT statement provides a detailed account of an RCT, it does not account for patient-reported outcomes (PRO). Patient-reported outcomes, in contrast with observer-reported outcomes, give a better idea about the health-related quality of life and satisfaction of the participants. Consequently, in 2013, the PRO extension was added to the CONSORT statement in the hopes of improving patient care (Calvert et al., 2013). Similarly, 2018 witnessed a CONSORT-SPI extension to cater to the social and psychological interventions in RCT (Montgomery et al., 2018). The reporting of RCT is a dynamic process that keeps witnessing new recommendations with ongoing changes in the world. In recent times, the CONSORT statement has been extended, with guidelines to analyze trials with interventions related to artificial intelligence, while some modifications were introduced to allow for rapid changes in trials during the COVID-19 pandemic (Liu et al., 2020; Orkin et al., 2021).

In recent years, registries have gained immense importance, as they have become the basis for improving the quality of subsequent research (Prang et al., 2022). Clinical trials are long-term; hence, financially exhaustive as well. In order to reduce the budget by maintaining the quality of the trial, registry-based randomized control trials (RRCT) are becoming increasingly popular. These are the trials that gain access to the patient's health information present in registries. It helps the researchers to enroll the patients for the study in comparatively lesser time, reducing the financial burden on the study and having a low cost with high generalizability of findings (G. Li et al., 2016). Some researchers advocate moving on to Phase III directly from the Phase I trial if the data supports adequate efficacy and safety, and if the resources are unlimited. Skipping Phase II trial should be based on a robust evaluation of all the aspects of the study. Some researchers also advocate combining Phase II and Phase III trials. This will allow Phase II data to be transferred to Phase III trials and reduce patient accrual in subsequent stages (Korn et al., 2012).

8.2.3   PHASE III

In Phase III clinical trial, the drug, treatment, or material is administered to a large group of participants to confirm its safety and effectiveness and to compare it to conventional materials/drugs available for the targeted treatment. A large group of volunteers are involved in Phase III clinical trials. The focus of this phase trial is to govern whether the intervention would be effective and safe for a diverse group of individuals (Bobo et al., 2016).

The regime aims at allotting contributors to treatment or control groups. If the intervention involves a combination of treatment plans, drugs, or components, there can be more than one study group. One group is provided with either the current standard of treatment or a placebo treatment. The inclusion of each volunteer into any of the two groups is purely by chance. The two groups are under the following:

- Control group—the group that gets the regular standard intervention
- Study group—the group that gets the innovative intervention being tested

Phase III of the clinical trial normally involves about 3,000 participants, on which the new material is to be tested. These trials can last up to several years. The objective of this experimental trial is to determine the effectiveness of new material and the way it performs its desired function in comparison to the already existing materials for the same purpose. The investigators need to demonstrate that the new material, at least, is as safe and effective as the existing materials (Costa, 2020). These trials compare conventional intervention with a completely new intervention or different dosages and frequency of the same intervention in order to assess the effectiveness of that treatment.

8.2.3.1   Clinical Trial Designs

Phase III trials are difficult to design and conduct. There are different trial designs for Phase III, as presented in Figure 8.3. Phase III trials are divided into phases IIIA and IIIB. Phase IIIA trials are performed after the drug or material has been determined as effective but prior to the submission for a New Drug Application (NDA), whereas phase IIIB trials are carried out after submission for an NDA but prior to their launch in the market (Mahan, 2014).

8.2.3.1.1   Randomization

Mostly, Phase III trials are randomized. Randomization is a process in which participants are assigned to one of two groups (i.e., control group and study group) randomly. The group that receives a standard treatment is called the control group. Participants in the other group receive a new treatment or a device that is to be tested. This is called the study group (Reardon et al., 2020).

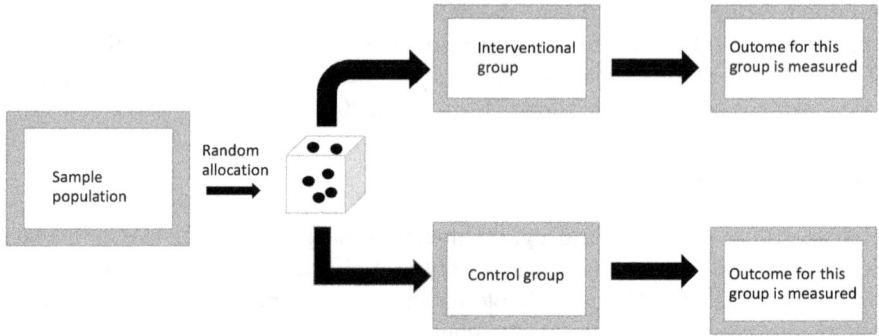

FIGURE 8.3   Designs for Phase III clinical trials.

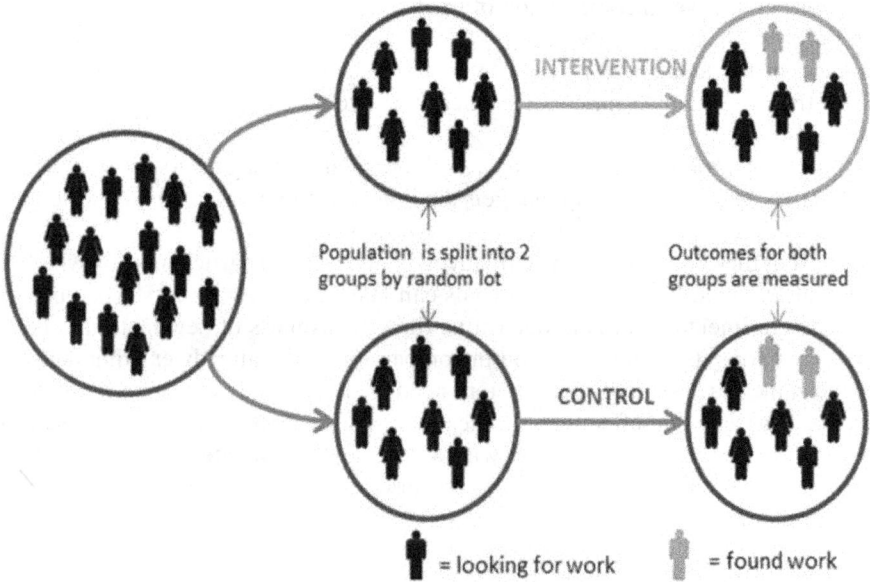

FIGURE 8.4   Design of a randomized controlled trial.

Randomized trials (Figure 8.4) are conducted to ensure the accuracy of tests and results. It is the most meticulous and vigorous method of associating the cause-effect relationship between intervention and outcome. The main advantage of randomized controlled trials is the elimination of bias. Bias is described as the propensity of any element within the study or intervention to deviate the outcome from its factual value. Random allocation of participants/individuals is the only way to eliminate bias. In RCTs, any participant receiving one intervention or the other is decided purely by chance (Wang et al., 2021).

Benefits of randomized controlled trial design: The main advantage of randomized controlled trials is the process of randomization. Many confounding factors are involved in every study design, but randomization limits the interference of known and unknown confounding variables. These variables are impossible to be controlled in non-randomized studies. With randomization, definitive conclusions with respect to treatment or intervention can be made. Randomization can be double-blind or single-blind (Gui et al., 2018).

Bias: Bias is defined as any statistical or operational modifications in the trial. The sources of bias can be categorized into four types:

i. Expected and controllable, changes in laboratory/diagnostic procedures
ii. Expected but not controllable, changes in dose or duration of study
iii. Unexpected but controllable, uncooperative patient/non-compliant patient
iv. Unexpected and uncontrollable, any random error in responses or outcomes

A perfect clinical trial aims at eliminating as many sources of bias as possible (Mylona et al., 2020).

Blinding: Blinding is a procedure done in randomized controlled trials to minimize detection and performance bias. Normally, a practitioner or a researcher may unconsciously favor the treatment/intervention of his choice and confidence and, consequently, will perceive an enhanced effect of the respective treatment. To reduce this type of bias, blinding is conducted in clinical trials. Blinding may be complete or partial, or only apply to the assessment of outcomes (Bodner & Kaul, 2021). Blinding can be of two types; single-blind or double-blind. In a single-blind study, the participants are unaware of the treatment or intervention being given to them. In double-blinding, both the participants and the provider are unaware of the treatment being assigned. The assignment is purely by chance. Double-blinding is the highest means of eliminating all bias from the study. It refers to the complete avoidance of performance bias by blinding both the participants and providers. It prevents outcomes to be influenced by the assignment of treatment. Blinding is not possible in other study designs, and this is the reason randomized controlled trials are considered the gold standard of all clinical trials (Kudrow et al., 2020).

Limitations of randomized controlled trial design: Although these trials are considered the gold standard verification for the endorsement of innovative drugs, a few problems have still been encountered in their use. There is a partial clinical advantage in large RCTs, an estimate of a fruitful phase trial from phase data is not possible, toxicity testing is not possible, studies including a combination of drugs cannot be conducted easily, and the cost of RCTs does not make it user-friendly (Vanneste et al., 2021).

8.2.3.1.2 Non-Randomized Concurrent Trial

This is a clinical trial in which the contestants are assigned haphazardly that is not by chance to different groups of treatment. Contributors themselves may opt for which group they want to be in, or they are allotted by the researchers. The methods used in this trial are not random, and the possibility of bias is always increased.

8.2.3.1.2.1 Uncontrolled Trials
Uncontrolled clinical trials are defined as trials with no control and all the patients are receiving the same intervention. These trials are

followed up for a certain period. Conducting uncontrolled clinical trials is thought to be more convenient, less expensive, and faster than that of randomized control trials (RCT). However, they are less reliable and biased as compared to randomized controlled trials (Mickenautsch & Yengopal, 2017).

8.2.3.2 Historical Control

A clinical trial intended to support a comparative conclusion regarding the treatment is known as a historical control trial. The comparator to the treated group is not a concurrent separate group of patients. The comparison is between two different times (Han, 2021).

8.2.3.3 Factorial Design

Factorial designs in clinical trials are the ones that allow the study of several interventions simultaneously. Factorial clinical trials are the ones that test the efficacy of two or more interventions at the same time. They are designed in such a way as to conduct the comparison of different interventions simultaneously using various combinations of interventions. This design allows the investigators to compare the investigational interventions with the control group, compare the investigational interventions with one other, and explore likely connections between them (Brittain & Wittes, 1989). Factorial designs may be used when the factors are regarded as being independent or the factors are thought to be complementary, and the specific aim is to investigate these interactions (Pandis et al., 2014).

8.2.3.4 Group Sequential Design

This is a type of clinical trial in which sample size is not predetermined; data is sequentially evaluated as collected. This trial can be terminated when desired effects are not achieved; otherwise, more participants are recruited during the trial. Group sequential investigation can reach a definitive inference much ahead of the one that would be probable with a traditional scheme. Therefore, this type of treatment design can reduce the exposure of participants to low-quality interventions and save resources and time for the patients (van Eijk et al., 2018).

8.2.3.5 Adaptive Clinical Trials

The adaptations made to statistical analysis or the main trial for the purpose of improvement of basic study design without negatively influencing the quality and validity of the trial is known as an adaptive clinical trial. These adaptations are denoted as alterations or amendments in order to improve the efficacy and safety of clinical trials.

In contrast, according to the FDA (Food and Drug Administration), adaptive design is a study that incorporates a prospectively planned opportunity for amendment of one or more definite features of the study design and assumptions based on investigation of (usually interim) data from participants in the study (Day, 2020). An adaptive design is also known as a flexible design by the European Medicines Agency (EMA) (Laage et al., 2017). Commonly used adaptive clinical designs are shown in Figure 8.5 (Day, 2020).

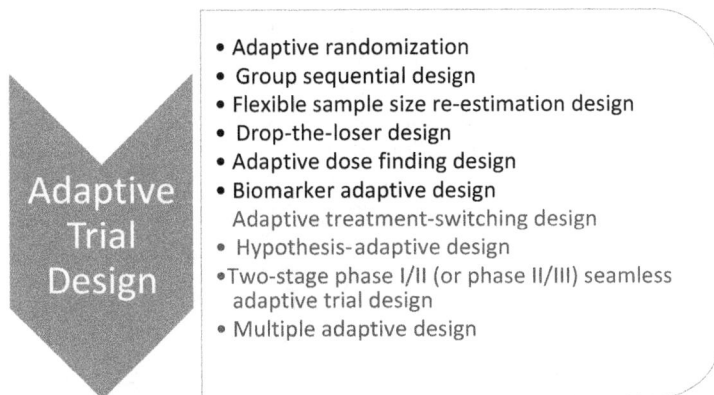

The figure shows a downward-pointing chevron labeled "Adaptive Trial Design" with a list of commonly used adaptive clinical trial designs:

- Adaptive randomization
- Group sequential design
- Flexible sample size re-estimation design
- Drop-the-loser design
- Adaptive dose finding design
- Biomarker adaptive design
  Adaptive treatment-switching design
- Hypothesis-adaptive design
- Two-stage phase I/II (or phase II/III) seamless adaptive trial design
- Multiple adaptive design

FIGURE 8.5 Commonly used adaptive clinical trial designs.

8.2.3.5.1 How Is a Randomized Clinical Trial Adaptive?

Significant study design constituents can be adapted during the trial, whereby the trial planning involves numerous sequences of replications. Before the commencement of this study design, the consequences and benefits of possible trial adaptations should be clear and well-understood. The statistical analysis plans are needed for both interim and final analyses. The research question may vary along with adaptations (for example, narrowing the population); however, multiple trials (such as phases II and III) can effortlessly be merged into one adaptive trial. Novel investigational management can be supplemented rather than commencing a new, separate trial.

The adaptive clinical trial design is beneficial because it aids in choosing the most reliable preference early, and it grants the researcher the ability to correct inappropriate declarations made at the commencement of the trial. It also provides the investigator the chance to react timely to any positive or negative thing. These designs allow continuous learning throughout the process. Adaptive designs can be finished earlier than trials with non-adaptive or conventional strategies. This design can make the development time shorter and, consequently, enhance the process. In short, this design allows the researcher to amend or modify the trial according to his needs. This trial is an innovative method that aims to decrease the number of resources used and completion time. A smaller number of patients are exposed to new interventions, and the possibility of analyzing treatment effects is greatly increased (Chow & Corey, 2011).

After the completion of Phase III clinical trials, patients getting diverse types of interventions are compared to the control group and evaluated for any improvement in their health conditions. If the results depict a deterioration in the patient's general health or any other adverse side effects encountered, the FDA will not give authorization for a request for a New Drug Application (NDA). In the other scenario, if there is a marked increase in the health of patients receiving trial treatment, FDA will approve the drug and give a hand up when applying for NDA (Faris, 2013).

Phase III trials are the complete assessment of any intervention designed in such a way that they compare the effectiveness of the experimental treatment with the standard treatment. Phase III trials are the most meticulous and broad investigation of a new material or device. They are intended to be precise and accurate in their outcomes. At the same time, these are the most time-consuming, painstaking, and expensive of all the phases of clinical trials. Phase III trials are also known as the premarketing phase of clinical trials (Marc, 2018). The outcome of Phase III trials should be improved clinical medicine, along with patient safety and secure data storage. A well-developed and well-conducted phase III trial leads to a successful next phase trial (Briggs & Ramer, 2017).

8.2.4 PHASE IV

A form of scientific experiment that "studies the side effects caused over time by a new treatment after it has been approved and is on the market" (NCI Dictionary of Cancer Terms, 2022). The purpose of this experiment is to observe undesirable outcomes caused by a particular drug that were not observed in the previous trials; this type of experiment is also used to study the success of a new drug over a specific time interval (NCI Dictionary of Cancer Terms, 2022). Phase IV trials are also used to assess the time frame for which the drug will remain active when it is being used by a large section of the population.

The various phases of drug testing are an essential part of drug development. For some drugs, Phase IV trials begin as soon as the first three phases have been completed, while for others, the process begins after the marketing campaign begins and continues till the end of the commercial life of the drug (Bourin, 2016). Phase IV trials are basically designed and conducted to provide more information and better insight in terms of the advantages of the drug as well as give more epidemiological data (Bourin, 2016).

8.2.4.1 Need for Phase IV Trials

8.2.4.1.1 Improving Scientific Data

Phase III trials are generally performed on a very meticulously picked cohort of the populace following strict inclusion and exclusion criteria. These will exclude patients that might become recipients of the drug when it is introduced to the general population. These may include children, teenagers, pregnant women, and other groups not included in the Phase III trials (Black, 2017). The scientific data regarding any new drug is not complete in most cases due to the small sample size for the trial, which has been mentioned already. While in Phase IV trials, the drug and its recommended dosage are administered to all patients without any consideration for any criteria (Bourin, 2016).

In real-world scenarios, the occurrence of the disease is not confined to specific criteria; therefore, the dosage and indications are modified per the situation. This may lead to different responses by the patient based on the different subcategories, which can be found in the general population based on age, sex, race, and ethnic origin (Buyse, 1995). All these have different effects on the thermodynamics and thermokinetics of the drug and can lead to a better understanding of the efficacy and adverse effects (Bourin, 2016). In order to get this data trials with a group consisting of a large section of the population, it is used with minimal to no interventions

(Kolitsopoulos et al., 2022). As drugs in general practice are usually prescribed in combination with other drugs, the combinations are infinite, which cannot be covered in a controlled trial, making it necessary to conduct Phase IV trials (Kolitsopoulos et al., 2022). Another important thing that needs to be assessed is the effect of various pathologies or system conditions on the drug, which could lead to possible side effects (Clayton et al., 2011).

8.2.4.1.2   Stakeholders/Economic Purposes

The main beneficiaries of Phase IV trials are health strategy designers in government and may also include supervisory bodies, medical physicians, patients, public society groups, and distributors of medicines. The authorities are continuously looking at the performance and adverse effects of any new drug in the market to assess its long-term safety (Black, 2017). Government bodies need high-quality Phase IV trial data to determine the long-term efficacy and cost-effectiveness of any particular drug. This data also provides health professionals with key information regarding any new drug when they are advising their patients (Black, 2017).

Another important stakeholder is the pharmaceutical company itself, which starts the marketing campaign for any new drug as they start to familiarize the maximum number of health practitioners with the new drug (Bourin, 2016; Rauf et al., 2022). The main goal of the pharmaceutical company is to obtain quantitative and qualitative data with regard to the therapeutic effects of the drug, which will in turn determine the true medicinal value of the drug. The main outcome required from Phase IV experiments is to launch a new treatment into mainstream medical use.

8.2.4.2   Types of Phase IV Trials

Phase IV clinical experiments are classified into the following types:

- Clinical research
- Seeding trials
- Pharmacovigilance
- Intervention effectiveness

8.2.4.2.1   Clinical Research

Clinical research studies can be initiated by pharmaceutical companies based on a line of inquiry to get the required data regarding the effectiveness and adverse effects of a new drug. The data collected can lead to further improvements in future versions of the drug. This data will also benefit public authorities, health insurance companies, and medical associations.

8.2.4.2.2   Seeding Trials

Seeding trials are used as a method of not only collecting data regarding a new drug but also promoting and acquainting physicians with a new product. These trials provide physicians with incentives on prescribing a specific drug, which is a gray area ethically. However, these trials are justifiable in cases where they are strictly monitored and scientifically significant (Bourin, 2016). As previously mentioned, pharmaceutical companies may incentivize physicians to prescribe a new drug to collect data from a large cross-section of the population. These incentives can include fees or other benefits and utilize promotional events and the use of medical representatives to push the new drug to physicians. Although this method is on the decline, it is still used as a viable option for the commercial development of a product and mass data collection.

8.2.4.2.3 Pharmacovigilance

"Pharmacovigilance" is defined as "the science and activities relating to the detection, assessment, understanding, and prevention of adverse effects or any other possible drug-related problems" (World Health Organization, 2006). These investigations are created to assess long- and short-term harmful reactions to any drug. Health authorities sometimes monitor specific drugs to identify the incidence of unusual or significant harmful reactions. Pharmacovigilance may involve observational or interventional studies, such as case-control studies, cohort studies, and passive reporting schemes. Mostly harmful effects of medicines are submitted by medical practitioners, which are collected by federal pharmacovigilance centers.

8.2.4.2.4 Intervention Effectiveness

Phase IV experiments can be used for intrusions that are comparatively well-recognized in the community health system. This may include medicines that are already being actively prescribed by health practitioners to patients; this data can be correlated with previous clinical effectiveness experiments, whether that data was extracted from controlled experiments. These experiments are planned to assess the decline of the effectiveness of any medicine or treatment from the perspective of the health structure mechanism. These may result from behavior related to specific patients or due to the general behavior of the population. This may also include access to the treatment, correct diagnostics and prescription of treatment, and cooperation by the patient.

8.2.4.3 Study Design

One of the primary goals of these experiments is to observe the effectiveness of a treatment in an objective environment. This means that the sample size of patients that are enrolled in such study designs should be calculated to be able to satisfy all the queries raised with a certain amount of confidence. Inclusion criteria for these trials are not as strict as phase III trials, and the subjects omitted from studies for various reasons can now be included. However, some criteria should be followed to create an optimal design (Buyse, 1995). Many new drugs must be evaluated against the placebo to be granted marketing authorization even though an effective therapy is already available. Yet the pertinent medical problem is not to demonstrate that the drug is biologically active in comparison to the placebo but rather to demonstrate that the treatment is better than what is being used currently by medical practitioners. The results of these clinical studies are not required for approval of the new treatment or drug but rather to assess and improve the effectiveness of the treatment or drug. Commonly conducted studies include additional drug-drug interaction, dose-response or safety studies, and studies designed to support use under the approved indication (e.g., mortality/morbidity studies and epidemiological studies).

The goal of these clinical experiments is to assess the side effects in a larger patient pool sample over an extended period, which was not assessed in the clinical trials conducted in Phase I–III (Phases of clinical trials I Cancer Research UK, 2014). In terms of study designs, pharmacovigilance studies, such as observational or interventional studies, are mostly used. These may include case-control studies, cohort studies, and passive monitoring schemes.

8.2.4.4 Ethical Considerations

Designers of Phase IV experiments also supervise the adequate delivery of the new treatment or drug regime so that the new process works correctly while also allowing for flexibility in the new regime, as advised by other stakeholders. Oversights of these trials require a balance between the requirements of the medical system already in place and the standards set by international scientific bodies. It is pertinent to establish a team that includes all the stakeholders to discuss, advise, and analyze the results as well as how to best use them in any given scenario (Black, 2017).

8.2.4.5 Data Collection and Analysis

Phase IV efficacy experiments can effectively use the medical service audience as well as the accumulated data by these systems and various other sources. Aspects of connecting large sample patient data to medical institutions' data should be explored; however, these are not integrated easily in most instances. Prospective studies provide greater chances than retrospective studies to gather essential additional data. One major issue in data collection is answering specific questions related to the effectiveness of the drug and its harmful reactions, which may need more diverse methods of data collection. This may be collected via household and hospital surveys, whereas longitudinal health studies and qualitative research can also prove beneficial in collecting data (Black, 2017).

8.2.4.6 Distribution of the Data

Although data reporting for Phase I to Phase III trials are widely accepted and practiced, the guidelines used for studies involved in Phase IV trials are more recent and follow the STROBE statement (Strengthening the Reporting of Observational Studies in Epidemiology) (Elm et al., 2008). The STROBE statement is a worksheet of items that should be identified and addressed in research papers, which discuss the major types of experimental designs related to analytical epidemiology: cohort, case-control, and cross-sectional studies. The purpose is to provide guidance on the results of these studies, which should be disseminated effectively: the suggestions are not stringent rules for planning or performing (Elm et al., 2008). The checklist is made up of 22 items that are essential for reporting observational studies used in Phase IV trials.

Phase IV trials, as discussed, are a very important tool in acquiring vital clinical data regarding newly released drugs and their effect on the general population, as well as in documenting adverse effects that may not have been observed during the previous phases of drug trials. Although randomized trials are still considered ideal for obtaining scientifically relevant data for new drugs, real-world trials with proper study designs and implantation can greatly improve the value of the data collected and benefit the general population and physicians (Freemantle & Strack, 2009).

REFERENCES

Abi Jaoude, J., Kouzy, R., Ghabach, M., Patel, R., Pasalic, D., Ghossain, E., Miller, A. B., Lin, T. A., Verma, V., Fuller, C. D., Subbiah, V., Minsky, B. D., Ludmir, E. B., & Taniguchi, C. M. (2021). Food and drug administration approvals in phase 3 cancer clinical trials. *BMC Cancer*, 21(1), 695. https://doi.org/10.1186/s12885-021-08457-5.

Aguilera-Márquez, J. D. R., de Dios-Figueroa, G. T., Reza-Saldivar, E. E., Camacho-Villegas, T. A., Canales-Aguirre, A. A., & Lugo-Fabres, P. H. (2022). Biomaterials: Emerging systems for study and treatment of glioblastoma. *Neurology Perspectives*, 2, S31–S42. https://doi.org/10.1016/J.NEUROP.2021.12.001.

Black, J. (2017). Field trials of health interventions: A toolbox. *Australian and New Zealand Journal of Public Health*, 41(4), 452–452. https://doi.org/10.1111/1753-6405.12577.

Blass, B. E. (2015). Basics of clinical trials. In: *Basic Principles of Drug Discovery and Development*. Elsevier, pp. 383–314. https://doi.org/10.1016/B978-0-12-411508-8.00009-8.

Bobo, D., Robinson, K. J., Islam, J., Thurecht, K. J., & Corrie, S. R. (2016). Nanoparticle-based medicines: A review of FDA-approved materials and clinical trials to date. *Pharmaceutical Research*, 33(10), 2373–2387. https://doi.org/10.1007/s11095-016-1958-5.

Bodner, J., & Kaul, V. (2021). A framework for in silico clinical trials for medical devices using concepts from model verification, validation, and uncertainty quantification (VVUQ). Proceedings of the 2021 ASME Verification and Validation Symposium, VVS 2021. https://doi.org/10.1115/VVS2021-65094.

Bourin, M. (2016). What value for the phase IV clinical trials? *SOJ Pharmacy & Pharmaceutical Sciences*, 3(2), 01–03. https://doi.org/10.15226/2374-6866/3/2/00138.

Briggs, R. P., & Ramer, L. (2017). Elements of a clinical trial protocol for medical devices. *Journal of Nursing Education and Practice*, 7(6), 65. https://doi.org/10.5430/jnep.v7n6p65.

Brittain, E., & Wittes, J. (1989). Factorial designs in clinical trials: The effects of non-compliance and subadditivity. *Statistics in Medicine*, 8(2), 161–171. https://doi.org/10.1002/sim.4780080204.

Buyse, M. (1995). Phase IV clinical trials purposes, design, and a limited place for good clinical practice. 29, 79–86. https://doi.org/10.1177/0092861595029001.

Calvert, M., Blazeby, J., Altman, D. G., Revicki, D. A., Moher, D., & Brundage, M. D. (2013). Reporting of patient-reported outcomes in randomized trials the CONSORT PRO extension. *JAMA*, 309(8), 814–822. 10.1001/jama.2013.879.

Chan-Tack, K. M., Struble, K. A., Morgensztejn, N., Murray, J. S., Gulick, R., Cheng, B., Weller, I., & Miller, V. (2008). HIV clinical trial design for antiretroviral development: Moving forward. *AIDS*, 22(18), 2419–2427. https://doi.org/10.1097/QAD.0B013E32831692E6.

Chow, S. C., & Corey, R. (2011). Benefits, challenges and obstacles of adaptive clinical trial designs. *Orphanet Journal of Rare Diseases*, 6(1), 79. https://doi.org/10.1186/1750-1172-6-79.

Clayton, A. H., Gommoll, C., Chen, D., & Nunez, R. (2011). Sexual dysfunction during treatment of major depressive disorder with vilazodone, citalopram, or placebo: Results from a phase IV clinical trial. 30(4), 216–223. https://doi.org/10.1097/YIC.0000000000000075.

Clinical Trial Startup Material. (2020). *In Definitions.* https://doi.org/10.32388/0jc1hh.

Costa, L. J. (2020). Clinical trial material. *The Lancet Haematology*, 7(5). https://doi.org/10.1016/S2352-3026(20)30118-6.

Day, S. (2020). Adaptive and platform trials. In *Innovation in Clinical Trial Methodologies: Lessons Learned during the Corona Pandemic*. https://doi.org/10.1016/B978-0-12-824490-6.00016-5.

Elm, E. Von, Altman, D. G., Egger, M., Pocock, S. J., Gøtzsche, P. C., & Vandenbroucke, J. P. (2008). The strengthening the reporting of observational studies in epidemiology (STROBE) statement : Guidelines for reporting observational studies. 61, 344–349. https://doi.org/10.1016/j.jclinepi.2007.11.008.

Faris, O. (2013). *Clinical Trials for Medical Devices: FDA and the IDE Process*. FDA.

Freemantle, N., & Strack, T. (2009). Real-world effectiveness of new medicines should be evaluated by appropriately designed clinical trials. *Journal of Clinical Epidemiology*, 63(10), 1053–1058. https://doi.org/10.1016/j.jclinepi.2009.07.013.

Gan, H. K., Grothey, A., Pond, G. R., Moore, M. J., Siu, L. L., & Sargent, D. (2010). Randomized phase II trials: Inevitable or inadvisable? *Journal of Clinical Oncology*, 28(15), 2641–2647. https://doi.org/10.1200/JCO.2009.26.3343.

Gottlieb, K., Dawson, J., Hussain, F., & Murray, J. A. (2015). Development of drugs for celiac disease: Review of endpoints for Phase 2 and 3 trials. *Gastroenterology Report*, 3(2), 91–102. https://doi.org/10.1093/GASTRO/GOV006.

Grayling, M. J., Dimairo, M., Mander, A. P., & Jaki, T. F. (2019). A review of perspectives on the use of randomization in phase II oncology trials. *JNCI: Journal of the National Cancer Institute*, 111(12), 1255–1262. https://doi.org/10.1093/JNCI/DJZ126.

Gui, G., Agusti, A., Twelves, D., Tang, S., Kabir, M., Montgomery, C., Nerurkar, A., Osin, P., & Isacke, C. (2018). INTEND II randomized clinical trial of intraoperative duct endoscopy in pathological nipple discharge. *British Journal of Surgery*, 105(12). https://doi.org/10.1002/bjs.10990.

Han, G. (2021). Designing historical control studies with survival endpoints using exact statistical inference. *Pharmaceutical Statistics*, 20(1), 4–14. https://doi.org/10.1002/pst.2050.

Hansen, A. R., Graham, D. M., Pond, G. R., & Siu, L. L. (2014). Phase 1 trial design: Is 3 + 3 the best? *Cancer Control*, 21(3), 200–208. https://doi.org/10.1177/107327481402100304.

Hay, M., Thomas, D. W., & Craighead, J. L. (2014). Clinical development success rates for investigational drugs. *Nature Biotechnology*, 32(1), 40–51. www.nature.com/articles/nbt.2786.

Hench, L. L. (1998). Biomaterials: A forecast for the future. *Biomaterials*, 19(16), 1419–1423. https://doi.org/10.1016/S0142-9612(98)00133-1.

Huebsch, N., & Mooney, D. J. (2009). Inspiration and application in the evolution of biomaterials. *Nature*, 462(7272), 426–432. www.nature.com/articles/nature08601.

Ivanova, A., Montazer-Haghighi, A., Mohanty, S. G., & Durham, S. D. (2003). Improved up-and-down designs for phase I trials. *Wiley Online Library*, 22(1), 69–82. https://doi.org/10.1002/sim.1336.

Ivy, S. P., Siu, L. L., Garrett-Mayer, E., & Rubinstein, L. (2010). Approaches to phase 1 clinical trial design focused on safety, efficiency, and selected patient populations: A report from the clinical trial design task force of the national cancer institute investigational drug steering committee. *Clinical Cancer Research*, 16(6), 1726–1736. https://doi.org/10.1158/1078-0432.CCR-09-1961.

Johnson, R. A., Rid, A., Emanuel, E., & Wendler, D. (2016). Risks of phase I research with healthy participants: A systematic review. *Clinical Trials*, 13(2), 149–160. https://doi.org/10.1177/1740774515602868.

Kolitsopoulos, F. M., Strom, B. L., Faich, G., Eng, S. M., Kane, J. M., & Reynolds, R. F. (2022). Lessons learned in the conduct of a global, large simple trial of treatments indicated for schizophrenia. *Contemporary Clinical Trials*, 34(2), 239–247. https://doi.org/10.1016/j.cct.2012.12.001.

Korn, E. L., Freidlin, B., Abrams, J. S., & Halabi, S. (2012). Design issues in randomized phase II/III trials. *Journal of Clinical Oncology*, 30(6), 667. https://doi.org/10.1200/JCO.2011.38.5732.

Kudrow, D., Krege, J. H., Hundemer, H. P., Berg, P. H., Khanna, R., Ossipov, M. H., & Pozo-Rosich, P. (2020). Issues impacting adverse event frequency and severity: Differences between randomized phase 2 and phase 3 clinical trials for lasmiditan. *Headache*, 60(3), 576–588. https://doi.org/10.1111/head.13731.

Laage, T., Loewy, J. W., Menon, S., Miller, E. R., Pulkstenis, E., Kan-Dobrosky, N., & Coffey, C. (2017). Ethical considerations in adaptive design clinical trials. *Therapeutic Innovation and Regulatory Science*, 51(2). https://doi.org/10.1177/2168479016667766.

Lattermann, C., Proffitt, M., Kraus, V. B., & Spindler, K. P. (2014). MOON-AAA GCP clinical trial: Early lessons from an early interventional trial in patients within 1 week after ACL tear. *Osteoarthritis and Cartilage*, 22, S199. https://doi.org/10.1016/j.joca.2014.02.380.

Leung, D. H. Y., & Wang, Y.-G. (2002). Isotonic designs for phase I trials. *Controlled Clinical Trials*, 22(2), 126–138. https://doi.org/10.1016/S0197-2456(00)00132-X.

Li, A., & Bergan, R. C. (2020). Clinical trial design: Past, present, and future in the context of big data and precision medicine. *Cancer*, 126(22), 4838–4846. https://doi.org/10.1002/cncr.33205.

Li, G., Sajobi, T. T., Menon, B. K., Korngut, L., Lowerison, M., James, M., Wilton, S. B., Williamson, T., Gill, S., Drogos, L. L., Smith, E. E., Vohra, S., Hill, M. D., & Thabane, L. (2016). Registry-based randomized controlled trials—what are the advantages, challenges, and areas for future research? *Journal of Clinical Epidemiology*, 80, 16–24. https://doi.org/10.1016/J.JCLINEPI.2016.08.003.

Liu, X., Rivera, S. C., Moher, D., Calvert, M. J., Denniston, A. K., & SPIRIT-AI and CONSORT-AI Working Group. (2020). Reporting guidelines for clinical trial reports for interventions involving artificial intelligence: The CONSORT-AI extension. *BMJ (Clinical Research Ed.)*, 370(9), m3164. https://doi.org/10.1136/bmj.m3164.

Longo, D., Jameson, J., & Kaspe, D. (2011). *Harrison's Principles of Internal Medicine* (vol. 2, 19th ed.). http://kubalibri.cz/files/198—Harrison-s-Principles-of-Internal-Medicine-2-Volumes.pdf.

Love, S. B., Brown, S., Weir, C. J., Harbron, C., Yap, C., Gaschler-Markefski, B., Matcham, J., Caffrey, L., Mckevitt, C., Clive, S., Craddock, C., Spicer, J., & Cornelius, V. (2017). Embracing model-based designs for dose-finding trials. *British Journal of Cancer*, 117(3), 332–339. https://doi.org/10.1038/bjc.2017.186.

Madorran, E., Stožer, A., Bevc, S., & Maver, U. (2020). In vitro toxicity model: Upgrades to bridge the gap between preclinical and clinical research. *Bosnian Journal of Basic Medical Sciences*, 20(2), 157. https://doi.org/10.17305/BJBMS.2019.4378.

Mahan, V. L. (2014). Clinical trial phases. *International Journal of Clinical Medicine*, 5(21), 1374–1383. https://doi.org/10.4236/ijcm.2014.521175.

Malik, L., & Lu, D. (2019). Eligibility criteria for phase I clinical trials: Tight vs loose? *Cancer Chemotherapy and Pharmacology*, 83(5), 999–1002. https://doi.org/10.1007/S00280-019-03801-W.

Mandrekar, S. J., & Sargeant, D. J. (2009). Clinical trial designs for predictive biomarker validation: Theoretical considerations and practical challenges. *Journal of Biopharmaceutical Statistics*, 19(3), 530–542. www.ncbi.nlm.nih.gov/pmc/articles/PMC2734400/.

Marc, A. R. (2018). *Clinical Trials—Medical Device Trials*. Genesis Research Services.

Massett, H. A., Mishkin, G., Rubinstein, L., Ivy, S. P., Denicoff, A., Godwin, E., DiPiazza, K., Bolognese, J., Zwiebel, J. A., & Abrams, J. S. (2016). Challenges facing early phase trials sponsored by the national cancer institute: An analysis of corrective action plans to improve accrual. *Clinical Cancer Research*, 22(22), 5408–5416. https://doi.org/10.1158/1078-0432.CCR-16-0338/274240/AM/CHALLENGES-FACING-EARLY-PHASE-TRIALS-SPONSORED-BY.

Mickenautsch, S., & Yengopal, V. (2017). Reports of uncontrolled clinical trials for directly placed restorations in vital teeth. *Brazilian Oral Research*, 31. https://doi.org/10.1590/1807-3107BOR-2017.vol31.0048.

Moher, D., Hopewell, S., Schulz, K. F., Montori, V., Gøtzsche, P. C., Devereaux, P. J., Elbourne, D., Egger, M., & Altman, D. G. (2010). CONSORT 2010 explanation and elaboration: Updated guidelines for reporting parallel group randomised trials. *Journal of Clinical Epidemiology*, 63(8), e1–e37. https://doi.org/10.1016/J.JCLINEPI.2010.03.004.

Moher, D., Pham, B., Jones, A., Cook, D. J., Jadad, A. R., Moher, M., Tugwell, P., & Klassen, T. P. (1998). Does quality of reports of randomised trials affect estimates of intervention efficacy reported in meta-analyses? *The Lancet*, 352(9128), 609–613. https://doi.org/10.1016/S0140-6736(98)01085-X.

Moher, D., Schulz, K. F., Altman, D. G., & Lepage, L. (2001). The CONSORT statement: Revised recommendations for improving the quality of reports of parallel-group randomised trials. *The Lancet*, 357(9263), 1191–1194. https://doi.org/10.1016/S0140-6736(00)04337-3.

Montgomery, P., Grant, S., Mayo-Wilson, E., Macdonald, G., Michie, S., Hopewell, S., Moher, D., Lawrence Aber, J., Altman, D., Bhui, K., Booth, A., Clark, D., Craig, P., Eisner, M., Sherman, L., Fraser, M. W., Gardner, F., Hedges, L., Hollon, S., & Yaffe, J. (2018). Reporting randomised trials of social and psychological interventions: The CONSORT-SPI 2018 extension. *Trials*, 19(1). https://doi.org/10.1186/S13063-018-2733-1.

Murray, P., García Godoy, C., & García Godoy, F. (2007). How is the biocompatibilty of dental biomaterials evaluated? *Medicina Oral, Patología Oral y Cirugía Bucal*, 12(3), 258–266. https://scielo.isciii.es/scielo.php?script=sci_arttext&pid=S1698-69462007000300017.

Mylona, V., Anagnostaki, E., Parker, S., Cronshaw, M., Lynch, E., & Grootveld, M. (2020). Laser-assisted aPDT protocols in randomized controlled clinical trials in dentistry: A systematic review. *Dentistry Journal*, 8(3), 107. https://doi.org/10.3390/dj8030107.

NCI Dictionary of Cancer Terms. (2022.). *National Cancer Institute*. Retrieved September 18, 2022, from www.cancer.gov/publications/dictionaries/cancer-terms/def/phase-iv-clinical-trial.

Nikkho, S., Fernandes, P., White, R. J., Deng, C., Farber, H. W., & Corris, P. A. (2020). Clinical trial design in phase 2 and 3 trials for pulmonary hypertension. *Pulmonary Circulation*, 10(4), 2045894020941491. https://doi.org/10.1177/2045894020941491.

Orkin, A. M., Gill, P. J., Ghersi, D., Campbell, L., Sugarman, J., Emsley, R., Steg, P. G., Weijer, C., Simes, J., Rombey, T., Williams, H. C., Wittes, J., Moher, D., Richards, D. P., Kasamon, Y., Getz, K., Hopewell, S., Dickersin, K., Wu, T., & Chan, A. W. (2021). Guidelines for reporting trial protocols and completed trials modified due to the COVID-19 pandemic and other extenuating circumstances: The CONSERVYE 2021 statement. *JAMA*, 326(3), 257–265. https://doi.org/10.1001/JAMA.2021.9941.

Pandis, N., Walsh, T., Polychronopoulou, A., Katsaros, C., & Eliades, T. (2014). Factorial designs: An overview with applications to orthodontic clinical trials. *European Journal of Orthodontics*, 36(3), 314–320. https://doi.org/10.1093/ejo/cjt054.

Phases of clinical trials | Cancer Research UK. (2014, October 21). *Cancer Research UK*. www.cancerresearchuk.org/about-cancer/find-a-clinical-trial/what-clinical-trials-are/phases-of-clinical-trials.

Prang, K.-H., Karanatsios, B., Verbunt, E., Wong, H.-L., Yeung, J., Kelaher, M., & Gibbs, P. (2022). Clinical registries data quality attributes to support registry-based randomised controlled trials: A scoping review. *Contemporary Clinical Trials*, 119, 106843. https://doi.org/10.1016/J.CCT.2022.106843.

Ratain, M. J., & Sargent, D. J. (2008). Optimising the design of phase II oncology trials: The importance of randomisation. *European Journal of Cancer*, 45(2), 275–280. https://doi.org/10.1016/j.ejca.2008.10.029.

Rauf, A., Abu-Izneid, T., Khalil, A. A., Hafeez, N., Olatunde, A., Rahman, M., Semwal, P., Al-Awthan, Y. S., Bahattab, O. S., Khan, I. N., Khan, M. A., & Sharma, R. (2022). Nanoparticles in clinical trials of COVID-19: An update. *International Journal of Surgery*, 104, 106818. https://doi.org/10.1016/J.IJSU.2022.106818.

Reardon, D. A., Brandes, A. A., Omuro, A., Mulholland, P., Lim, M., Wick, A., Baehring, J., Ahluwalia, M. S., Roth, P., Bähr, O., Phuphanich, S., Sepulveda, J. M., de Souza, P., Sahebjam, S., Carleton, M., Tatsuoka, K., Taitt, C., Zwirtes, R., Sampson, J., & Weller, M. (2020). Effect of nivolumab vs bevacizumab in patients with recurrent glioblastoma: The checkmate 143 phase 3 randomized clinical trial. *JAMA Oncology*, 6(7). https://doi.org/10.1001/jamaoncol.2020.1024.

Rock, E. P., Molloy, V. J., & Humphrey, J. S. (2010). GCP data quality for early clinical development. *Clinical Cancer Research*, 16(6). https://doi.org/10.1158/1078-0432.CCR-09-3267.

Rogatko, A., Schoeneck, D., Jonas, W., Tighiouart, M., Khuri, F. R., & Porter, A. (2007). Translation of innovative designs into phase I trials. *Journal of Clinical Oncology*, 25(31), 4982–4986. https://doi.org/10.1200/JCO.2007.12.1012.

Rubinstein, L., Sargent, D., & Shi, Q. (2014). Phase II design: History and evolution. *Chinese Clinical Oncology*, 3(4), 48. https://doi.org/10.3978/j.issn.2304-3865.2014.02.02.

Sargent, D., & Oncol, S. G. (2010). Clinical trials data collection: When less is more. *Journal of Clinical Oncology*, 28(34), 5019–5021. www.academia.edu/download/44068565/Clinical_Trials_Data_Collection_When_Les20160324-30468-2xzxjc.pdf.

Simon, R. (1989). Optimal two-stage designs for phase II clinical trials. *Controlled Clinical Trials*, 10(1), 1–10. www.researchgate.net/publication/288264333.

Simon, R., Freidlin, B., Rubinstein, L., Arbuck, S. G., Collins, J., & Christian, M. C. (1997). Accelerated titration designs for phase I clinical trials in oncology. *JNCI: Journal of the National Cancer Institute*, 89(15), 1138–1147. https://doi.org/10.1093/JNCI/89.15.1138.

Siu, L. L., Le Tourneau, C., & Lee, J. J. (2009). Dose escalation methods in phase I cancer clinical trials. *Journal of the National Cancer Institute*, 101(10), 708–720. https://doi.org/10.1093/jnci/djp079.

Torres-Saavedra, P. A., & Winter, K. A. (2022). An overview of phase 2 clinical trial designs. *International Journal of Radiation Oncology Biology Physics*, 112(1), 22–29. https://doi.org/10.1016/J.IJROBP.2021.07.1700.

van Brummelen, E. M. J., Huitema, A. D. R., van Werkhoven, E., Beijnen, J. H., & Schellens, J. H. M. (2016). The performance of model-based versus rule-based phase I clinical trials in oncology: A quantitative comparison of the performance of model-based versus rule-based phase I trials with molecularly targeted anticancer drugs over the last 2 years. *Journal of Pharmacokinetics and Pharmacodynamics*, 43(3), 235–242. https://doi.org/10.1007/S10928-016-9466-0/FIGURES/2.

van Eijk, R. P. A., Nikolakopoulos, S., Ferguson, T. A., Liu, D., Eijkemans, M. J. C., & van den Berg, L. H. (2018). Increasing the efficiency of clinical trials in neurodegenerative disorders using group sequential trial designs. *Journal of Clinical Epidemiology*, 98. https://doi.org/10.1016/j.jclinepi.2018.02.013.

Van Norman, G. A. (2021). Data safety and monitoring boards should be required for both early—and late-phase clinical trials. *JACC: Basic to Translational Science*, 6(11), 887–896. https://doi.org/10.1016/J.JACBTS.2021.09.005.

Vanneste, B. G. L., van Limbergen, E. J., Reynders, K., & de Ruysscher, D. (2021). An overview of the published and running randomized phase 3 clinical results of radiotherapy in combination with immunotherapy. *Translational Lung Cancer Research*, 10(4). https://doi.org/10.21037/tlcr-20-304.

Wang, S., Liu, H., Zhao, S. Y., & Peng, C. F. (2021). A randomized clinical trial of two bioceramic materials in primary molar pulpotomies. *Zhonghua Kou Qiang Yi Xue Za Zhi = Zhonghua Kouqiang Yixue Zazhi = Chinese Journal of Stomatology*, 56(2). https://doi.org/10.3760/cma.j.cn112144-20200520-00287.

World Health Organization. (2006, February 22). The safety of medicines in public health programmes: pharmacovigilance an essential tool. From www.who.int/publications/i/item/9241593911

9 Business and Market of Material Products for Medical Applications— Material-Based Products, Business and Profits of Products, Major Market Players, Global Trends, Investments, and Future Opportunities

Firdos Alam Khan

9.1 INTRODUCTION

The term 'nanotechnology' was first coined by K. Eric Drexler in 1986 (Eric, 1986), and his concept was based on the initial idea given by Nobel laureate Richard Feynman (Feynman, 1960). Thereafter, the nanotechnology field has progressed well, and various types, shapes, and sizes of biomaterials and nanomaterials have been synthesized. The unique properties of nanomaterials not only attracted technologists and engineers fields but also attracted the biologist and physicians globally. The different types of nanomaterials have been applied in the biomedical field, especially for the treatment of different types of diseases and also in the diagnosis of various types of diseases, including cancers. One of the main advantages of nanomaterials is their small size, better surface area, better drug conjugation capability, better bioavailability, and specific tissue targeting. The use of nanomaterials is not only limited to in vitro and preclinical studies but also applied in clinical conditions in treating human diseases. Presently, different types of nano-based products have been produced for therapeutic and diagnosis purposes (Farjadian et al., 2019).

DOI: 10.1201/9781003317715-9

9.2   LIST OF NANOMATERIAL-BASED PRODUCTS

A summary of various types of nano-based products, which are specially produced for the treatment of human diseases, is as follows.

9.2.1   Emend®

This is a nano-based product that has been specially named Emend® and was produced by Merck & Co. Inc., New Jersey, USA. This product is available in nanocrystalline form as an anti-emetic drug approved by the US FDA in 2003. This drug is used in the prevention of nausea and vomiting in cancer patients who undergo chemotherapy, and it has a high dose of cisplatin. Emend or aprepitant is a specific antagonist human substance P ligand with binding affinity to neurokinin-1 receptors, which are called vomiting centers in the brain (Andrews et al., 2001; Merck & Co Inc., NJ, USA, 2015). The prime advantage of Emend over other available drugs is that it has no binding affinity to serotonin, corticosteroids, or dopamine receptors, and has specific targets (Merck & Co. Inc., NJ, USA, 2015; Maggi, 1995). The absorption of Emend or aprepitant generally occurs in the upper gastrointestinal tract (Junghanns and Müller, 2008), and it is not soluble in water (Merck & Co Inc., NJ, USA, 2015). The non-solubility issue is solved by developing new technology, which is called Elan Drug Delivery Nanocrystals®, and orally produced nano-based Emend possesses better water solubility and is found to have greater absorption capacity in the upper part of the gastrointestinal tract and with higher bioavailability (Junghanns and Müller, 2008). Interestingly, the US FDA approved the intravenous injectable form of Emend in 2008, where the active ingredient was fosaprepitant dimeglumine, a pro-drug of aprepitant that is water-soluble and can be easily converted to aprepitant within 30 minutes after intravenous injection (Merck & Co Inc., NJ, USA, 2015; Roila et al., 2010).

9.2.2   Ostim®

The nano-based drug Ostim® is produced by Osartis GmbH and Company, based in Germany. This drug is a nanocrystalline paste (20 nm) containing calcium hydroxyapatite. In 2004, this drug was approved by the US FDA. The structure of calcium hydroxyapatite resembles natural bone minerals, which has the ability to induce osteo-conduction, thus making this product highly biocompatibility (Brandt et al., 2010). Ostim has been used as a bone-grafting material in many biomedical conditions, such as in orthopedic and dental surgical procedures. Ostim paste contains 25% water, with dispersed nanosized calcium hydro-xyapatite crystals (Brandt et al., 2010; Huber et al., 2006; Tadic and Epple, 2004).

9.2.3   Rapamune®

This nanoformulation is called Rapamune®, which was produced by Wyeth Pharmaceuticals Inc., which is a supplementary company associated with Pfizer, USA. In 2010, sirolimus or rapamycin is known as the first nanocrystalline drug approved by the US FDA (Narayan et al., 2017). This drug is generally used in patients who usually undergo kidney transplantation to prevent rejection. The active ingredient of Rapamune is a *macrocyclic triene* antibiotic; this acts as an immunosuppressant to prevent rejection of kidney transplants. This antibiotic is derived from the bacteria *Streptomyces hygroscopicus*. The drug delivery can be improved by the application of Elan Drug Delivery Nanocrystals Technology, which involves bead milling, which improves drug bio-availability (Bobo et al., 2016; Shegokar and Müller, 2010). The nanoformulation improves drug storage and is suitable for oral administration (Kesisoglou et al., 2007). It has been found that Rapamune blocks T-lymphocyte cell proliferation (Sehgal, 1998), which results in improving a deteriorated immune system to prevent the rejection of a transplanted organ. Rapamune was approved in 2015 for the clinical management of rare progressive lung disease.

9.2.4 VITOSS®

The product Vitoss® is produced by Orthovita Inc. USA and is considered the best-selling synthetic bone graft substitute. This product consists of 100 nm β--tricalcium phosphate nanocrystals approved by the US FDA in 2003 (Marya et al., 2017). It has been reported that Vitoss is able to simulate the behavior of the spongy appearance of bone, which helps to fill holes in the skeletal muscles. The product Vitoss is manufactured by the calcination process and comprises porous granules with a diameter of 1–4 mm (Tadic and Epple, 2004; Campion et al., 2013). There is another formulation of this product, known as Vitoss Bioactive, which contains Vitoss plus a bioactive agent to improve bone regeneration speed (Bajwa et al., 2017). Another company named Stryker Company was acquired by Orthovita Inc. in 2011 (Behabtu et al., 2013).

9.2.5 RITALIN®

This nano-formulated product Ritalin® was produced by Novartis, Basel, Switzerland. This product is called methylphenidate nanocrystals and was approved by the US FDA in 1955 for the clinical management of hyperactivity disorders in children (Swanson et al., 2004; Harris, 2006). This nanodrug is mainly used in patients who have attention deficit hyperactivity disorder (Diller, 1996). This drug is mostly prescribed for attention deficit hyperactivity disorder since 1990 (Lange et al., 2010). It has been reported that this drug has been prescribed to 420,000 patients in the UK in the year 2007, and 657,000 was prescribed to patients in 2012 (Doward and Craig, 2012). Attention deficit hyperactivity disorder is mostly linked to the dysregulation of dopamine and norepinephrine (Hunt et al., 2006; Arnsten and Li, 2005). In attention deficit hyperactivity disorder patients, after the drug treatment, there was an increase in the levels of dopamine and norepinephrine in the synaptic cleft, which subsequently increased the cognitive functions of the brain (Markowitz et al., 2009; Volkow et al., 2001). Treatment with the drug increases the alertness of the brain, which results in short-term benefits as a cost-effective therapy (Steele et al., 2006; Mott and Leach, 2004). This drug Ritalin also displays many side effects in attention deficit hyperactivity disorder patients (Alagona, 2010).

9.2.6 TriCor®

The nanoformulation TriCor® is produced by Abbott Laboratories, Illinois, USA. The generic name of this drug is fenofibrate, which was approved by the US FDA in 2004. This drug is mainly used to prevent the development of atherosclerosis by reducing triglyceride and cholesterol levels. This drug also decreased the formation of plaques on artery walls, thus preventing strokes and heart attacks. This drug can be orally administered, and after administration, this drug is metabolized into fenofibric acid in the intestine (Alagona, 2010; Adedoyin, 2018). It has been reported that treatment with fenofibric acid is responsible for the activation of peroxisome proliferator-activated receptor α, and after lipoprotein lipase activation, it has been found that the apolipoprotein C-III levels decrease (Abbott Laboratories, IL, USA, 2010). This procedure finally causes the decline in the total cholesterol and triglyceride levels in blood circulation and also increases high-density lipoprotein and apolipoproteins I and II production (Abbott Laboratories, IL, USA, 2010). The water solubility of this drug can be improved by using the Elan drug delivery nanocrystals technology, and it has been found that fenofibrate becomes more water-soluble in TriCor. Previously, using Elan drug delivery nanocrystals technology, fenofibrate is usually recommended to be taken along with food because food allows surfactants and lipids to be easily emulsified in the food for better drug action (Junghanns and Müller, 2008). Interestingly, this drug also possesses higher water solubility, which is good for better drug delivery (Abbott Laboratories Press Release, 2004).

9.2.7 Doxil®

This nano-formulated drug Doxil is produced by Alza, Pakistan, which is also called Caelyx® or Evacet® or Lipodox®. This drug received US FDA approval in 1995 for clinical application. This drug is used for the treatment of different types of cancers (Lasic, 1996; Gill et al., 1996; Andreopoulou et al., 2007). This drug is produced by encapsulating the anticancer drug doxorubicin or Adriamycin with liposomes covered with polyethylene glycol (PEG). The size of these nanoformulations falls between 80 and 90 nm. The drug encapsulation increases the circulation of the drug, which leads to an improvement in drug bioavailability (Pillai and Ceballos-Coronel, 2013; Park, 2002; Biggers and Scheinfeld, 2008). Doxil is a first-generation injectable where doxorubicin hydrochloride combined in liposomes was produced by Sun Pharma Global FZE, India, which was approved by the US FDA in 2013 (Pillai and Ceballos-Coronel, 2013). The mechanism of Doxil's action has been studied, and it has been found that it acts in two ways: (1) by disrupting topoisomerase and (2) by inducing intracellular production of reactive oxygen species (Gordon et al., 2000). The second-generation drugs Doxil and Lipodox PEGylated liposomal doxorubicin generally act on the cancer tumor cells (Gabizon et al., 2006). One of the significant advantages of liposomal doxorubicin drug nanoformulation is a reduction in the adverse effects of the drug.

9.2.8 DaunoXome®

The liposomal-formulated daunorubicin drug, which is also known as DaunoXome®, is produced by Galen, UK, and the US FDA approval was given in 1996. The anthrax-cycline anticancer drug can be used in the treatment of cancers as a chemo-therapy drug (Gill et al., 1996). Furthermore, based on various clinical trials, it has been found that daunorubicin has been effectively used in different types of leukemia (Murphy and Yee, 2017; Greenwald et al., 2003). The liposomes with a diameter of 45 nm comprise lipid bilayers, which are composed of cholesterol (Fassas and Anagnostopoulos, 2005). Per preclinical studies, it has been found that DaunoXome increased the concentration of doxorubicin in the tumor tissues (Yarmolenko et al., 2010; Fosså et al., 1998).

9.2.9 ONIVYDE®

The nanoformulation Onivyde® was produced by Merrimack Pharmaceuticals, USA, and this product is known as MM-398 or PEP02. This liposomal nanoformulation of irinotecan was approved in 2015 for the management of metastatic pancreatic cancer (Passero et al., 2016; FDA, 2015; Handen et al., 1991). This product is used with other anticancer agents; for example, FOLFIRINOX, which is a chemother-apeutic drug, is used in patients associated with pancreatic cancer, and this drug formulation contains irinotecan + 5-fluorouracil + oxaliplatin + folinic acid and showed better anticancer action on patients than gemcitabine treatments (Conroy et al., 2011; Zhang, 2016). Additionally, the treatment of the nanoliposomal formula-tion of irinotecan gives extra advantages; for example, better improvements in drug circulation time, better drug biodistribution, and better accumulation in the tumor tissues (Zhang, 2016).

9.2.10 DEPOCYT®

This nano-formulated drug DepoCyt® was produced by Pacira Pharmaceuticals, USA, and approved by the US FDA in 1999. This drug is basically a liposo-mal formulation of cytarabine, as produced by using Depofoam® technology (Mantripragada, 2002), which was approved by the US FDA in 2007. This drug is used to treat lymphomatous meningitis (Pillai and Ceballos-Coronel, 2013). This liposomal cytarabine drug is delivered to the patients by intrathecal administration; in this case, systemic treatment of cytarabine is trivial (Jaeckle et al., 2002; Pearce et al., 1990). The liposomal cytarabine formulation basically contains (dipalmi-toyl phosphatidyl glycerol + dioleoyl phosphatidyl choline + triolein + cholesterol) (Kim et al., 1993). Additionally, a new drug named DepoCyt, which is basically a sustained-release formulation that contains cytarabine, is used in the treatment of cerebrospinal fluid disease (Takayama et al., 2002). This drug induces antineoplas-tic action on the cancerous cells of the S-phase of cell division and inhibits DNA polymerase (Galmarini et al., 2002).

9.2.11 MARQIBO®

This nano-formulated drug is basically liposome vincristine sulfate, marketed in the name of Marqibo®, and this US FDA product is approved and produced by Talon Therapeutics, USA. Vincristine is used as an anticancer agent, where Marqibo is encapsulated in sphingomyelin or cholesterol liposomes, which bind to tubulin and interferes with cancer cell division (Dawidczyk et al., 2014). The treatment with Marqibo showed good anticancer action in Philadelphia chromosome-negative chronic myelogenous leukemia (Harrison and Lyseng-Williamson, 2013). It has been reported that liposomal vincristine shows slower blood circulation clearance (Yang et al., 2012). This drug also offers additional advantages; for example, improved drug circulation time in blood and better drug accumulation in cancer tumors (Boman et al., 1994; Weissig et al., 2014). This drug comes with several side effects, such as constipation, nausea, fatigue, diarrhea, and insomnia (Thomas et al., 2006).

9.2.12 AmBisome®

This drug named AmBisome® is produced by NeXstar Pharmaceuticals, USA. This drug is a liposomal form of amphotericin B or L-amphotericin, which possesses antifungal capabilities used in the treatment of fungal infections. Since this drug does not act through enzyme inhibition, amphotericin B does not lead to the appearance of resistant fungus compared with additional antifungal agents (Takemoto and Kanazawa, 2016; Torres, 2010). The undesirable dose-limiting toxicity, like nephrotoxicity by using a conventional formulation of amphotericin B, Fungizone, can be solved by an injectable formulation of water-insoluble amphotericin B (Clemons and Stevens, 2004). The drug has been extensively examined to study better stability and lower toxicity with the combination containing (phosphatidylcholine + cholesterol + distearoylphosphatidylglycerol containing amphotericin B) (Takemoto and Kanazawa, 2016). It has been found that this drug has many advantages, such as better pharmacokinetic properties, better drug stability, reduced drug accumulation in non-cancerous tissues, and reduced drug toxicity (Takemoto and Kanazawa, 2016). Additionally, the mechanism of action of amphotericin B allows the drug to penetrate the fungus membrane and eventually cause the death of the fungal cells (Stone et al., 2016).

9.2.13 Vyxeos®

This drug is basically daunorubicin and cytarabine, which is encapsulated in liposomes. This drug is marketed as Vyxeos® by Jazz Pharmaceutics, Dublin, Ireland. This drug has been approved by the US FDA in 2017 (FDA, 2017) for the clinical management of patients suffering from acute myeloid leukemia (Crain, 2018; Allen, 2016). The drug was produced by loading cytarabine and daunorubicin into a liposomal (Waknine, 2011). It has been reported that treatment with this drug develops complexes with cancer cell DNA, where daunorubicin impacts the synthesis of DNA, which results in cancer cell death (Crain, 2018). Treatment with the drug Vyxeos strikingly improves the drug circulation in plasma and reduces the delivery to non-cancerous tissues (Mayer et al., 2016). Vyxeos was prescribed to 309 patients with acute myeloid leukemia, and the results showed an improvement in the survival of the patients (Crain, 2018). This drug also comes with several side effects, such as hypersensitivity reaction, cardio-toxicity, and tissue necrosis (Crain, 2018).

9.2.14 ABELCET®

This is another amphotericin B-lipid-complex drug (Abelcet), which is produced by Defiante Farmaceutica, Funchal, Portugal. This drug was approved in 1965 for the clinical management of serious leishmaniasis and fungal infections (Wu, 1994; Camarata et al., 1992). This drug contains amphotericin B and two phospholipids (Veerareddy and Vobalaboina, 2004). This drug also produces fewer side effects compared with amphotericin B treatment.

9.2.15 VISUDYNE®

This drug Visudyne® was produced by QLT Phototherapeutics, Canada. This drug is a liposomal formulation of the photosensitizer benzo-porphyrin-derivative mono-acid ring A (Bressler, 2001). This drug was approved by the US FDA in 2001 for the clinical management of choroidal neo-vascularization in age-related macular degeneration (Liu, 1998). It has been learned that the growth of unwanted blood vessels in the back of the eye is one of the leading causes of blindness in patients. The drug Visudyne can be injected intravenously into the eye, and this drug stops unwanted growth of the blood and reverses the progressive loss of vision. This drug is also used for macular degeneration, and a combination of Visudyne photodynamic therapy + immunosuppression is useful in treatment (Rogers et al., 2003; Parodi et al., 2006; Wachtlin et al., 2003; Hogan et al., 2005). This drug also induces side effects, such as minor changes in vision, dryness, redness or swelling in the eyes, and headache.

9.2.16 CIMZIA®

This drug Cimzia® was produced by UCB, Belgium, and is also called certolizumab pegol. This drug was approved in 2008 by the US FDA. This drug is used as a PEGylated blocker for TNF-α (tumor necrosis factor alpha). It has been reported that Cimzia is a PEGylated, which recognizes and binds to the TNF-α of cancer cells, consequently defusing its action (Nesbitt et al., 2007). The drug Cimzia is used for the clinical management of patients with rheumatoid arthritis (Connock et al., 2010), Crohn's disease (Sandborn et al., 2007), psoriatic arthritis (Mease et al., 2013), and ankylosing spondylitis (Landewé et al., 2013). The majority of these mentioned diseases are related to autoimmunity; however, Crohn's disease is not an autoimmune disease (Casanova and Abel, 2009). It has been reported that TNF-α is a pro-inflammatory cytokine and is responsible for autoimmune occurrence (Nesbitt et al., 2007; Mease et al., 2013; Landewé et al., 2013).

9.2.17 ADAGEN®

The drug Adagen® was produced by Enzon Inc., USA (Enzon Pharmaceuticals Inc, 2006) and this drug is PEGylated adenosine deaminase (ADA) and was approved by the US FDA in 1990 as the first PEGylated-formulated protein in the market. It has been reported that ADA deficiency is caused by gene mutations (Stephan et al., 1993). It has been found that a shortage of ADA causes a deposit of adenosine and

2'-deoxyadenosine, and this additional deposit results in metabolic disorders (Sigma-Tau Pharmaceuticals, Inc., MD, USA, 2014). Before the discovery of the drug Adagen, ADA immunodeficiency disorder was treated with bone marrow transplantations (Joralemon et al., 2010; Davis et al., 1981) since treatment of the native enzyme was not effective. It has been learned that naked ADA has a short blood circulation time and also induces an immunogenic response (Davis et al., 1981). The PEGylation of ADA solves these issues, and it has been shown that PEGylated ADA has a longer circulation time (Davis et al., 2008).

9.2.18 Neulasta®

The drug Neulasta® was produced by Amgen Inc., USA, and in 2002, this drug was approved by the FDA with the general name PEG-filgrastim. This drug is a PEGylated arrangement of filgrastim. Chemotherapy produces several side effects, where a low white blood cell count is very common (Sheridan et al., 1992). Neulasta® is used for the clinical management of febrile neutropenia, and resulting infections develop due to the absence of neutrophils. Moreover, Filgrastim is a recombinant methionyl human granulocyte colony-stimulating factor that was produced from *E. coli* (Curran and Goa, 2002). Neulasta is manufactured by the attachment of a mono-methoxy-PEG aldehyde chain to the N-terminal methionine residue of filgrastim (Alconcel et al., 2011; Piedmonte and Treuheit, 2008). It has been reported that PEGylation of filgrastim results in an increased drug circulation time (Piedmonte and Treuheit, 2008).

9.2.19 Oncaspar®

The drug Oncaspar® was produced by Enzon Pharmaceuticals Inc., USA, which is also commonly known as PEGylated-L-asparaginase, and the drug was approved by the US FDA. This drug is clinically used in patients with acute lymphoblastic leukemia and chronic myelogenous leukemia conditions. This is an alternative drug used in patients with leukemia who show a hypersensitivity reaction to *E. coli*–derived L-asparaginase (Milton and Chess, 2003; Graham, 2003). It has been recommended that Oncaspar can be administered every two weeks to reduce hypersensitivity (Graham, 2003) and be an economical approach for patients (Duncan, 2003; Peters et al., 1995).

9.2.20 Pegasys®

Pegasys was produced by Genentech USA Inc., California, USA, and this drug is commonly known as peginterferon alfa-2a, and in 2002, this drug was approved. It has been reported that Pegasys is produced by recombinant DNA technology, where human alfa-2a interferon was conjugated with PEG (Duncan, 2014). This drug is used for the treatment of hepatitis C (Fried et al., 2002) and positive chronic hepatitis B (Lau et al., 2005). The long half-life of Pegasys is due to PEGylation, which makes it easy to administer every 12 weeks (Davis et al., 2008). Additionally, it has been recommended that a combination of Pegasys with ribavirin improves hepatitis

C therapy (Fried et al., 2002). Moreover, the combination of lamivudine and Pegasys improves the treatment of chronic hepatitis B condition (Lau et al., 2005).

9.2.21 SOMAVERT®

The drug Somavert® was produced by Pfizer Pharmaceuticals, Connecticut, USA. The generic name of this drug is pegvisomant, which is basically the PEGylated analog of the human growth hormone, which is used in patients with acromegaly disease where the pituitary gland secretes disproportionate quantities of the growth hormone. This drug was approved by FDA in 2003. It has been reported that patients with a successive production of the growth hormone may lead to abnormal enlargement of their forehead, jaw, hands, and feet. Treatment with the drug Somavert, which is an antagonist of growth hormone receptors, reduces the serum concentration of the growth hormone (Roelfsema et al., 2006; Van der Lely et al., 2001). The PEGylation with Somavert reduces drug clearance with an increased half-life of the drug in the patients (Leonart et al., 2018).

9.2.22 MACUGEN®

Pegatinib sodium is an ocular therapeutic drug produced by EyeTech Pharmaceuticals. In 2004, this drug received US FDA approval, and the brand name of this drug is Macugen®, which was used in the neo-vascular form for age-related macular degeneration patients (Gragoudas et al., 2004). The drug Macugen is based on nanovectors used for the treatment of human diseases (Shukla et al., 2007). The aptamer is composed of RNA/DNA that binds to a specific target site on cancer cells (Bunka et al., 2010). It has been reported that pegatinib is an aptamer with 28 nucleotides conjugated to two PEG and applied as an anti-angiogenesis agent. Macugen can be used in injection form with a desirable dosage every 42 days (Ng et al., 2006). Diarrhea, eye irritation, headache, and nausea are a few side effects of Macugen treatment.

9.2.23 MIRCERA®

The drug Mircera®, which is also called epoetin β (EPO), is conjugated to methoxy-PEG. This drug is generally for the treatment of anemia (Mcgahan, 2008; Association, 2008). The European Commission and US FDA gave their approval in 2007 for the clinical application of treating anemia patients. The drug Mircera is a recombinant erythropoietin produced by using recombinant DNA technology. It has been reported that erythropoietin can stimulate erythropoiesis by acting on the erythropoietin receptors located on the surface of the bone marrow progenitor cells (Frimat et al., 2013). To produce Mircera, the PEG is first connected with butanoic acid, and the NHS-modified structure is linked to the lysine structure of the epoetin β. This formulation helps to deliver the drug in a sustained-release manner with 135 hours of half-life compare with naked EPO, with 7 to 20 hours of half-life (Association, 2008). Mircera can be administered through intravenous (IV) or subcutaneous routes (SC) every 14 days (Association, 2008).

9.2.24 PEG-INTRON®

PEG interferon® alfa-2b is a nanoformulation, which possesses alpha interferon molecule conjugated to a mono-PEG chain via succinimidyl-carbonate (Glue et al., 2000). It has a long half-life in the bloodstream, with slower drug elimination, and due to these properties, this drug needs less frequent administration compared to the standard interferon molecule (Glue et al., 2000). In 2001, this product was approved by the US FDA and clinically applied alone or in combination with the drug ribavirin for the treatment of chronic hepatitis C (Jacobson et al., 2007; Manns et al., 2013).

9.2.25 KRYSTEXXA®

Krystexxa® is produced by Savient Pharmaceuticals, USA, and this drug is used with patients who are suffering from refractory chronic gout (US FDA, 2009). It has been found that treatment with this drug causes a reduction in uric acid and a reduction in uric acid crystals formation in bone joints and soft tissues. The US FDA has given the approval in 2010 (Food and Drug Administration (FDA), 2010), and approval was also received from EMA in 2013 for the clinical treatment of tophaceous gout disorder (US FDA, 2009; Alconcel et al., 2011). This nanoformulation is produced by recombinant technology, where porcine-like uricase can metabolize uric acid to allantoin. Pegloticase is composed of four uniform chains of about 300 amino acids (Alconcel et al., 2011). In addition, the PEG molecules in pegloticase can enhance the drug's half-life period to 10 days (Alconcel et al., 2011). Infusion, allergic reactions, sore throat, vomiting, nausea, and chest pain are a few side effects of Krystexxa, (US FDA, 2009).

9.2.26 PLEGRIDY®

This nanoformulation is known as Plegridy®, which comprises the active molecules where IFN-β-1a is conjugated with PEG (Centonze et al., 2016). In 2014, this nanoformulation received approval from the US FDA for clinical application in patients with multiple sclerosis (Chaplin and Gnanapavan, 2015). It has been reported that Plegridy causes an increase in the levels of hepatic enzymes and also causes liver injury, and it's important to avoid the use of Plegridy if patients show any signs of hepatic damage (Idec, 2015).

9.2.27 ADYNOVATE®

This nanoformulation is known as Adynovate®, a recombinant pegylated antihemophilic factor, which is in patients who are suffering from hemophilia A (Turecek et al., 2016). It has been reported that treatment with Adynovate causes an increase in the blood-clotting factor VIII level for a brief duration. Moreover, Adynovate has a longer circulation time in the bloodstream for better drug bioavailability. Adynovate® comprises coagulation factor VIII, which is conjugated to PEG (Konkle et al., 2015). The Adynovate® drug has been tested in many patients who are suffering from hemophilia; and diarrhea, vomiting, rash, nausea, headache, and allergic reactions are a few side effects of Adynovate® drug treatment (Turecek et al., 2016).

9.2.28 COPAXONE®

This unique formulation known as Copaxone is a synthetic polymer containing L-alanine + L-glutamic acid + L-tyrosine + L-lysine (Grewal, 2009). The US FDA gave its approval for the clinical application in patients who are suffering from multiple sclerosis (Grewal, 2009). Even though the mechanism of action of this drug is not known, nevertheless, it has been found that Copaxone suppresses inflammatory action by blocking MHC II receptors and also causes a change in the T-cell population (Wolinsky et al., 2007; Johnson, 2012). Considering its effective therapeutic characteristics, this drug has been approved in several countries, such as the USA, Canada, and some European countries (Mckeage et al., 2015; Arnon and Aharoni, 2004). There are side effects observed related to the heart, eyes, skin, and gastrointestinal and immune systems after treatment with Copaxone (Weber et al., 2007).

9.2.29 ELIGARD®

Eligard® is a nanoformulation used as an injectable nanosuspension agent in the treatment of prostate cancer, and this drug received its US FDA approval in 2002 (Berges, 2005). Eligard® consists of leuprolide acetate, where Lupron is a synthetic peptide analog of the gonadotropine-releasing hormone (GRH). The decrease in GRH secretion is reported to decrease the level of the luteinizing hormone (LH) and follicle-stimulating hormone (FSH), respectively. In the hypogonadism condition, it has been found that estradiol and testosterone levels were decreased. Eligard® is a polymer mixture of poly-lactic and poly-glycolide (Sartor, 2003; Wex et al., 2013), which is used as an advanced drug delivery system for Lupron. Eligard® drug is available in an injectable liquid form, and upon injecting inside the human body, this drug slowly solidifies and starts releasing the drug for about 30 days (Sartor, 2003). Eligard® also causes a few side effects, like erythema and irritation (Berges, 2005).

9.2.30 RENAGEL®

This unique formulation known as Renagel® received US FDA approval in 2000 for the treatment of patients who have high serum levels of phosphorus (Slatopolsky et al., 1999). This formulation is usually prescribed in patients with hyper-phosphatemia caused by chronic kidney disease (Rosenbaum et al., 1997; Oka et al., 2008). This drug has a polymeric structure, which can be cross-linked with poly-allylamine hydrochloride and epichlorohydrin, respectively. It has been recommended that starting treatment dosage completely relies on the levels of serum levels of phosphorus (Spaia, 2011).

9.2.31 ESTRASORB®

This nanoformulated drug is known as Estrasorb®, which is produced by Novavax Inc., USA. This is a micellar-encapsulated emulsion of estradiol hemihydrate, which was approved by the US FDA in 2003 for clinical application in patients with moderate vasomotor symptoms caused by menopause. The major clinical symptoms of vasomotor symptoms are getting hot flushes, night sweats and disrupted sleep patterns, loss of memory, and fatigue; and it has been reported that Estradiol shows a role in decreasing these symptoms (Buster, 2010). It has been found that treatment with Estrasorb shows a reduced number of hot flashes in randomized and double-blind clinical trials (Simon, 2006). Estrasorb is available in a foil pouch, which can be applied on the skin as a lotion (Prausnitz and Langer, 2008).

9.2.32 ZILRETTA®

This is another unique nanoformulation where triamcinolone acetonide was conjugated with PLGA hydrogel. This nanoformulation also known as Zilretta® received its US FDA approval in 2017 for the treatment of knee osteoarthritis (Rai and Pham, 2018; Taylor, 2018; Byers-Kraus et al., 2017). This drug is produced by Flexion Therapeutics, USA. This drug can be delivered to patients through the intra-articular route to decrease knee osteoarthritis pain (Adedoyin, 2018).

9.2.33 ABRAXANE®

Abraxane® is produced by Celgene Pharmaceutical Co. Ltd, which is also known as ABI-007, which consists of albumin nanoparticles bound to paclitaxel. The US FDA approved this product for the treatment of metastatic breast cancer in 2005, lung cancer in 2012, and metastatic pancreatic adenocarcinoma in 2013 (Celgene Pharmaceutical Co, NJ, USA, 2005), respectively. It has been reported that the drug paclitaxel interferes with cellular mitosis and prevents microtubule depolymerization, which finally decreases the concentration of tubulin (Celgene Pharmaceutical Co, NJ, USA, 2005; Schwab et al., 2014).

9.2.34 ONTAK®

This formulation is called denileukin diftitox, also known as Ontak®, which was produced by Eisai Company, Japan. In 1999, US FDA has given its approval for the treatment of T-cell lymphoma (Mann et al., 2007; Manoukian and Hagemeister, 2009). Ontak® contains recombinant diphtheria toxin protein, which is conjugated to IL-2 to successfully bind to the IL 2 receptor. It's used in patients who are suffering from leukemia and lymphoma. This drug selectively delivers diphtheria toxin in the target cells, which are known to express interleukin 2 receptors (Kaminetzky and Hymes, 2008). There are a few reports that show that Ontak can also be used in mycosis fungoides treatment (Foss, 2006; Duvic, 2000). This drug also causes many side effects, such as fever, shortness of breath, nausea, low blood pressure, back pain, vomiting, and liver problems (Foss, 2006). In addition, a serious problem with loss of vision was reported in 2006, and considering its major health issues, the FDA finally discontinued this drug in the USA (Schwab et al., 2014).

9.2.35 REBINYN®

Rebinyn® is produced by Novo Nordisk, Bagsværd, Denmark. This drug is a PEG-conjugated glycol-protein drug that received its US FDA approval in 2017. This product is for the treatment of factor IX deficiency or hemophilia (Woods et al., 2018). This formulation contains PEG attached to recombinant DNA-derived coagulation factor IX (Peters and Harris, 2018; Curran and Goa, 2002).

9.2.36 FERAHEME®

This formulation is known as ferumoxytol/Feraheme®/Rienso® made by AMAG Pharmaceuticals, USA. In 2009, the product was approved by the US FDA for the clinical treatment of anemia by intravenous injection (Coyne, 2009; Schwenk, 2010). This drug is generally prescribed in adult patients with signs of iron overload (Curtis et al., 2007). It has been shown that treatment of 510 mg of ferumoxytol through an intravenous is well-accepted in patients (Landry et al., 2005; Spinowitz et al., 2005). There are a few side effects of this drug, such as nausea, diarrhea, hypotension, constipation, dizziness, and peripheral edema (Mccormack, 2012).

9.3 GLOBAL MARKET OF NANO-BASED PRODUCTS

The global nanotechnology market was $1.76 billion in 2020 and is expected to grow to $33.63 billion by 2030 (Allied Market Research, 2022). Nano-based formulations or drugs generally have a high added value compared with traditional pharmaceutical drugs. As this field of nanomedicine is emerging, there is a disparity that has been found regarding its name, like nanotechnology and nanopharmaceutical products have followed different regulatory guidelines in different countries, which makes it difficult to estimate accurate data on the global nanomedicine market size. In 2015, the total market size for nanomedicine was $1 trillion (ETPN—Nanomedicine European Technology Platform). There is a progressive growth rate of some nanopharmaceuticals for treating different types of diseases, such as cancer, immune and nervous system diseases, and infectious diseases, such as AIDS. It has been predicted that the global market is expected to grow by 22% for nanopharmaceutical products (BCC Research, 2014). The market for protein-based nanopharmaceuticals will be about $14 billion; for nucleic acid–based nanopharmaceuticals, it will be $7 ± 3 billion; and for small molecule–based nanopharmaceuticals, it will be $3 ± 3 billion by 2020 (Moghimi et al., 2011).

9.4 MARKET TRENDS OF NANOMEDICINE PRODUCTS

As the field of nanotechnology keeps expanding, there is a great deal of interest among academicians in university laboratories to synthesize various types of novel nanomaterials that have potential applications in the biomedical field (Bajwa et al., 2017). Nanomedicine is extensively used in the treatment of chronic diseases, like (1) cardiovascular diseases, (2) diabetes, (3) cancer, (4) dementia, and others, where it aids in the rapid metabolism of medications in the body. There is an overall increase in scientific research publications and also an increase in patent applications. Only a few patents usually move to the production phase, as the cost of testing in clinical phases of trials is a highly expensive affair and needs a lot of investments and funding. It has been predicted that the worldwide nanomedicine market will reach

$350.8 billion by 2025 per Grand View Research Inc. (Bowman et al., 2017). In another report, it has been reported that the worldwide nanomedicine market was esteemed at $171 billion in 2020, and it's expected to grow to $393 billion by 2030 (Allied Market Research, 2022a). The key market applications, indications, and market players are listed in Figure 9.1. North America remains the most attractive market for the nanomedicine market due to an increase in the number of lethal diseases, an increase in the demand for nanomedicine, the availability of better healthcare and trained medical professionals, a rise in the number of research and development activities, and most importantly, a continuous increase in both government and private company investments. The Asia-Pacific region is also showing a promising increase in nanomedicine application, production, and research developments; and among different Asia-Pacific regions, China and Japan are the most attractive market for nanomedicine products.

9.4.1 KEY DEVELOPMENTS IN THE NANOMEDICINE MARKET

The development of nanomedicine products can meet the global demand for the treatments of various diseases. In 2022, NaNotics LLC, in collaboration with May Clinics, produced NaNot, which is used to target cancer cells. In 2020, Innovasis Inc. received US FDA approval for the 3D implant to be used in spinal cord injury

Key market application	Key market indication	Key market players
Drug delivery	Clinical oncology	Abbott Laboratories
Diagnostics imaging	Infectious diseases	DiaSorin, S.p.A
Regenerative medicine	Clinical cardiology	General Electric
Implants	Orthopedics	Company
Vaccines	Neurology	Invitae Corporation
Others	Urology	Johnson & Johnson
	Ophthalmology	Leadient BioSciences
	Immunology	Inc.
	Others	Mallinckrodt Plc.
		Merck & Co. Inc.
		Pfizer Inc.
		Teva Pharmaceuticals
		Ltd
		Sigma-Tau
		Pharmaceuticals, Inc.
		GE Healthcare
		UCB SA
		Nanosphere, Inc.
		CombiMatrix Corp
		Celgene Corporation

FIGURE 9.1   Key market applications, indications, and players in nanomedicine.

patients, and in 2019, Nanobiotix received approval for the treatment of metastatic tumors (Transparency Market Research, 2021).

9.5 CHALLENGES IN THE NANOMEDICINE MARKET

Recently, there has been a huge number of reports and studies that are related to the nanoformulation of drugs; only a handful of such nanosystems have advanced to market-related assessment. It has been reported that the success of the translation of basic science to clinical application has been less than 10% (Adams, 2012). Consequently, the drug manufacturing process is a time-consuming, expensive, and ineffective series of investigations, which escalates healthcare costs as a whole. One of the main challenges concerns the in vivo behavior of nanoformulations, which is likely to be very different from their in vitro behavior. There are major issues, such as drug-cell interactions, drug transportation, drug diffusion, and drug biocompatibility, which need to be carefully examined in animal models. Additional challenges, particularly for tumor-targeted nanoformulations, are the intricacy and heterogeneous nature of tumor tissues. There are also differences in tumors gene expression, molecular patterns, and degree of drug resistance, which are also main obstacles for poor drug penetration (Park, 2013; Prabhakar et al., 2013; Rosenblum and Peer, 2014; Roointan et al., 2018). Despite promising preclinical data in animals, this effort could lead to an ineffective clinical trial of the tested nanoformulations.

Drug penetration into cancer tissues or tumors can be improved by better targeting the cancer cells where drug-loaded nanomaterials are found to be very effective in both in vitro and in vivo experimentations (Park, 2013). Another aspect is the economic front, where all in vitro and in vivo experimentations and analyses need a large amount of financing. The variation in the multistructure nanoformulations may also pose a challenge to nano-formulation approvals. It has been reported that nanoformulations possess a hybrid structure that may affect the diagnostic and therapeutic results. In addition, more comprehensive experiments are needed to demonstrate the safety and long-term biocompatibility of these nanoformulations (Bregoli et al., 2016; Eetezadi et al., 2015). There are regulatory authority restrictions that may also be time-consuming and expensive affairs to get the approvals for the theranostic nanoformulations. Additionally, most of the nano-formulation production or synthesis is primarily based on chemical reactions, which also need improvements and automation to produce better-quality and pure-quality nanomaterials. For example, batch-to-batch variation is an additional test that can obstruct the manufacture of adequate shares of nanoformulations. The current method of nanomaterial upscaling and characterizations are very laborious, time-consuming, and costly processes (Bregoli et al., 2016; Gabizon et al., 2014; Lammers, 2013).

Some challenges that restrict the market entry of nanomedicine products can be classified as (1) financial challenges, (2) ethical challenges, and (3) regulatory challenges (Satalkar et al., 2016). Regarding financial challenges, most educational or academic research laboratories don't provide funding to produce quality materials (Satalkar et al., 2016). The objective of academic research laboratories is to produce nanomaterials for research purposes only, which leads to either academic and research publications or patent applications. Hence, these academic institutes or universities don't produce nanomaterials that can be used in clinical trials, as these institutes or universities don't have the fund to produce quality or clinical-grade materials. These are challenges that current institutes or universities are facing (Satalkar et al., 2016).

Besides financial and regulatory issues, there are ethical issues that also affect the business and market of nanomaterial-based products. It has been reported that most clinical trials using nanomaterials have been performed on patients who are suffering from incurable diseases or patients who have received many different treatments (Kimmelman, 2012). Despite the outcome of these clinical trials, most of the clinical participants are doubtful to get clinical improvement in their disease condition. The main challenge is the first phase of clinical trials, where the benefit or harm ratio on the health of patients caused by the nanoformulation is still well understood (Satalkar et al., 2016; Kimmelman, 2012; Van De Poel, 2008).

The recognized regulations laid down by drug authorities in different countries across the globe are another challenge on the road to new nanoformulations. The regulations by EMA and the US FDA are different from each other, and these regulations are always undergoing some periodical changes. Therefore, such regulations can meaningfully affect the whole process of clinical trials (Satalkar et al., 2016). Once it has been decided that the clinical trial needs to be planned and executed for a new nanoformulation, different drug authorities with their strict regulations will arrive on the scene. Although they can provide a source of valuable information and advice, especially in the design and development of clinical trials, their regulations usually involve differences between national and ethnic groups, and occasionally, there is a request for different clinical trials on individuals from different national or ethnic groups. Delivery of precise and detailed information about the nanocharacterization and safety of the nanomedicine to the drug authorities could also be another roadblock (Satalkar et al., 2016).

REFERENCES

Abbott Laboratories. *Tricor® Fenofibrate Tablet*. Prescribing Information. 2010. [Google Scholar].

Abbott Laboratories Press Release. *Nanoparticle Technology Now Allows TriCor(R) to be Taken with or Without Food*. 2004. www.abbottinvestor.com/news-releases/news-release-details/abbott-receives-fda-approval-new-formulation-tricorr-fenofibrate [Google Scholar].

Adams DJ. The valley of death in anticancer drug development: A reassessment. *Trends Pharmacol. Sci.* 2012;33(4):173–180. [PMC free article] [PubMed] [Google Scholar].

Adedoyin AA. *Development of Injectable, Stimuli-Responsive Biomaterials as Active Scaffolds for Applications in Advanced Drug Delivery and Osteochondral Tissue Regeneration*. Doctoral dissertation, Northeastern University. 2018.

Alagona P, Jr. Fenofibric acid: A new fibrate approved for use in combination with statin for the treatment of mixed dyslipidemia. *Vasc. Health Risk Manag.* 2010;6(1):351–362. [PMC free article] [PubMed] [Google Scholar].

Alconcel SNS, Baas AS, Maynard HD. FDA-approved poly (ethylene glycol)-protein conjugate drugs. *Polym. Chem.* 2011;2(7):1442–1448. [Google Scholar]

Allen C. Why I'm holding onto hope for nano in oncology. *Mol. Pharm.* 2016;13(8): 2603–2604. [PubMed] [Google Scholar].

Allied Market Research. 2022a. www.alliedmarketresearch.com/nanomedicine-market#:~:-text=The%20global%20nanomedicine%20market%20size,prevention%20and%20 treatment%20of%20diseases.

Allied Market Research. 2022b. www.alliedmarketresearch.com/nanotechnology-market.

Andreopoulou E, Gaiotti D, Kim E et al. Pegylated liposomal doxorubicin HCL (PLD; Caelyx/ Doxil®): Experience with long-term maintenance in responding patients with recurrent epithelial ovarian cancer. *Ann. Oncol.* 2007;18(4):716–721. [PubMed] [Google Scholar].

Andrews PLR, Kovacs M, Watson JW. The anti-emetic action of the neurokinin₁ receptor antagonist CP-99,994 does not require the presence of the area postrema in the dog. *Neurosci. Lett.* 2001;314(1–2):102–104. [PubMed] [Google Scholar].

Arnon R, Aharoni R. Mechanism of action of glatiramer acetate in multiple sclerosis and its potential for the development of new applications. *Proc. Natl Acad. Sci. USA.* 2004;101(Suppl. 2):14593–14598. [PMC free article] [PubMed] [Google Scholar].

Arnsten AF, Li B-M. Neurobiology of executive functions: Catecholamine influences on pre-frontal cortical functions. *Biol. Psychiatry.* 2005;57(11):1377–1384. [PubMed] [Google Scholar].

Association EM. *Scientific Discussion: Summary of Product Characteristics: MIRCERA (Methoxy Polyethyl-Ene Glycol-Epoetin Beta).* 2008. https://www.ema.europa.eu/en/ documents/scientific-discussion/mircera-epar-scientific-discussion_en.pdf

Bajwa S, Munawar A, Khan W. Nanotechnology in medicine: Innovation to market. *Pharm. Bioprocess.* 2017;5(2):11–15. [Google Scholar]

BCC Research. *Global Markets for Nanoparticle Size Analysis Instrumentation in the Life Sciences.* 2014. www.bccresearch.com/market-research/biotechnology/nanoparticle-size-analysis-instrumentation-life-sciences-report-bio114b.html.

Behabtu N, Young CC, Tsentalovich DE et al. Strong, light, multifunctional fibers of carbon nanotubes with ultrahigh conductivity. *Science.* 2013;339(6116):182–186. [PubMed] [Google Scholar].

Berges R. Eligard®: Pharmacokinetics, effect on testosterone and PSA levels and tolerability. *Eur. Urol. Suppl.* 2005;4(5):20–25. [Google Scholar].

Biggers K, Scheinfeld N. Pegloticase, a polyethylene glycol conjugate of uricase for the potential intravenous treatment of gout. *Curr. Opin. Investig. Drugs.* 2008;9(4):422–429. [PubMed] [Google Scholar]

Bobo D, Robinson KJ, Islam J, Thurecht KJ, Corrie SR. Nanoparticle-based medicines: A review of FDA-approved materials and clinical trials to date. *Pharm. Res.* 2016;33(10):2373–2387. [PubMed] [Google Scholar].

Boman NL, Masin D, Mayer LD, Cullis PR, Bally MB. Liposomal vincristine which exhibits increased drug retention and increased circulation longevity cures mice bearing P388 tumors. *Cancer Res.* 1994;54(11):2830–2833. [PubMed] [Google Scholar].

Bowman D, Marino AD, Sylvester DJ. The patent landscape of nanomedicines. *Med. Res. Arch.* 2017;5(9). [Google Scholar].

Brandt J, Henning S, Michler G, Hein W, Bernstein A, Schulz M. Nanocrystalline hydroxyapa-tite for bone repair: An animal study. *J. Mater. Sci. Mater. Med.* 2010;21(1):283–294. [PubMed] [Google Scholar].

Bregoli L, Movia D, Gavigan-Imedio JD, Lysaght J, Reynolds J, Prina-Mello A. Nanomedicine applied to translational oncology: A future perspective on cancer treatment. *Nanomed. Nanotechnol. Biol. Med.* 2016;12(1):81–103. [PubMed] [Google Scholar].

Bressler NM. Treatment of age-related macular degeneration with photodynamic therapy study G. Photodynamic therapy of subfoveal choroidal neovascularization in age-related mac-ular degeneration with verteporfin: Two-year results of 2 randomized clinical trials-tap report 2. *Arch. Ophthalmol.* 2001;119(2):198–207. [PubMed] [Google Scholar].

Bunka DHJ, Platonova O, Stockley PG. Development of aptamer therapeutics. *Curr. Opin. Pharmacol.* 2010;10(5):557–562. [PubMed] [Google Scholar].

Buster JE. Transdermal menopausal hormone therapy: Delivery through skin changes the rules. *Expert Opin. Pharmacother.* 2010;11(9):1489–1499. [PubMed] [Google Scholar].

Byers-Kraus V, Aazami H, Mehra P et al. Synovial and systemic pharmacokinetics of triamcinolone acetonide following intra-articular injection of an extended release formulation (FX006) or standard crystalline suspension in patients with knee osteoarthritis. *Osteoarthr. Cartil.* 2017;25:S431. [PubMed] [Google Scholar].

Camarata PJ, Dunn DL, Farney AC, Parker RG, Seljeskog EL. Continual intracavitary administration of amphotericin B as an adjunct in the treatment of aspergillus brain abscess: Case report and review of the literature. *Neurosurgery.* 1992;31(3):575–579. [PubMed] [Google Scholar].

Campion CR, Ball SL, Clarke DL, Hing KA. Microstructure and chemistry affects apatite nucleation on calcium phosphate bone graft substitutes. *J. Mater. Sci. Mater. Med.* 2013;24(3):597–610. [PubMed] [Google Scholar].

Casanova JL, Abel L. Revisiting Crohn's disease as a primary immunodeficiency of macrophages. *J. Exp. Med.* 2009;206(9):1839–1843. [PMC free article] [PubMed] [Google Scholar].

Celgene Pharmaceutical Co. *Abraxane® for Injectable Suspension.* Prescribing Information. 2005. [Google Scholar].

Centonze D, Puma E, Saleri C et al. Pegylation and interferons in multiple sclerosis. *Farmeconomia.* 2016;17(Suppl. 2):5–11. [Google Scholar].

Chaplin S, Gnanapavan S. Plegridy for the treatment of RRMS in adults. *Prescriber.* 2015;26(9):29–31. [Google Scholar].

Clemons KV, Stevens DA. Comparative efficacies of four amphotericin B formulations—Fungizone, Amphotec (Amphocil), AmBisome, and Abelcet—against systemic murine aspergillosis. *Antimicrob. Agents Chemother.* 2004;48(3):1047–1050. [PMC free article] [PubMed] [Google Scholar].

Connock M, Tubeuf S, Malottki K et al. Certolizumab pegol (CIMZIA®) for the treatment of rheumatoid arthritis. *Health Technol. Assess.* 2010;14(Suppl 2):1–10. [PubMed] [Google Scholar].

Conroy T, Desseigne F, Ychou M et al. FOLFIRINOX versus gemcitabine for metastatic pancreatic cancer. *N. Engl. J. Med.* 2011;364(19):1817–1825. [PubMed] [Google Scholar].

Coyne DW. Ferumoxytol for treatment of iron deficiency anemia in patients with chronic kidney disease. *Expert Opin. Pharmacother.* 2009;10(15):2563–2568. [PubMed] [Google Scholar].

Crain ML. Daunorubicin & CYTARABINE LIPOSome (Vyxeos™). *Oncology Times.* 2018;40(10):30. [Google Scholar].

Curran MP, Goa KL. Pegfilgrastim. *Drugs.* 2002;62(8):1207–1213. [PubMed] [Google Scholar]

Curtis BM, Barrett BJ, Djurdjev O, Singer J, Levin A, Group C-CI. Evaluation and treatment of CKD patients before and at their first nephrologist encounter in Canada. *Am. J. Kidney Dis.* 2007;50(5):733–742. [PubMed] [Google Scholar].

Davis ME, Chen Z, Shin DM. Nanoparticle therapeutics: An emerging treatment modality for cancer. *Nat. Rev. Drug Discov.* 2008;7(9):771–782. [PubMed] [Google Scholar].

Davis S, Abuchowski A, Park YK, Davis FF. Alteration of the circulating life and antigenic properties of bovine adenosine deaminase in mice by attachment of polyethylene glycol. *Clin. Exp. Immunol.* 1981;46(3):649–652. [PMC free article] [PubMed] [Google Scholar].

Dawidczyk CM, Kim C, Park JH et al. State-of-the-art in design rules for drug delivery platforms: Lessons learned from FDA-approved nanomedicines. *J. Control. Rel.* 2014;187:133–144. [PMC free article] [PubMed] [Google Scholar].

Diller LH. The run on Ritalin: Attention deficit disorder and stimulant treatment in the 1990s. *Hastings Cent. Rep.* 1996;26(2):12–18. [PubMed] [Google Scholar]

Doward J, Craig E. Ritalin use for ADHD children soars fourfold. *Observer.* 2012:6. [Google Scholar].

Duncan R. The dawning era of polymer therapeutics. *Nat. Rev. Drug Discov.* 2003;2(5):347–360. [PubMed] [Google Scholar].

Duncan R. Polymer therapeutics: Top 10 selling pharmaceuticals–what next? *J. Control. Release.* 2014;190:371–380. [PubMed] [Google Scholar].

Duvic M. Bexarotene and DAB389IL-2 (Denileukin Diftitox, ONTAK) in treatment of cutaneous T-cell lymphomas: Algorithms. *Clin. Lymphoma.* 2000;1:S51–S55. [PubMed] [Google Scholar].

Eetezadi S, Ekdawi SN, Allen C. The challenges facing block copolymer micelles for cancer therapy: *in vivo* barriers and clinical translation. *Adv. Drug Del. Rev.* 2015;91:7–22. [PubMed] [Google Scholar]

Enzon Pharmaceuticals Inc. *Oncaspar® (Pegaspargase) Intravenous or Intramuscular Injection* [Prescribing Information]. 2006. [Google Scholar]

Eric DK. *Engines of Creation. The Coming Era of Nanotechnology.* Doubleday, 1986. [Google Scholar].

ETPN—Nanomedicine European Technology Platform. *Src, Ncpm, Ncrd. Strategic Agenda for EuroNanoMed.* https://etp-nanomedicine.eu/about-nanomedicine/strategic-research-and-innovation-agenda/.

Farjadian F, Ghasemi A, Gohari O, Roointan A, Karimi M, Hamblin MR. Nanopharmaceuticals and nanomedicines currently on the market: Challenges and opportunities. *Nanomedicine (Lond).* 2019 Jan;14(1):93–126. doi: 10.2217/nnm-2018-0120. Epub 2018 Nov 19. PMID: 30451076; PMCID: PMC6391637.

Fassas A, Anagnostopoulos A. The use of liposomal daunorubicin (DaunoXome) in acute myeloid leukemia. *Leuk. Lymphoma.* 2005;46(6):795–802. [PubMed] [Google Scholar].

FDA, *FDA Approves Irinotecan Liposome to Treat Pancreatic Cancer.* 2015. https://www.cancer.gov/news-events/cancer-currents-blog/2015/irinotecan-liposome-pancreatic#:~:text=On%20October%2022%2C%20the%20U.S.,progressed%20after%20gemcitabine%2Dbased%20chemotherapy.

FDA. *Rebinyn: Coagulation Factor IX (Recombinant), GlycoPEGylated.* 2017. [Google Scholar].

FDA approves DaunoXome as first-line therapy for Kaposi's sarcoma. Food and Drug Administration. *J. Int. Assoc. Phys. AIDS Care.* 1996;2(5):50–51. [PubMed] [Google Scholar].

Feynman RP. There's plenty of room at the bottom. *Eng. Sci.* 1960;23(5):22–36. [Google Scholar] The very first inkling of what would become the nanotechology revolution.

Food and Drug Administration (FDA). Label and Approval History KRYSTEXXA BLA 125293 Savient Pharm. 2010.

Foss F. Clinical experience with denileukin diftitox (ONTAK). *Semin. Oncol.* 2006;33(1 Suppl. 3):S11–S16. [PubMed] [Google Scholar].

Fosså S, Aass N, Parö G. A phase II study of DaunoXome® in advanced urothelial transitional cell carcinoma. *Eur. J. Cancer.* 1998;34(7):1131–1132. [PubMed] [Google Scholar].

Fried MW, Shiffman ML, Rajender Reddy K et al. Peginterferon alfa-2a plus ribavirin for chronic hepatitis C virus infection. *N. Engl. J. Med.* 2002;347(13):975–982. [PubMed] [Google Scholar].

Frimat L, Mariat C, Landais P, Koné S, Commenges B, Choukroun G. Anaemia management with CERA in routine clinical practice: OCEANE (Cohorte Mircera patients non-dialyses), a national, multicenter, longitudinal, observational prospective study, in patients with chronic kidney disease not on dialysis. *BMJ Open.* 2013;3(3):e001888. [PMC free article] [PubMed] [Google Scholar].

Gabizon A, Bradbury M, Prabhakar U, Zamboni W, Libutti S, Grodzinski P. Cancer nanomedicines: Closing the translational gap. *Lancet.* 2014;384(9961):2175–2176. [PMC free article] [PubMed] [Google Scholar].

Gabizon AA, Shmeeda H, Zalipsky S. Pros and cons of the liposome platform in cancer drug targeting. *J. Liposome Res.* 2006;16(3):175–183. [PubMed] [Google Scholar].

Galmarini CM, Thomas X, Calvo F et al. *In vivo* mechanisms of resistance to cytarabine in acute myeloid leukaemia. *Br. J. Haematol.* 2002;117(4):860–868. [PubMed] [Google Scholar].

Gill PS, Wernz J, Scadden DT et al. Randomized phase III trial of liposomal daunorubicin versus doxorubicin, bleomycin, and vincristine in AIDS-related Kaposi's sarcoma. *J. Clin. Oncol.* 1996;14(8):2353–2364. [PubMed] [Google Scholar].

Glue P, Fang JW, Rouzier-Panis R et al. Pegylated interferon-α2b: Pharmacokinetics, pharmacodynamics, safety, and preliminary efficacy data. *Clin. Pharmacol. Ther.* 2000;68(5):556–567. [PubMed] [Google Scholar].

Gordon AN, Granai C, Rose PG et al. Phase II study of liposomal doxorubicin in platinum-and paclitaxel-refractory epithelial ovarian cancer. *J. Clin. Oncol.* 2000;18(17):3093–3100. [PubMed] [Google Scholar].

Gragoudas ES, Adamis AP, Cunningham ETJ, Feinsod M, Guyer DR. Pegaptanib for neovascular age-related macular degeneration. *N. Engl. J. Med.* 2004;351(27):2805–2816. [PubMed] [Google Scholar].

Graham ML. Pegaspargase: A review of clinical studies. *Adv. Drug Del. Rev.* 2003;55(10): 1293–1302. [PubMed] [Google Scholar].

Greenwald RB, Choe YH, Mcguire J, Conover CD. Effective drug-delivery by PEGylated drug conjugates. *Adv. Drug Del. Rev.* 2003;55(2):217–250. [PubMed] [Google Scholar]

Grewal IS. *Emerging Protein Biotherapeutics*. CRC Press, Boca Raton, 2009. [Google Scholar]

Handen BL, Feldman H, Gosling A, Breaux AM, Mcauliffe S. Adverse side effects of methylphenidate among mentally retarded children with ADHD. *J. Am. Acad. Child Adolesc. Psychiatry.* 1991;30(2):241–245. [PubMed] [Google Scholar]

Harris G. Warning urged on stimulants like Ritalin. *New York Times.* 2006:10. [Google Scholar].

Harrison TS, Lyseng-Williamson KA. Vincristine sulfate liposome injection. *Biodrugs.* 2013;27(1):69–74. [PubMed] [Google Scholar]

Hogan A, Behan U, Kilmartin DJ. Outcomes after combination photodynamic therapy and immunosuppression for inflammatory subfoveal choroidal neovascularisation. *Br. J. Ophthalmol.* 2005;89(9):1109–1111. [PMC free article] [PubMed] [Google Scholar].

Huber FX, Belyaev O, Hillmeier J et al. First histological observations on the incorporation of a novel nanocrystalline hydroxyapatite paste OSTIM® in human cancellous bone. *BMC Musculoskelet. Disord.* 2006;7(50). [PMC free article] [PubMed] [Google Scholar].

Hunt RD. Functional roles of norepinephrine and dopamine in ADHD. *Medscape Psychiatr.* 2006;11(1):2006. [Google Scholar].

Idec B. *Plegridy Prescribing Information.* 2015. https://www.accessdata.fda.gov/drugsatfda_docs/label/2014/125499lbl.pdf

Jacobson IM, Brown RS, Freilich B et al. Peginterferon alfa-2b and weight-based or flat-dose ribavirin in chronic hepatitis C patients: A randomized trial. *Hepatology.* 2007;46(4):971–981. [PubMed] [Google Scholar].

Jaeckle KA, Batchelor T, O'day SJ et al. An open label trial of sustained-release cytarabine (DepoCyt™) for the intrathecal treatment of solid tumor neoplastic meningitis. *J. Neurooncol.* 2002;57(3):231–239. [PubMed] [Google Scholar].

Johnson KP. Glatiramer acetate for treatment of relapsing-remitting multiple sclerosis. *Expert Rev. Neurother.* 2012;12(4):371–384. [PubMed] [Google Scholar].

Joralemon MJ, Mcrae S, Emrick T. PEGylated polymers for medicine: From conjugation to self-assembled systems. *Chem. Commun.* 2010;46(9):1377–1393. [PubMed] [Google Scholar].

Junghanns jUaH, Müller RH. Nanocrystal technology, drug delivery and clinical applications. *Int. J. Nanomed.* 2008;3(3):295–309. [PMC free article] [PubMed] [Google Scholar]

Kaminetzky D, Hymes KB. Denileukin diftitox for the treatment of cutaneous T-cell lymphoma. *Biologics.* 2008;2(4):717–724. [PMC free article] [PubMed] [Google Scholar].

Kesisoglou F, Panmai S, Wu Y. Nanosizing—oral formulation development and biopharmaceutical evaluation. *Adv. Drug Del. Rev.* 2007;59(7):631–644. [PubMed] [Google Scholar]

Kim S, Chatelut E, Kim JC et al. Extended CSF cytarabine exposure following intrathecal administration of DTC 101. *J. Clin. Oncol.* 1993;11(11):2186–2193. [PubMed] [Google Scholar].

Kimmelman J. Beyond human subjects: Risk, ethics, and clinical development of nanomedicines. *J. Law Med. Ethics.* 2012;40(4):841–847. [PubMed] [Google Scholar].

Konkle BA, Stasyshyn O, Chowdary P et al. Pegylated, full-length, recombinant factor VIII for prophylactic and on-demand treatment of severe hemophilia A. *Blood.* 2015;126(9):1078–1085. [PMC free article] [PubMed] [Google Scholar].

Lammers T. Smart drug delivery systems: Back to the future vs. clinical reality. *Int. J. Pharm.* 2013;454(1):527–529. [PMC free article] [PubMed] [Google Scholar]

Landewé R, Braun J, Deodhar A et al. Efficacy of certolizumab pegol on signs and symptoms of axial spondyloarthritis including ankylosing spondylitis: 24-week results of a double-blind randomised placebo-controlled Phase 3 study. *Ann. Rheum. Dis.* 2013;73(1):39–47. [PMC free article] [PubMed] [Google Scholar].

Landry R, Jacobs PM, Davis R, Shenouda M, Bolton WK. Pharmacokinetic study of ferumoxytol: A new iron replacement therapy in normal subjects and hemodialysis patients. *Am. J. Nephrol.* 2005;25(4):400–410. [PubMed] [Google Scholar].

Lange KW, Reichl S, Lange KM, Tucha L, Tucha O. The history of attention deficit hyperactivity disorder. *Atten. Defic. Hyperact. Disord.* 2010;2(4):241–255. [PMC free article] [PubMed] [Google Scholar].

Lasic DD. Doxorubicin in sterically stabilized liposomes. *Nature.* 1996;380(6574):561. [PubMed] [Google Scholar].

Lau GKK, Piratvisuth T, Kang XL et al. Peginterferon Alfa-2a, lamivudine, and the combination for hBeAg-positive chronic hepatitis B. *N. Engl. J. Med.* 2005;352(26):2682–2695. [PubMed] [Google Scholar].

Leonart LP, Tonin FS, Ferreira VL et al. Effectiveness and safety of pegvisomant: A systematic review and meta-analysis of observational longitudinal studies. *Endocrine.* 2018;63:18–26.

Liu R. Methods of making liposomes containing hydro-monobenzoporphyrin photosensitizer. *US Patent.* 1998:5707608.

Maggi CA. The mammalian tachykinin receptors. *Gen. Pharmacol.* 1995;26(5):911–944. [PubMed] [Google Scholar].

Mann BS, Johnson JR, Cohen MH, Justice R, Pazdur R. FDA approval summary: Vorinostat for treatment of advanced primary cutaneous T-cell lymphoma. *Oncologist.* 2007;12(10):1247–1252. [PubMed] [Google Scholar].

Manns M, Pockros P, Norkrans G et al. Long-term clearance of hepatitis C virus following interferon α-2b or peginterferon α-2b, alone or in combination with ribavirin. *J. Viral Hepat.* 2013;20(8):524–529. [PubMed] [Google Scholar].

Manoukian G, Hagemeister F. Denileukin diftitox: A novel immunotoxin. *Expert Opin. Biol. Ther.* 2009;9(11):1445–1451. [PubMed] [Google Scholar]

Mantripragada S. A lipid based depot (DepoFoam® technology) for sustained release drug delivery. *Prog. Lipid Res.* 2002;41(5):392–406. [PubMed] [Google Scholar].

Markowitz J, Devane C, Ramamoorthy S, Zhu H-J. The psychostimulant d-threo-(R,R)-methylphenidate binds as an agonist to the 5HT1A receptor. *Die Pharmazie.* 2009;64(2):123–125. [PubMed] [Google Scholar].

Marya S, Ariyanayagam T, Chatterjee B, Toms AP, Crawford R. A prospective study of the efficacy of vitoss (beta tricalcium phosphate) as a bone graft substitute for instrumented posterolateral lumbar fusions. *Spine J.* 2017;17(3):S23. [Google Scholar].

Mayer L, Liboiron B, Xie S, Tardi P, Paulsen K, Chiarella M. *VYXEOS™(CPX-351) Significantly Improves Overall Survival in Phase 3 High-Risk AML Trial, Validating the CombiPlex Technology and Opening Opportunities for Novel Combinations Lawrence*

Mayer, Barry Liboiron, Sherwin Xie and Paul Tardi, Kim Paulsen, Michael Chiarella and Arthur Louie. 2016. www.controlledreleasesociety.org/meetings/Documents/2016%20 Abstracts/33.pdf

Mccormack PL. Ferumoxytol. *Drugs.* 2012;72(15):2013–2022. [PubMed] [Google Scholar].

Mcgahan L. Continuous erythropoietin receptor activator (Mircera) for renal anemia. *Issues Emerg. Health Technol.* 2008;(113):1–6. [PubMed] [Google Scholar].

Mckeage K. Glatiramer acetate 40 mg/mL in relapsing-remitting multiple sclerosis: A review. *CNS Drugs.* 2015;29(5):425–432. [PubMed] [Google Scholar].

Mease P, Fleischmann R, Deodhar AA et al. Effect of certolizumab pegol on signs and symptoms in patients with psoriatic arthritis: 24 week results of a Phase 3 double-blind randomised placebo-controlled study (RAPID-PsA). *Ann. Rheum. Dis.* 2013;73(1):48–55. [PMC free article] [PubMed] [Google Scholar].

Merck & Co., Inc., NJ, USA. *Emend® (Aprepitant) Capsules, for Oral Use and Oral Suspension.* Prescribing Information. 2015. [Google Scholar].

Milton HJ, Chess RB. Effect of pegylation on pharmaceuticals. *Nat. Rev. Drug Discov.* 2003;2(3):214–221. [PubMed] [Google Scholar].

Moghimi SM, Peer D, Langer R. Reshaping the future of nanopharmaceuticals: Adiudicium. *ACS Nano.* 2011;5(11):8454–8458. [PubMed] [Google Scholar].

Mott TF, Leach L. Is methylphenidate useful for treating adolescents with ADHD? *J. Fam. Pract.* 2004;53(9):650–663. [PubMed] [Google Scholar].

Murphy T, Yee KW. Cytarabine and daunorubicin for the treatment of acute myeloid leukemia. *Expert Opin. Pharmacother.* 2017;18(16):1765–1780. [PubMed] [Google Scholar].

Narayan R, Pednekar A, Bhuyan D, Gowda C, Koteshwara K, Nayak UY. A top-down technique to improve the solubility and bioavailability of aceclofenac: *in vitro* and *in vivo* studies. *Int. J. Nanomed.* 2017;12:4921. [PMC free article] [PubMed] [Google Scholar].

Nesbitt A, Fossati G, Bergin M et al. Mechanism of action of certolizumab pegol (CDP870): *In vitro* comparison with other anti-tumor necrosis factor α agents. *Inflamm. Bowel Dis.* 2007;13(11):1323–1332. [PubMed] [Google Scholar].

Ng EWM, Shima DT, Calias P, Cunningham ET, Guyer DR, Adamis AP. Pegaptanib, a targeted anti-VEGF aptamer for ocular vascular disease. *Nat. Rev. Drug Discov.* 2006;5(2): 123–132. [PubMed] [Google Scholar].

Oka Y, Miyazaki M, Takatsu S et al. A review article: Sevelamer hydrochloride and metabolic acidosis in dialysis patients. *Cardiovasc. Hematol. Disord. Drug Targets.* 2008;8(4): 283–286. [PubMed] [Google Scholar].

Park JW. Liposome-based drug delivery in breast cancer treatment. *Breast Cancer Res.* 2002;4(3):95. [PMC free article] [PubMed] [Google Scholar]

Park K. Facing the truth about nanotechnology in drug delivery. *ACS Nano.* 2013;7(9): 7442–7447. [PMC free article] [PubMed] [Google Scholar].

Parodi MB, Iacono P, Spasse S, Ravalico G. Photodynamic therapy for juxtafoveal choroidal neovascularization associated with multifocal choroiditis. *Am. J. Ophthalmol.* 2006;141(1):123–128. [PubMed] [Google Scholar].

Passero FC, Jr, Grapsa D, Syrigos KN, Saif MW. The safety and efficacy of Onivyde (irinotecan liposome injection) for the treatment of metastatic pancreatic cancer following gemcitabine-based therapy. *Expert Rev. Anticancer Ther.* 2016;16(7):697–703. [PubMed] [Google Scholar].

Pearce H, Winter M, Beck WT. Structural characteristics of compounds that modulate P-glycoprotein-associated multidrug resistance. *Adv. Enzyme Regul.* 1990;30:357–373. [PubMed] [Google Scholar]

Peters BG, Goeckner BJ, Ponzillo JJ, Velasquez WS, Wilson AL. Pegaspargase versus asparaginase in adult ALL: A pharmacoeconomic assessment. *Formulary.* 1995;30(7): 388–393. [PubMed] [Google Scholar].

Peters R, Harris T. Advances and innovations in haemophilia treatment. *Nat. Rev. Drug Discov.* 2018;17(7):493–508. [PubMed] [Google Scholar].

Piedmonte DM, Treuheit MJ. Formulation of Neulasta®(pegfilgrastim) *Adv. Drug Del. Rev.* 2008;60(1):50–58. [PubMed] [Google Scholar].

Pillai G, Ceballos-Coronel ML. Science and technology of the emerging nanomedicines in cancer therapy: A primer for physicians and pharmacists. *SAGE Open Med.* 2013;1 [PMC free article] [PubMed] [Google Scholar].

Prabhakar U, Maeda H, Jain RK et al. Challenges and key considerations of the enhanced permeability and retention effect for nanomedicine drug delivery in oncology. *Cancer Res.* 2013;73(8):2412–2417. [PMC free article] [PubMed] [Google Scholar].

Prausnitz MR, Langer R. Transdermal drug delivery. *Nat. Biotechnol.* 2008;26(11):1261–1268. [PMC free article] [PubMed] [Google Scholar]

Rai MF, Pham CT. Intra-articular drug delivery systems for joint diseases. *Curr. Opin. Pharmacol.* 2018;40:67–73. [PMC free article] [PubMed] [Google Scholar]

Roelfsema F, Biermasz NR, Pereira AM, Romijn J. Nanomedicines in the treatment of acromegaly: Focus on pegvisomant. *Int. J. Nanomed.* 2006;1(4):385–398. [PMC free article] [PubMed] [Google Scholar].

Rogers AH, Duker JS, Nichols N, Baker BJ. Photodynamic therapy of idiopathic and inflammatory choroidal neovascularization in young adults. *Ophthalmology.* 2003;110(7):1315–1320. [PubMed] [Google Scholar].

Roila F, Herrstedt J, Aapro M et al. Guideline update for MASCC and ESMO in the prevention of chemotherapy-and radiotherapy-induced nausea and vomiting: Results of the Perugia consensus conference. *Ann. Oncol.* 2010;21(Suppl. 5) [PubMed] [Google Scholar].

Roointan A, Kianpour S, Memari F, Gandomani M, Gheibi Hayat SM, Mohammadi-Samani S. Poly(lactic-*co*-glycolic acid): The most ardent and flexible candidate in biomedicine! *Int. J. Polym. Materi. Polym. Biomater.* 2018;67(17):1028–1049. [Google Scholar].

Rosenbaum DP, Holmes-Farley SR, Mandeville WH, Pitruzzello M, Goldberg DI. Effect of RenaGel, a non-absorbable, cross-linked, polymeric phosphate binder, on urinary phosphorus excretion in rats. *Nephrol. Dial. Transplant.* 1997;12(5):961–964. [PubMed] [Google Scholar].

Rosenblum DP, Peer D. Omics-based nanomedicine: The future of personalized oncology. *Cancer Lett.* 2014;352(1):126–136. [PubMed] [Google Scholar].

Sandborn WJ, Feagan BG, Stoinov S et al. Certolizumab pegol for the treatment of Crohn's disease. *N. Engl. J. Med.* 2007;357(3):228–238. [PubMed] [Google Scholar].

Sartor O. Eligard: Leuprolide acetate in a novel sustained-release delivery system. *Urology.* 2003;61(2):25–31. [PubMed] [Google Scholar].

Satalkar P, Elger BS, Hunziker P, Shaw D. Challenges of clinical translation in nanomedicine: A qualitative study. *Nanomedicine.* 2016;12(4):893–900. [PubMed] [Google Scholar].

Schwab CL, English DP, Roque DM, Pasternak M, Santin AD. Past, present and future targets for immunotherapy in ovarian cancer. *Immunotherapy.* 2014;6(12):1279–1293. [PMC free article] [PubMed] [Google Scholar]

Schwenk MH. Ferumoxytol: A new intravenous iron preparation for the treatment of iron deficiency anemia in patients with chronic kidney disease. *Pharmacotherapy.* 2010;30(1):70–79. [PubMed] [Google Scholar].

Sehgal SN. Rapamune® (RAPA, rapamycin, sirolimus): Mechanism of action immunosuppressive effect results from blockade of signal transduction and inhibition of cell cycle progression. *Clin. Biochem.* 1998;31(5):335–340. [PubMed] [Google Scholar].

Shegokar R, Müller RH. Nanocrystals: Industrially feasible multifunctional formulation technology for poorly soluble actives. *Int. J. Pharm.* 2010;399(1–2):129–139. [PubMed] [Google Scholar]

Sheridan WP, Fox RM, Begley CG et al. Effect of peripheral-blood progenitor cells mobilised by filgrastim (G-CSF) on platelet recovery after high-dose chemotherapy. *Lancet.* 1992;339(8794):640–644. [PubMed] [Google Scholar]

Shukla D, Namperumalsamy P, Goldbaum M, Cunningham E Jr, Pegaptanib sodium for ocular vascular disease. *Indian J. Ophthalmol.* 2007;55(6):427–430. [PMC free article] [PubMed] [Google Scholar].

Sigma-Tau Pharmaceuticals, Inc., MD, USA. *Adagen®* *(Pegademase Bovine) Injection*. Pre-scribing Information. 2014. [Google Scholar].

Simon JA, Group FTES. Estradiol in micellar nanoparticles: The efficacy and safety of a novel transdermal drug-delivery technology in the management of moderate to severe vasomo-tor symptoms. *Menopause*. 2006;13(2):222–231. [PubMed] [Google Scholar]

Slatopolsky EA, Burke SK, Dillon MA. RenaGel, a nonabsorbed calcium—and aluminum-free phosphate binder, lowers serum phosphorus and parathyroid hormone. The RenaGel Study Group. *Kidney Int*. 1999;55(1):299–307. [PubMed] [Google Scholar].

Spaia S. Phosphate binders: Sevelamer in the prevention and treatment of hyperphosphatae-mia in chronic renal failure. *Hippokratia*. 2011;15(Suppl. 1):22–26. [PMC free article] [PubMed] [Google Scholar].

Spinowitz BS, Schwenk MH, Jacobs PM et al. The safety and efficacy of ferumoxytol ther-apy in anemic chronic kidney disease patients. *Kidney Int*. 2005;68(4):1801–1807. [PubMed] [Google Scholar].

Steele M, Weiss M, Swanson J, Wang J, Prinzo RS, Binder CE. A randomized, controlled effectiveness trial of OROS-methylphenidate compared to usual care with immediate-release methylphenidate in attention deficit-hyperactivity disorder. *Can. J. Clin. Phar-macol*. 2006;13(1):e50–e62. [PubMed] [Google Scholar].

Stephan J, Vlekova V, Le Deist F et al. Severe combined immunodeficiency: A retrospective single-center study of clinical presentation and outcome in 117 patients. *J. Pediatrics*. 1993;123(4):564–572. [PubMed] [Google Scholar].

Stone NRH, Bicanic T, Salim R, Hope W. Liposomal Amphotericin B (AmBisome®): A review of the pharmacokinetics, pharmacodynamics, clinical experience and future directions. *Drugs*. 2016;76(4):485–500. [PMC free article] [PubMed] [Google Scholar].

Swanson JM, Wigal SB, Wigal T et al. A comparison of once-daily extended-release methyl-phenidate formulations in children with attention-deficit/hyperactivity disorder in the laboratory school (the Comacs Study). *Pediatrics*. 2004;113(3):e206–e216. [PubMed] [Google Scholar].

Tadic D, Epple M. A thorough physicochemical characterisation of 14 calcium phosphate-based bone substitution materials in comparison to natural bone. *Biomaterials*. 2004;25(6):987–994. [PubMed] [Google Scholar].

Takayama N, Sato N, O'Brien SG, Ikeda Y, Okamoto SI. Imatinib mesylate has limited activity against the central nervous system involvement of Philadelphia chromosome-positive acute lymphoblastic leukaemia due to poor penetration into cerebrospinal fluid. *Br. J. Haematol*. 2002;119(1):106–108. [PubMed] [Google Scholar].

Takemoto K, Kanazawa K. AmBisome: Relationship between the pharmacokinetic char-acteristics acquired by liposomal formulation and safety/efficacy. *J. Liposome Res*. 2016;27(3):1–9. [PubMed] [Google Scholar].

Taylor N. Nonsurgical management of osteoarthritis knee pain in the older adult: An update. *Rheum. Dis. Clin. North Am*. 2018;33(4):41–51. [Google Scholar].

Thomas DA, Sarris AH, Cortes J et al. Phase II study of sphingosomal vincristine in patients with recurrent or refractory adult acute lymphocytic leukemia. *Cancer*. 2006;106(1):120–127. [PubMed] [Google Scholar].

Torres C. Rare opportunities appear on the horizon to treat rare diseases. *Nat. Med*. 2010;16(3):241–241. [PubMed] [Google Scholar]

Transparency Market Research. 2021. www.transparencymarketresearch.com/nanomedicine-market.html.

Turecek PL, Bossard MJ, Schoetens F, Ivens IA. PEGylation of biopharmaceuticals: A review of chemistry and nonclinical safety information of approved drugs. *J. Pharm. Sci*. 2016;105(2):460–475. [PubMed] [Google Scholar]

Turecek PL, Romeder-Finger S, Apostol C et al. A world-wide survey and field study in clinical haemostasis laboratories to evaluate FVIII: C activity assay variability of ADYNO-VATE and OBIZUR in comparison with ADVATE. *Haemophilia.* 2016;22(6):957–965. [PubMed] [Google Scholar].

US Food and Drug Administration (US FDA). *Prescribing Information for KRYST-EXXAI): Savient Pharmaceuticals.* 2 009. www.accessdata.fda.gov/drugsatfda_docs/label/2010/125293s0000lbl.pdf.

Van De Poel I. How should we do nanoethics? A network approach for discerning ethical issues in nanotechnology. *Nanoethics.* 2008;2(1):25–38. [Google Scholar].

Van der Lely AJ, Hutson RK, Trainer PJ et al. Long-term treatment of acromegaly with peg-visomant, a growth hormone receptor antagonist. *Lancet.* 2001;358(9295):1754–1759. [PubMed] [Google Scholar]

Veerareddy PR, Vobalaboina V. Lipid-based formulations of amphotericin B. *Drugs of Today.* 2004;40(2):133–146. [PubMed] [Google Scholar].

Volkow ND, Wang G, Fowler JS et al. Therapeutic doses of oral methylphenidate significantly increase extracellular dopamine in the human brain. *J. Neurosci.* 2001;21(2):RC121. [PMC free article] [PubMed] [Google Scholar].

Wachtlin J, Heimann H, Behme T, Foerster MH. Long-term results after photodynamic therapy with verteporfin for choroidal neovascularizations secondary to inflammatory chorioretinal diseases. *Graefes Arch. Clin. Exp. Ophthalmol.* 2003;241(11):899–906. [PubMed] [Google Scholar].

Waknine Y. *Medscape. FDA Approves New Drug for Hereditary Angioedema.* 2 011. www.medscape.com/viewarticle/748570.

Weber MS, Hohlfeld R, Zamvil SS. Mechanism of action of glatiramer acetate in treatment of multiple sclerosis. *Neurotherapeutics.* 2007;4(4):647–653. [PMC free article] [PubMed] [Google Scholar].

Weissig V, Pettinger TK, Murdock N. Nanopharmaceuticals (part 1): Products on the market. *Int. J. Nanomed.* 2014;9:4357. [PMC free article] [PubMed] [Google Scholar]

Wex J, Sidhu M, Odeyemi I, Abou-Setta AM, Retsa P, Tombal B. Leuprolide acetate 1-, 3—and 6-monthly depot formulations in androgen deprivation therapy for prostate cancer in nine European countries: Evidence review and economic evaluation. *Clinicoecon. Outcomes Res.* 2013;5:257–269. [PMC free article] [PubMed] [Google Scholar].

Wolinsky JS, Narayana PA, O'Connor P et al. Glatiramer acetate in primary progressive multiple sclerosis: Results of a multinational, multicenter, double-blind, placebo-controlled trial. *Ann. Neurol.* 2007;61(1):14–24. [PubMed] [Google Scholar].

Woods GM, Dunn MW, Dunn AL. Emergencies in hemophilia. *Clin. Pediatr. Emerg. Med.* 2018;19(2):110–121. [Google Scholar].

Wu TC. On the development of antifungal agents: Perspective of the US Food and Drug Administration. *Clin. Infect. Dis.* 1994;19(Suppl. 1):S54–S58. [PubMed] [Google Scholar].

Yang S-H, Lin C-C, Lin Z-Z, Tseng Y-L, Hong R-L. A phase I and pharmacokinetic study of liposomal vinorelbine in patients with advanced solid tumor. *Invest. New Drugs.* 2012;30(1):282–289. [PubMed] [Google Scholar].

Yarmolenko PS, Zhao Y, Landon C et al. Comparative effects of thermosensitive doxorubicin-containing liposomes and hyperthermia in human and murine tumours. *Int. J. Hyperthermia.* 2010;26(5):485–498. [PMC free article] [PubMed] [Google Scholar].

Zhang H. Onivyde for the therapy of multiple solid tumors. *Onco Targets Ther.* 2016;9:3001. [PMC free article] [PubMed] [Google Scholar].

10 Development of Material Products for Medical Applications — Product Development and Approval Process, Patents Trends, US FDA Approval Process, WHO Guidelines, World Global Regulations

Firdos Alam Khan

10.1 PRODUCT DEVELOPMENT PROCESS

The product development process for nanomaterials usually follows similar processes followed in pharmaceutical products. The various phases are (1) synthesis and characterization of nanomaterials and in vitro biological assay; (2) preclinical testing of nanomaterials in different animals models, where the effectiveness of nanomaterials are examined, along with their cytotoxic effects in diseased and normal animals; (3) clinical phase I trials, where the safety of the nanomaterials are examined in normal humans; (4) clinical phase II trials, where the effectiveness of the nanomaterials are examined in patients with a certain disease, and this is usually done in a small population of 10–100 patients; and (5) clinical phase III trials, which is the last phase of trials, where the effectiveness of the nanomaterials are examined in patients with a certain disease, and this is usually done in a big population of 100–1,000 patients. If the nanomaterials are successfully tested in all phases, then FDA or country-concerned regulatory agencies will approve the nanomaterials for clinical applications, and the manufacturers of the nanomaterials can now proceed with large-scale production of nanomaterials per the good manufacturing practice

 DOI: 10.1201/9781003317715-10

(GMP) or clean room specifications. During trials, if the nanomaterials showed any side effects in human patients (phase I, phase II, and phase III trials) that cannot be treated and may have implications on the patient's health, then the FDA or country regulatory agencies will halt the trials, and such nanomaterials will be rejected for clinical applications. In case nanomaterials are successfully approved by the FDA, then the nano-based drugs or formulations will be available for human consumption. The manufacturer of the nanomaterials will continue to examine the effectiveness and safety of the nanomaterials, which is called clinical phase IV trials. This phase IV clinical trials ensure that nanomaterials produced and marketed don't produce any unknown side effects that may harm the patients (Figure 10.1). Phase IV clinical trials are usually conducted as long as the product is available in the market. The quality of the product is usually monitored or regulated by internal quality assurance and quality control departments and externally by US FDA or countries regulatory agencies where the product is produced.

During the production phase, the manufacturer needs to apply for an Investigational New Drug (IND) application before starting phase I of the clinical trial; once they receive the approval from the US FDA, they can start the clinical trial. After the completion of phase III of the clinical trial, the manufacturer needs to apply for a New Drug Application (NDA) to market the product. Upon receiving approval from the US FDA, the manufacturer can now successfully launch the product in the market for human consumption. It's important to know the time required to complete the process of production. Like other pharmaceutical products, nanoproducts also follow a similar time frame for work to complete the process. About 10–15 years are generally required to complete the nano-based product development, as shown in Figure 10.2. The cost of the product is also very critical to know how much fund is needed to develop a nano-based product. It's a very expensive process; the total cost of development of a nano-based product is about $300–425 million, as shown in Figure 10.3.

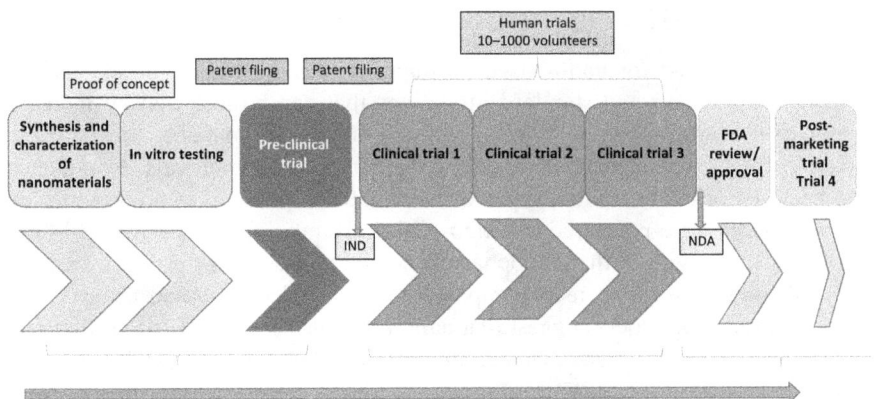

FIGURE 10.1 Diagrammatic illustration of nano-based product development, IND (Investigational New Drug), and NDA (New Drug Application).

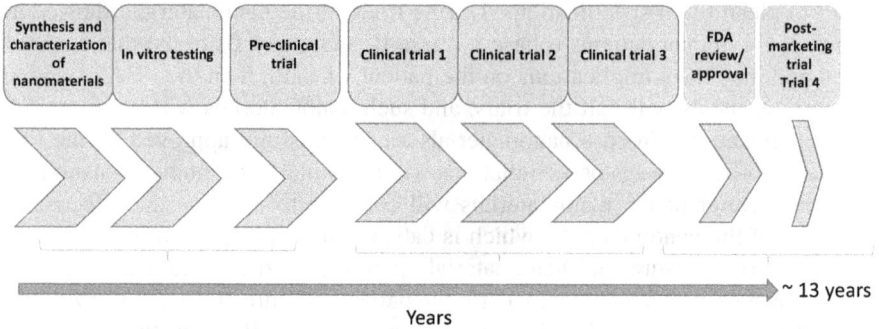

FIGURE 10.2 Diagrammatic illustration of the work timeframe for the nano-based product development.

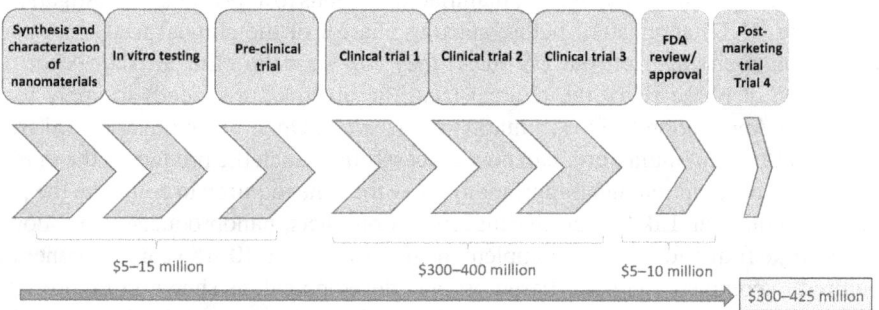

FIGURE 10.3 Diagrammatic illustration of funds required for nano-based product development.

10.2 NANO-BASED PRODUCT APPROVAL PROCESS

The approval process for nano-based products is very long and time-consuming, and there are no clear and standard guidelines that can be followed by industrial and manufacturing companies. The US FDA so far has not published any dedicated policies for nanopharmaceutical product development and approvals. Nonetheless, general regulations for different types of nanomaterial products and cosmetics and food ingredients were presented in August 2016 (Hamburg, 2012). The US FDA is basically really convinced that nanopharmaceutical products may produce some different and unexpected responses compare to small molecule–based drugs (Bawa, 2013). However, researchers suggest that nanomaterials are not only dissimilar from the same bulk material in size, shape, and surface area, but they also vary in biodistribution, cell toxicity, pharmacokinetic, and pharmacodynamic aspects (Zolnik et al., 2011).

Some of the major difficulties for nanopharmaceuticals are environmental factors and conditions in which the nanomaterials are injected or tested. These injected nanomaterials may give different results in both in vitro and in vivo conditions, and many times, it has been observed that testing results of in vitro studies are different when nanomaterials are tested in vivo conditions or in animal trials. The lack of availability of standard testing methods may discourage investors or financial companies not to support such research. This makes it difficult for companies to fund such projects, where methods of testing give varied results. Moreover, getting the necessary approval for such is also difficult. To be able to get successful approval, the pharmaceutical product must be assessed for its final application. For example, an injectable drug must be examined in animals or human bloodstream, and in the same way, tablets must be examined in a suitable medium to imitate the digestive tract of the animal or human.

Another issue is the poor classification of the product by the US FDA, and it has been found that the US FDA categorizes its regulations on drugs, medical devices, blood products, and biological agents similarly (Hamburg, 2012). The guideline is generally applied for the categorization of a combination of materials depending on the mode of drug action. For example, nanomaterials will be categorized in both devices and drug categories in case prosthetic bone cement is supported by nanomaterials or nanotherapeutics; occasionally, the primary mode of action is not completely clear; therefore, the selected product then falls into a category of combination products. Besides, the safety of the nanomaterials may pose not only serious health risks but also environmental risks, as it has been found that nanomaterials interact with both living cells and tissues and may enter the human body through the air (Nowack et al., 2012). To take it seriously, the US National Research Council has decided to develop a system to correctly evaluate the environmental risks that are based on the critical elements of nanomaterial interactions, which may pose potential environmental risks and health risks (Louie et al., 2012). It must be kept in mind that the developmental process for any pharmaceutical agents or drugs takes approximately 10 to 15 years to be available for human consumption. There is a need to study the long-term effects of nanomaterials on the human body and the environment to better understand the safety of nanomaterials per the US FDA guidelines (Bawa, 2011). There is another aspect of non-biological complex drugs (Gaspar et al., 2012), which basically contain nanomaterials that also need to be properly evaluated in both in vitro and in vivo conditions to ensure that nanomaterials do not cause any harmful side effects to the human body (European Medicines, 2012). There is a great need for standardized guidelines for the approval of nanomaterials (Schellekens et al., 2014).

Every day, many patients utilize a variety of nanopharmaceuticals that are available in the market, and these products are manufactured by various companies all around the globe. There is a bright future for different nanomaterials as therapeutic agents. There are many nanopharmaceutical products that are available globally, and these products are categorized based on the type of nanoformulations. These nanoformulations are nanocrystals, liposomes and lipid-based, polymeric, pegylated biologics, gels and emulsions, protein-based, and metallic nanoparticles. Nanomedicine can be defined as the science of using materials with a size of 1 to 100 nm to achieve better drug targeting, reduced cell toxicity, and improved efficacy. These nanoformulations can be administered orally or intravenously routes. Estrasorb™, a nanoformulated product, can be administered by the transdermal delivery route. Nanomaterials can be conjugated to existing anticancer drugs in order to alter the pharmacokinetic or pharmacodynamic properties for better drug action. In many cases, these nanomaterials are conjugated with the drug to achieve better targeting and help to penetrate inside cancer tumor cells or tissues. It has been reported that anticancer drug that is conjugated with nanomaterials showed better tumor permeability and also showed better circulation time and better bioavailability (Duncan and Sat, 1998). Other prominent features of nanomaterials are that they can also be linked or conjugated with specific cells that overexpress certain cell-surface receptors, such as proteins, antibodies, and small molecules, to the surface of the materials, which finally cause better drug penetration and accumulation inside tumor cells. Ontak®, which is based on the antibody-drug conjugates–nanoparticles combination product (Casi and Neri, 2012; Diamantis and Banerji, 2016), is applied in cancer therapy.

Presently, the US FDA approval process for nanomedicine products takes about 10 to 15 years, which is basically the same as other existing regulated drugs in humans (Eifler and Thaxton, 2011). The whole process of making one drug is estimated to cost over $1 billion. The approval process involves the testing of nanomaterials through various phases, such as in vitro testing, preclinical or animal testing, phase I, phase II, phase III, and phase IV to check the drug efficacy, drug safety, and drug toxicity. Over time, the nanomedicine field has advanced with new techniques and new machines, which help researchers to better understand the physicochemical properties of nanomaterials, and the reproducibility and scalability of the manufacturing process. Guidelines related to the nanoformulation were prepared by the Nanotechnology Characterization Laboratory, National Cancer Institute, USA. These guidelines are available for researchers who need nanomaterials testing and validations (Tinkle et al., 2014; Dobrovolskaia, 2015; Nanotechnology Characterization Laboratory, 2016; Bobo et al., 2016). There is also a need for further study to understand how nanomaterials behave with living cells or organisms, which may include the development of advanced assays to predict the impact of the nanomaterials on human cells, tissues, and organisms. The question of nanomaterial characterization per the guidelines of the US FDA has been continuously improved over the years, and now researchers better understand the material synthesis for biomedical applications. The nanomaterial's efficacy, toxicity, and physicochemical capabilities can now be prepared and documented per the guidelines of the Investigational New Drug (IND) for US FDA approval. After obtaining IND approval, different phases of human clinical trials can be started to examine the safety profile and efficacy profile of the new nanoformulations. Clinical phases can be categorized as Phase I, where dosing, toxicity, and excretion of nanomaterials can be studied in healthy subjects; and in Phase II, the safety and efficacy of nanomaterials will be studied in a larger group of patients with the target illness. Phase III, which is conducted through multicenter, randomized, placebo-controlled trials, a large population of patients is involved and assessed for drug efficacy and drug toxicity. Once this is done, the manufacturer can file a New Drug Application (NDA) with the US FDA, asking for approval to market the products. There is also Phase IV trials, which is also called post-marketing trial, undertaken at the request of the US FDA for checking the efficacy and toxicity of the drug throughout the shelf-life.

10.3   PATENTS TRENDS FOR MATERIAL/NANOMATERIAL-BASED PRODUCTS

There has been a continuous surge in the number of patents granted by the US patent office. During the search on the US patent office website (www.uspto.gov) by using the keyword "Nanomaterials and Medical Applications", we found that as of May 2022, the total number of patents issued was 603. These patents have been issued for their inventions in the medical applications of different types of nanomaterials, and most of the patents were focused on diagnosis, therapeutics, bio-imaging, and biosensor applications.

10.3.1   PATENTS GRANTED IN THE FIELD OF NANOMATERIALS FOR CANCER DIAGNOSIS

When we searched patents status at www.uspto.gov using the keywords "nanomaterials cancer diagnosis", we found 200 patents that have been granted to date. There are a number of patents that have mentioned both diagnosis and treatments of cancers (Table 10.1).

TABLE 10.1

Patents Issued for the Application of Nanomaterials for Cancer Diagnosis

PAT. NO.	Titles
11,311,631	Paclitaxel-albumin-binding agent compositions and methods for using and making the same
11,305,020	Methods for reducing the toxicity of a chemotherapeutic drug
11,298,428	Nanocarrier for selective fluorescence labeling of cancer cells and the preparation method thereof
11,285,221	Treating myelomas
11,246,946	Methods of treatment using ultrasmall nanoparticles to induce cell death of nutrient-deprived cancer cells via ferroptosis
11,242,532	Self-assembled 3D RNA cage nanoparticles
11,241,387	Carrier-binding agent compositions and methods of making and using the same
11,202,837	Biological materials and uses thereof
11,197,615	Noninvasive electroactive photonic protein nanosensor with polymer photovoltaic optics for memory transduction using organic and inorganic elements as platforms
11,174,465	pH-sensitive and bioreducible polymer-virus complex for cancer treatment
11,156,582	Systems for detecting and quantifying nucleic acids
11,155,584	Unstructured non-repetitive polypeptides having LCST behavior
11,135,309	Poly(vinyl alcohol) nanocarriers
11,135,301	Triblock polypeptide–based nanoparticles for the delivery of hydrophilic drugs
11,103,599	Nanocarriers for prostate cancer cell–targeted therapy and/or diagnosis thereof
11,103,529	Zero-valent gold nanoparticles as cancer therapy
11,090,385	Early cancer detection and enhanced immunotherapy

(Continued)

TABLE 10.1 *(Continued)*
Patents Issued for the Application of Nanomaterials for Cancer Diagnosis

PAT. NO.	Titles
11,083,807	Miniaturized device to sterilize from COVID-19 and other viruses
11,077,191	Multimodal therapy for cancer cell destruction
11,072,681	Compositions and methods of making polymerizing nucleic acids
11,054,428	Inhalable nanosensors with volatile reporters and uses thereof
11,045,874	Bipyramid-templated synthesis of monodisperse noble metal nanocrystals
11,045,548	Methods for inhibiting cancer cell migration with gold nanomaterials and photothermal therapy
11,022,610	Integrated dual-modality microfluidic sensor for biomarker detection using lithographic plasmonic crystal
11,020,740	Microfluidic biochip with enhanced sensitivity
11,016,089	Nanocomposites and nanoagents for the detection and treatment of a target of interest and methods of making and using the same
11,007,286	Compositions and methods for treatment and imaging using nanoparticles
10,993,912	Carrier-antibody compositions and methods of making and using the same
10,993,911	Carrier-antibody compositions and methods of making and using the same
10,980,744	High-density peptide polymers
10,966,923	Carrier-antibody compositions and methods of making and using the same
10,953,110	Dual emissive metal nanoparticles as ratiometric pH indicators
10,942,140	Morphology engineering of conductive metallic nanoparticles capped with an organic coating
10,901,051	Ferromagnetic particles as ultra-sensitive non-linear response labels for magnetic particles imaging (MPI) and sensing applications
10,883,998	Methods and products for in vivo enzyme profiling
10,878,936	Integrated biosensor and simulation system for diagnosis and therapy
10,876,955	Optical configuration methods for spectral scatter flow cytometry
10,874,609	Cyclodextrin-based star-shaped polymer, a preparation method thereof, and an integrated unimolecular micelle system for diagnosis and treatment thereof
10,866,242	System and method for protein corona sensor array for early detection of diseases
10,851,169	Conjugates of IL13R.alpha.2 binding agents and use thereof in cancer treatment
10,837,061	Enrichment and detection of nucleic acids with ultra-high sensitivity
10,830,716	Nanoparticle-assisted scanning focusing X-ray fluorescence imaging and enhanced treatment
10,824,925	Transponders and sensors for implantable medical devices and methods of use thereof
10,815,520	Nanovesicles, methods, and systems for diagnosis and prognosis of cancer
10,814,021	Paramagnetic boron-doped graphene quantum dots and their application for safe magnetic resonance imaging
10,799,604	Biopolymer-nanoparticle composite implant for tumor cell tracking
10,799,587	Ion implantation of neutron capture elements into nanodiamond particles to form composition for neutron capture therapy usage
10,788,486	Graphene oxide–based nanolab and methods of detecting exosomes
10,780,050	Lyophilized compositions comprising albumin-EGFR paclitaxel nanoparticle complexes
10,780,049	Lyophilized compositions comprising albumin-rankl or albumin-GD2 paclitaxel nanoparticle complexes

TABLE 10.1 *(Continued)*
Patents Issued for the Application of Nanomaterials for Cancer Diagnosis

PAT. NO.	Titles
10,772,833	Albumin-CTLA-4 paclitaxel nanoparticle complex compositions and methods of making and using the same
10,765,741	Methods for treating VEGF-expressing cancer using preformed nanoparticle complexes comprising albumin-bound paclitaxel and bevacizumab
10,759,878	Method of crosslinking of polysaccharides using photoremovable protecting groups
10,753,941	Biocompatible nanoparticles with aggregation-induced emission characteristics as fluorescent bioprobes and methods of using the same for in vitro and in vivo imaging
10,736,972	Methods of treatment using ultrasmall nanoparticles to induce cell death of nutrient-deprived cancer cells via ferroptosis
10,736,848	Vaccine nanotechnology
10,689,464	Self-supporting, biodegradable film based on hydrophobized hyaluronic acid, method of preparation and use thereof
10,670,592	Detection of analytes using metal nanoparticle probes and dynamic light scattering
10,670,581	Nanobubbles
10,668,151	Nanoparticle complexes of albumin, paclitaxel, and panitumumab for treatment of cancer
10,668,024	Mesoporous silica nanoparticles for biomedical applications
10,667,749	Device, method, and system for implementing a physical area network for cancer immunotherapy
10,663,420	Morphology engineering of conductive metallic nanoparticles capped with an organic coating
10,660,565	Device, method, and system for implementing a physical area network for cancer immunotherapy
10,653,357	Device, method, and system for implementing a physical area network for cancer immunotherapy
10,624,846	Lyophilized compositions comprising albumin-antibody paclitaxel nanoparticle complexes
10,618,984	Unsaturated derivatives of polysaccharides, method of preparation thereof and use thereof
10,618,969	Carrier-binding agent compositions and methods of making and using the same
10,617,711	Antitumor composition based on hyaluronic acid and inorganic nanoparticles, method of preparation thereof and use thereof
10,610,484	Methods of using albumin-CD20 paclitaxel nanoparticle complex compositions for treating cancer
10,605,630	Tactile sensor, method for manufacturing the same, three-dimensional mapping method
10,598,658	Reduced graphene oxide–based biosensor and use thereof
10,596,112	Methods of using albumin-antibody nanoparticle complex compositions for treating cancer
10,596,111	Methods of making lyophilized compositions comprising albumin-VEGF paclitaxel nanoparticle complexes
10,561,726	Methods of treating cancer using compositions of antibodies and carrier proteins with antibody pretreatment
10,548,998	Multimodal silica-based nanoparticles
10,548,993	Metal-encapsulated carbonaceous dots
10,548,959	Compositions and methods for modified dendrimer nanoparticle delivery
10,517,961	Drug formulation based on particulates comprising polysaccharide-vitamin conjugate

(Continued)

TABLE 10.1 *(Continued)*
Patents Issued for the Application of Nanomaterials for Cancer Diagnosis

PAT. NO.	Titles
10,512,691	Systems and methods for targeted imaging and ablation of cardiac cells
10,507,243	Nanoparticle complexes of rituximab, albumin, and paclitaxel
10,493,150	Nanoparticle complexes of paclitaxel, alemtuzumab, and albumin
10,478,495	Methods for treating cancer using nanoparticle complexes of paclitaxel, cetuximab, and albumin
10,471,145	Methods for treating cancer using nanoparticle complexes of paclitaxel, rituximab, and albumin
10,463,298	Device, method, and system for implementing a physical area network for cancer immunotherapy
10,441,656	Nanoparticle complexes of paclitaxel, cetuximab, and albumin, and methods of making the same
10,420,839	Methods for treating CD52-expressing cancers using compositions comprising nanoparticle complexes of paclitaxel, alemtuzumab, and albumin
10,414,832	Derivatives of sulfated polysaccharides, method of preparation, modification, and use thereof
10,413,609	Artificial bacteriophage based on carbon nanostructures for supplying medicaments
10,413,606	Methods for treating cancer with nanoparticle complexes of albumin-bound paclitaxel and anti-VEGF antibodies
10,406,224	Nanoparticle complexes of paclitaxel, trastuzumab, and albumin
10,400,289	Polynucleotide probe, method for detecting a target nucleic acid by using the same, and kit comprising the same
10,391,055	Carrier-antibody compositions and methods of making and using the same
10,376,580	Methods of treating cancer with antibody-albumin nanoparticle complexes comprising albumin, trastuzumab, and paclitaxel
10,376,579	Nanoparticle complexes of albumin, paclitaxel, and anti-VEGF antibody for the treatment of cancer
10,358,680	Nanoplasmonic molecular probes for plasmonics coupling interference
10,343,903	Cationic polymer coated mesoporous silica nanoparticles and uses thereof
10,322,084	Carrier-antibody compositions and methods of making and using the same
10,308,719	IL13R.alpha.2 binding agents and use thereof in cancer treatment
10,307,489	Organic anion transporting peptide–based cancer imaging and therapy
10,307,482	Nanoparticle complexes of paclitaxel, cetuximab, and albumin
10,300,121	Early cancer detection and enhanced immunotherapy
10,300,016	Carrier-antibody compositions and methods of making and using the same
10,292,956	Cancer starvation therapy
10,279,036	Antibody-albumin nanoparticle complexes comprising albumin, bevacizumab, and paclitaxel, and methods of making and using the same
10,279,035	Nanoparticle complexes of paclitaxel, trastuzumab, and albumin
10,265,017	Device, method, and system for implementing a physical area network for cancer immunotherapy
10,220,004	Method of controlled delivery using sub-micron-scale machines
10,213,513	Treating myelomas

TABLE 10.1 *(Continued)*
Patents Issued for the Application of Nanomaterials for Cancer Diagnosis

PAT. NO.	Titles
10,191,041	Detection of analytes using metal nanoparticle probes and dynamic light scattering
10,176,412	Transponders and sensors for implantable medical devices and methods of use thereof
10,136,820	Method to visualize very early stage neoplasm or other lesions
10,118,834	Superparamagnetic colloidal photonic structures
10,094,793	Nanomaterial-based photothermal immunosensing for quantitative detection of disease biomarkers
10,039,847	Multimodal silica-based nanoparticles
10,034,743	Breast implant with analyte sensors responsive to an external power source
9,999,694	Multimodal silica-based nanoparticles
9,993,437	Mesoporous silica nanoparticles for biomedical applications
9,987,427	Diagnostic/drug delivery "sense-respond" devices, systems, and uses thereof
9,974,870	Compositions and methods for treatment and imaging using nanoparticles
9,968,688	Shielded targeting agents, methods, and in vivo diagnostic system
9,910,035	Polyvalent functionalized nanoparticle-based in vivo diagnostic system
9,902,997	Kit comprising a polynucleotide probe for detecting a target nucleic acid
9,869,666	Electrical cell-substrate impedance sensor (ECIS)
9,851,343	Electrical cell-substrate impedance sensor (ECIS)
9,849,092	Early cancer detection and enhanced immunotherapy
9,821,060	Heat-sensitive nanoparticle system
9,808,526	Pharmaceutical kit and methods for cancer treatment via intracavity delivery and for preparing metal nanoparticle-antibody fragment conjugate
9,802,050	Energy-releasing carbon nanotube transponder and method of using the same
9,731,034	Protease assay
9,719,147	Integrated biosensor and simulation systems for diagnosis and therapy
9,682,155	Protease assay
9,675,556	Biodegradable stealth polymeric particles fabricated using the macromonomer approach by free radical dispersion polymerization
9,539,210	Vaccine nanotechnology
9,526,702	Vaccine nanotechnology
9,493,513	Polypeptides and their use
9,482,616	Methods, kits, and systems for signal amplification for bioassays using zinc nanoparticles
9,474,717	Vaccine nanotechnology
9,439,859	Adjuvant incorporation in immunoanotherapeutics
9,417,170	High-resolution, high-speed multifrequency dynamic study of visco-elastic properties
9,415,238	Pharmaceutical kit and methods for cancer treatment via intracavity delivery and for preparing metal nanoparticle-antibody fragment conjugate
9,402,926	Fluorescent magnetic nanoprobes, methods of making, and methods of use
9,402,911	Multifunctional small molecules
9,358,211	Stealth polymeric particles for delivery of bioactive or diagnostic agents
9,354,170	NIR fluorescence of heavy water
9,339,372	Breast implant with regionalized analyte sensors responsive to an external power source

(Continued)

TABLE 10.1 *(Continued)*
Patents Issued for the Application of Nanomaterials for Cancer Diagnosis

PAT. NO.	Titles
9,333,071	Breast implant with regionalized analyte sensors and internal power source
9,326,730	Breast implant with covering and analyte sensors responsive to an external power source
9,308,280	Targeting of antigen-presenting cells with immunonanotherapeutics
9,302,114	Energy-releasing carbon nanotube transponder and method of using same
9,233,072	Adjuvant incorporation in immunonanotherapeutics
9,220,917	Systems for autofluorescent imaging and target ablation
9,211,185	Breast implant with analyte sensors and internal power source
9,167,983	Imaging method for obtaining a spatial distribution of nanoparticles in the body
9,144,489	Breast implant with covering, analyte sensors, and internal power source
9,144,488	Breast implant with analyte sensors responsive to an external power source
9,127,293	Receptor-mediated delivery: compositions and methods
9,111,026	Integrated biosensor and simulation system for diagnosis and therapy
9,110,836	Integrated biosensor and simulation system for diagnosis and therapy
9,109,249	Microbe detection via hybridizing magnetic relaxation nanosensors
8,954,131	Magnetic particle imaging (MPI) system and method for use of iron-based nanoparticles in imaging and diagnosis
8,945,508	Dendrimer compositions and methods of synthesis
8,936,629	Autofluorescent imaging and target ablation
8,932,595	Nicotine immunonanotherapeutics
8,923,595	Method of identification of cancerous and normal cells
8,921,429	Biodegradable stealth polymeric particles fabricated using the macromonomer approach by free-radical dispersion polymerization
8,906,381	Immunonanotherapeutics that provide IGG humoral response without T-cell antigen
8,883,094	Detection of analytes using metal nanoparticle probes and dynamic light scattering
8,808,373	Breast implant with regionalized analyte sensors responsive to an external power source
8,795,359	Breast implant with regionalized analyte sensors and internal power source
8,790,400	Breast implant with covering and analyte sensors responsive to an external power source
8,788,033	Energy-releasing carbon nanotube transponder and method of using the same
8,778,411	Heat generating nanomaterials
8,772,355	Stealth polymeric particles for delivery of bioactive or diagnostic agents
8,722,017	Fluorescent magnetic nanoprobes, methods of making, and methods of use
8,637,028	Adjuvant incorporation in immunonanotherapeutics
8,591,905	Nicotine immunonanotherapeutics
8,562,998	Targeting of antigen-presenting cells with immunonanotherapeutics
8,423,298	Integrated biosensor and simulation system for diagnosis and therapy
8,374,796	Integrated biosensor and simulation system for diagnosis and therapy
8,370,078	Integrated biosensor and simulation system for diagnosis and therapy
8,370,073	Integrated biosensor and simulation system for diagnosis and therapy
8,370,072	Integrated biosensor and simulation system for diagnosis and therapy
8,370,071	Integrated biosensor and simulation system for diagnosis and therapy
8,370,070	Integrated biosensor and simulation system for diagnosis and therapy
8,370,068	Integrated biosensor and simulation system for diagnosis and therapy
8,364,413	Integrated biosensor and simulation system for diagnosis and therapy

TABLE 10.1 *(Continued)*
Patents Issued for the Application of Nanomaterials for Cancer Diagnosis

PAT. NO.	Titles
8,364,411	Integrated biosensor and simulation system for diagnosis and therapy
8,346,482	Integrated biosensor and simulation system for diagnosis and therapy
8,343,498	Adjuvant incorporation in immunonanotherapeutics
8,343,497	Targeting of antigen-presenting cells with immunonanotherapeutics
8,277,812	Immunonanotherapeutics that provide IgG humoral response without T-cell antigen
8,180,436	Systems for autofluorescent imaging and target ablation
8,160,680	Autofluorescent imaging and target ablation
8,145,295	Methods and systems for untethered autofluorescent imaging, target ablation, and movement of an untethered device in a lumen
7,829,348	Raman-active reagents and the use thereof
7,812,190	Derivatization and solubilization of fullerenes for use in therapeutic and diagnostic applications
7,557,070	Multiplexed cell analysis system
7,393,924	Smart bionanoparticle elements
7,354,871	Nanowires comprising metal nanodots and method for producing the same

10.3.2 PATENTS GRANTED IN THE FIELD OF NANOMATERIALS FOR CANCER TREATMENTS

When we searched the patents using the keywords "nanomaterials cancer treatments", we found 135 patents that have been granted to date (Table 10.2).

10.3.3 PATENTS GRANTED IN THE FIELD OF NANOMATERIALS FOR OTHER BIOMEDICAL APPLICATIONS

When we searched the patents using the keywords "nanomaterials anti-bacterial and antibacterial", we found 193 and 872 patents granted to date. When we searched the patents using the keywords "nanomaterials anti-viral and antiviral", we found 212 and 553 patents granted to date. When we searched the patents using the keywords "nanomaterials anti-biofilm and antibiofilm", we found 22 and 16 patents granted to date. When we searched the patents using the keywords "nanomaterials anti-fungus and antifungus", we found three patents granted to date.

10.4 APPLICATIONS OF SOME PATENTS ISSUED FOR MEDICAL APPLICATIONS

In this section, we have discussed some of the patents that have been granted to understand the various biomedical applications of the different nanomaterials. We have summarized the medical applications of various types of nanomaterials in tabular form (Table 10.3). These nanomaterials have been either used alone or in combination or in conjugation with drug molecules to get a better therapeutic response.

TABLE 10.2

Patents Issued for the Application of Nanomaterials for Cancer Treatments

PAT No.	Titles
11,324,773	Compounds, compositions, and methods for inhibiting a pathogen and/or modifying mucus
11,318,214	Iron oxide mesoporous microparticle drug carrier
11,181,519	System and method for differential diagnosis of diseases
11,155,584	Unstructured non-repetitive polypeptides having LCST behavior
11,135,301	Triblock polypeptide-based nanoparticles for the delivery of hydrophilic drugs
11,119,099	Nanocomposites and methods of making the same
11,110,181	Virus-like particle conjugates for diagnosis and treatment of tumors
11,110,168	Nanoparticles, controlled-release dosage forms, and methods for delivering an immunotherapeutic agent
11,096,950	Compounds, methods, and treatments for abnormal signaling pathways for prenatal and postnatal development
11,091,516	Synthetic binder of breast cancer stem cells
11,077,214	Multimodal CT/optical agents
10,946,075	Radioprotection, radiomitigation, and radiorecovery
10,888,227	Raman-triggered ablation/resection systems and methods
10,864,161	Systems and methods for targeted breast cancer therapies
10,836,735	Compositions and methods for treating cancers
10,830,767	Nanocomposites, methods of making same, and applications of same for multicolor surface-enhanced Raman spectroscopy (SERS) detections
10,822,355	Ultralow-power near-infrared lamp light operable targeted organic nanoparticle photodynamic therapy
10,799,462	Peptide-polypeptide co-assembled nanoparticles for drug delivery
10,688,189	Modulated guanidine-containing polymers or nanoparticles
10,668,151	Nanoparticle complexes of albumin, paclitaxel, and panitumumab for the treatment of cancer
10,667,749	Device, method, and system for implementing a physical area network for cancer immunotherapy
10,660,565	Device, method, and system for implementing a physical area network for cancer immunotherapy
10,653,357	Device, method, and system for implementing a physical area network for cancer immunotherapy
10,591,462	Electrochemical method and device for detecting the effect of anticancer drugs
10,588,984	Virus-like particle conjugates for diagnosis and treatment of tumors
10,543,171	Dermal drug delivery using amphiphilic dendron-coil micelles
10,537,640	Ultrasound delivery of nanoparticles
10,500,164	Nanoparticle-based combinatorial therapy
10,500,156	Multicompartmental macrophage delivery
10,463,298	Device, method, and system for implementing a physical area network for cancer immunotherapy

TABLE 10.2 *(Continued)*
Patents Issued for the Application of Nanomaterials for Cancer Treatments

PAT No.	Titles
10,398,661	Methods for classifying cancer as susceptible to TMEPAI-directed therapies and treating such cancers
10,392,611	Polymer conjugates having reduced antigenicity and methods of using the same
10,392,446	Compositions and methods to modify cells for therapeutic objectives
10,385,115	Fibronectin type III domain-based fusion proteins
10,376,580	Methods of treating cancer with antibody-albumin nanoparticle complexes comprising albumin, trastuzumab, and paclitaxel
10,364,451	Polymer conjugates having reduced antigenicity and methods of using the same
10,328,160	Hollow silica nanospheres and methods of making the same
10,286,075	Embolization particle
10,279,036	Antibody-albumin nanoparticle complexes comprising albumin, bevacizumab, and paclitaxel, and methods of making and using the same
10,279,035	Nanoparticle complexes of paclitaxel, trastuzumab, and albumin
10,266,505	Compositions and methods for treating cancers
10,265,017	Device, method, and system for implementing a physical area network for cancer immunotherapy
10,226,511	Memory or learning improvement using a peptide and other compositions
10,213,457	Brain and neural treatments comprising peptides and other compositions
10,188,603	Topical systems and methods for treating sexual dysfunction
10,155,048	Methods and systems for treating or preventing cancer
10,124,075	Bionanofluid for use as a contrast, imaging, disinfecting, and/or therapeutic agent
10,117,947	Virus-like particle conjugates for diagnosis and treatment of tumors
10,080,768	Systems and methods for delivery of peptides
10,071,117	Immune modulation using peptides and other compositions
10,064,955	Cardiovascular disease treatment and prevention
10,034,944	Wound healing using topical systems and methods
10,034,914	Brain and neural treatments comprising peptides and other compositions
10,034,828	Hair treatment systems and methods using peptides and other compositions
10,029,997	Compositions and methods for treating cancers
10,028,994	Memory or learning improvement using peptide and other compositions
9,956,290	Peptide systems and methods for metabolic conditions
9,943,562	Wound healing using topical systems and methods
9,937,221	Systems and methods for delivery of peptides
9,931,370	Peptide systems and methods for metabolic conditions
9,913,793	Treatment of skin, including aging skin, to improve appearance
9,872,818	Treatment of skin, including aging skin, to improve appearance
9,869,666	Electrical cell-substrate impedance sensor (ECIS)
9,851,343	Electrical cell-substrate impedance sensor (ECIS)
9,849,160	Methods and systems for treating or preventing cancer

(Continued)

TABLE 10.2 *(Continued)*
Patents Issued for the Application of Nanomaterials for Cancer Treatments

PAT No.	Titles
9,844,506	Compositions and methods for affecting mood states
9,827,316	Cardiovascular disease treatment and prevention
9,810,687	Nanocomposites and methods of making same
9,802,050	Energy-releasing carbon nanotube transponder and method of using same
9,789,159	Diagnosis and treatment of prostate cancer
9,784,737	Nanocomposites, methods of making same, and applications of same for multicolor surface-enhanced Raman spectroscopy (SERS) detections
9,770,419	Methods and compositions of camel-derived products
9,770,413	Amphiphilic dendron coils, micelles thereof, and uses
9,757,467	Cardiovascular disease treatment and prevention
9,750,787	Memory or learning improvement using peptides and other compositions
9,724,423	Thixotropic alpha-lactalbumin hydrogels, method for preparing same, and uses thereof
9,724,419	Peptide systems and methods for metabolic conditions
9,717,680	Topical systems and methods for treating sexual dysfunction
9,700,626	Wound healing using topical systems and methods
9,694,083	Methods and systems for treating or preventing cancer
9,694,029	Immune modulation using peptides and other compositions
9,687,520	Memory or learning improvement using peptide and other compositions
9,687,504	Brain and neural treatments comprising peptides and other compositions
9,682,102	Systems and methods for delivery of peptides
9,642,805	Aptamer-loaded, biocompatible nanoconstructs for nuclear-targeted cancer therapy
9,636,291	Hair treatment systems and methods using peptides and other compositions
9,585,931	Cardiovascular disease treatment and prevention
9,585,817	Treatment of skin, including aging skin, to improve appearance
9,572,880	Ultrasound delivery of nanoparticles
9,572,815	Methods and compositions of p27KIP1 transcriptional modulators
9,512,043	Ceramic powders coated with a nanoparticle layer and process for obtaining thereof
9,498,535	Wound healing using topical systems and methods
9,480,642	Compositions and methods for affecting mood states
9,446,126	Thermal treatment of acne with coated metal nanoparticles
9,442,115	Method of analyzing binding efficiency of adhesive nanoparticles
9,439,965	Thermal treatment of the skin surface with metal nanoparticles in surfactant-containing solutions
9,439,964	Thermal treatment of the skin surface with coated metal nanoparticles
9,439,926	Topical systems and methods for treating sexual dysfunction
9,433,678	Thermal treatment of acne with metal nanoparticles in surfactant-containing solutions
9,433,677	Thermal treatment of a pilosebaceous unit with metal nanoparticles in surfactant-containing solutions
9,433,676	Hair removal with nanoparticles with coatings that facilitate selective removal from the skin surface

TABLE 10.2 *(Continued)*
Patents Issued for the Application of Nanomaterials for Cancer Treatments

PAT No.	Titles
9,427,467	Hair removal with metal nanoparticles in surfactant-containing solutions
9,421,261	Thermal treatment of the skin surface with nanoparticles with coatings that facilitate selective removal from the skin surface
9,421,260	Thermal treatment of acne with nanoparticles with coatings that facilitate selective removal from the skin surface
9,421,259	Hair removal with coated metal nanoparticles
9,393,265	Wound healing using topical systems and methods
9,393,264	Immune modulation using peptides and other compositions
9,387,159	Treatment of skin, including aging skin, to improve appearance
9,387,036	Apparatus and method for selectively heating a deposit in fatty tissue in a body
9,375,790	Continuous flow reactor and method for nanoparticle synthesis
9,339,457	Cardiovascular disease treatment and prevention
9,320,758	Brain and neural treatments comprising peptides and other compositions
9,320,706	Immune modulation using peptides and other compositions
9,314,433	Methods and systems for treating or preventing cancer
9,314,423	Hair treatment systems and methods using peptides and other compositions
9,314,422	Peptide systems and methods for metabolic conditions
9,314,417	Treatment of skin, including aging skin, to improve appearance
9,302,114	Energy-releasing carbon nanotube transponder and method of using the same
9,295,647	Systems and methods for delivery of peptides
9,295,637	Compositions and methods for affecting mood states
9,295,636	Wound healing using topical systems and methods
9,241,899	Topical systems and methods for treating sexual dysfunction
9,220,685	Hollow silica nanospheres and methods of making the same
9,212,258	Amphiphilic dendron coils, micelles thereof, and uses
9,187,501	Nitric oxide–releasing nanorods and their methods of use
8,945,508	Dendrimer compositions and methods of synthesis
8,788,033	Energy-releasing carbon nanotube transponder and method of using the same
8,697,181	Multifunctional Fe3O4 cored magnetic-quantum dot fluorescent nanocomposites for RF nanohyperthermia of cancer cells
8,557,290	Multifunction nanoconjugates for imaging applications and targeted treatment
8,440,229	Hollow silica nanospheres and methods of making the same
8,423,152	Apparatus and method for selectively heating a deposit in fatty tissue in a body
8,333,874	Flexible apparatus and method for monitoring and delivery
7,897,181	Method for photothermal therapy using porous silicon and near-infrared radiation
7,671,230	Derivatization and solubilization of insoluble classes of fullerenes
7,557,070	Multiplexed cell analysis system

TABLE 10.3

Patents Issued for Medical Applications of Nanomaterials

Patent title	Applications	US Patent Number	Reference
Compounds, compositions, and methods for inhibiting a pathogen and/or modifying mucus	Provided herein are compounds, compositions, and methods for modifying mucus, including modifying mucus using nitric oxide–releasing biopolymers (e.g., NO-releasing chitosan oligosaccharides). In some embodiments, a compound, composition, and/or method of the present invention modifies one or more properties of mucus to increase mucus clearance in a subject and/or prevent the growth or kill one or more pathogens present in the mucus of a subject.	11,324,773	Schoenfisch and Reighard, 2022
Production of nanoscale powders of embedded nanoparticles	The invention provides a liquid-dispersible powder comprising nanoscale grains of matrix embedded with one or more isolated nanoparticles and a composition for the magnetic nanoparticle hyperthermia (MNH) treatment of tumors comprising nanoscale grains of matrix material containing one or more isolated nanoparticles. The invention also provides a method of production of a liquid-dispersible powder described herein; the method comprising the steps of providing nanoparticles prepared under ultra-high vacuum (UHV) gas phase conditions; co-depositing the nanoparticles within a matrix material under UHV gas phase conditions; and grinding the film to a fine powder comprising grains of groups of matrix material isolated nanoparticles. The invention also provides a method of reducing the agglomeration of nanoparticles in liquid, the method comprising isolating nanoparticles in nanoscale grains of the matrix material, and the use of a liquid-dispersible powder comprising nanoscale grains of matrix material containing one or more isolated nanoparticles in the manufacture of a medicament for the MNH treatment of tumors.	11,318,203	Binns and Kinmont, 2022
Methods of making and bio-electronic applications of metalized graphene fibers	The present disclosure provides methods of making and applying metalized graphene fibers in bioelectronics applications. For example, platinized graphene fibers may be used as an implantable conductive suture for neural and neuromuscular interfaces in chronic applications. In some embodiments, an implantable electrode includes a multilayer graphene-fiber core, an insulative coating surrounding the multilayer graphene-fiber core, and a metal layer disposed between the multilayer graphene-fiber core and the insulative coating.	11,311,720	Romero-Ortega et al., 2019
Antimicrobial compositions	Storage-stable compositions for generating antimicrobial activity are described. The compositions comprise an enzyme that is able to convert a substrate to release hydrogen peroxide and an unrefined natural substance, such as honey, that includes a substrate for the enzyme. In certain embodiments,	11,311,017	Patton et al., 2022

Title	Description	Patent No.	Reference
	the enzyme is a purified enzyme. In other embodiments, the substrate lacks catalase activity, and the enzyme is additional to any enzyme activity able to convert the substrate to release hydrogen peroxide that may be present in the unrefined natural substance. The storage-stable compositions do not include sufficient free water to allow the enzyme to convert the substrate. The use of the compositions to treat microbial infections and wounds is described, as well as methods for their production.		
Templated assembly of collagen fibers and uses thereof	The present invention relates to a biomaterial fabrication process for the manufacture of a collagen-based fabric for an aligned collagen fiber network.	11,299,630	Frampton and Paul, 2022
Methods for treating metabolic disorder	Provided are a self-nano-emulsifying 3D printer ink composition and a method of using such composition to manufacture a 3D-printed tablet having compartmentalized active pharmaceutical ingredients. In particular, the 3D-printed tablet composition includes glimepiride and/or rosuvastatin in a curcuma oil–based self-nano-emulsifying drug delivery system (SNEDDS). The disclosure also provides a method of treating a metabolic disorder or disease by administering a therapeutically effective amount of the 3D-printed tablet to a subject in need thereof.	11,298,321	El-Say et al., 2022
Small volume self-metered blood separation device	The invention is directed to devices and methods for low-cost and convenient separation of plasma from whole blood. In some embodiments, devices of the invention comprise an integrated collection of channels and chambers in a body that permits the acquisition of a blood sample by capillary action, centrifugal separation of cells from plasma, and manual dispensing of purified plasma by simple pinching of a bellows chamber to force air into plasma-holding channels, which thereby expels a predetermined volume of the purified plasma.	11,266,988	Kirakossian and Tan, 2022
Method of local exposure to biological tissues, tissue-substitute applicator, and use of porous poly-tetrafluoroethylene	The invention concerns medical applications and can be used in oncology as well as in neurosurgery, traumatology, neurology, and rehabilitation. The aim of the inventions claimed is the creation of a new method of local exposure on biological tissues and a new tissue-substitute applicator that benefits both the destruction and replacement of tumor tissue by a restored biological tissue with no external exposure applied (alternating magnetic field, heating, etc.) The aim set is solved by using porous poly-tetrafluoroethylene as a cytostatic material. The aim set is also achieved by using porous poly-tetrafluoroethylene in the production of a tissue-substitute applicator for treating or replacing tumor tissues. The aim set for the method of local exposure to biological tissues, including the placement of a tissue-substitute polymeric applicator in direct contact with the biological tissue to be exposed, is solved by using porous poly-tetrafluoroethylene for the constituent polymeric material.	11,266,682	Dosta, 2022

(Continued)

TABLE 10.3 (Continued)
Patents Issued for Medical Applications of Nanomaterials

Patent title	Applications	US Patent Number	Reference
Chelating platform for delivery of radionuclides	Siderocalin-metal chelator combinations that bind metallic radioisotopes used in nuclear medicine with high affinity are described. The high-affinity siderocalin-metal chelator combinations include a number of chelator backbone arrangements with functional groups that coordinate with metals. The siderocalin-metal chelator combinations can be used to deliver radionuclides for imaging and therapeutic purposes.	11,235,076	Strong et al., 2022
Targeted cancer therapy	Some embodiments of the present disclosure are directed to methods that include delivering to a subject a nucleic acid encoding an antigen, wherein the nucleic acid is delivered via a tumor-selective vehicle or via intra-tumoral injection, and delivering to the subject an immune cell expressing a receptor that binds to the antigen.	11,207,339	Lobb et al., 2021
Biovessels for use in tissue engineering	Described herein are bioengineered constructs and methods of producing the same. The constructs and methods disclosed herein can be applied toward, for example, the generation of vascular grafts to treat cardiovascular disease.	11,197,945	Ali, 2021
Antimicrobial compositions	Storage-stable compositions for generating antimicrobial activity are described. The compositions comprise an enzyme that is able to convert a substrate to release hydrogen peroxide and an unrefined natural substance, such as honey, that includes a substrate for the enzyme. In certain embodiments, the enzyme is a purified enzyme. In other embodiments, the substrate lacks catalase activity, and the enzyme is additional to any enzyme activity able to convert the substrate to release hydrogen peroxide that may be present in the unrefined natural substance. The storage-stable compositions do not include sufficient free water to allow the enzyme to convert the substrate. The use of the compositions to treat microbial infections and wounds is described as well as methods for their production.	11,185,080	Patton et al., 2021
System and method for differential diagnosis of diseases	The present invention further provides a method of diagnosing, screening, or monitoring a disease based on the determination of levels of volatile organic compounds (VOCs) from a universal biomarker set, including 2-ethylhexanol, 3-methylhexane, 5-ethyl-3-methyl-octane, acetone, ethanol, ethyl acetate, ethylbenzene, isononane, isoprene, nonanal, styrene, toluene, and undecane.	11,181,519	Haick and Nakhleh, 2021

Method for biological or biomimetic channel-based membrane fabrications using layer-by-layer structure	The present disclosure describes membrane compositions and methods for preparing membrane compositions. In particular, the methods employ a layer-by-layer approach to membrane preparation. The membrane compositions provide significantly enhanced membrane performance over existing commercial membranes, particularly in terms of permeability and selectivity.	11,154,822	Kumar et al., 2021
Method and system for thermal stimulation of targeted neural circuits for neurodegenerative disorders	A method and system for noninvasively treating a neurodegenerative disorder can involve determining characteristics indicative of physical attributes of a central nervous system and the characteristics including parameters for diminishing adverse impacts of a magnetothermal stimulation treatment for a neurodegenerative disorder with respect to the central nervous system, and applying as a part of the magnetothermal stimulation treatment and based on the characteristics of the physical attributes of the central nervous system, a magnetic field to the brain for a thermal stimulation of neuron cells within the brain.	11,147,982	Vafai and Kosari, 2021
X-ray interferometric imaging system	An X-ray interferometric imaging system in which the X-ray source comprises a target having a plurality of structured coherent sub-sources of X-rays embedded in a thermally conducting substrate. The system additionally comprises a beam-splitting grating G1 that establishes a Talbot interference pattern, which may be a pi-phase-shifting grating, and an X-ray detector to convert two-dimensional X-ray intensities into electronic signals. The system may also comprise a second analyzer grating G2 that may be placed in front of the detector to form additional interference fringes, a means to translate the second grating G2 relative to the detector. The system may additionally comprise an antiscattering grid to reduce signals from scattered X-rays. Various configurations of dark-field and bright-field detectors are also disclosed.	RE48,612	Yun et al., 2021
Spatiotemporal delivery system embedded in 3D-printing	Provided herein is a 3D-printing system and related compositions, and a method of using such that can produce a polymeric microfiber having embedded microspheres encapsulating an active agent with micron precision and high spatial and temporal resolution. One aspect of the present disclosure provides a method for forming a biocompatible scaffold. Another aspect provides a method of forming a polymeric fiber having a microencapsulated agent distributed in the polymeric fiber. Another aspect provides a composition including a polymeric microfiber produced by 3D printing.	11,045,585	Lee, 2021

10.5 WHO GUIDELINES FOR MATERIALS AND NANOMATERIAL-BASED PRODUCTS

The increased production of nanomaterials and their use in consumer products also produce an impact on the health of front-line workers and researchers who are exposed to various types of nanomaterials on a daily basis. The WHO has classified these nanomaterials with diameters less than 100 nanometers, which usually pose health hazards to people. The unique properties of MNMs may result in highly desirable behavior, including but not limited to increased reactivity or higher conductivity. As such, the past decade has witnessed the exploitation of these unique properties for industrial and consumer applications, and various types of nanomaterials have found their way into a plethora of sectors, including aerospace, cosmetics, foods, electronics, construction, and medicine, among others. Significant academic and industrial resources have been dedicated to the field of nanotechnology, increasing the scope and number of nanomaterials that will be available for future use. However, nanomaterials may also present health hazards that differ from those of the substance in bulk form and require different test methods for hazard, exposure, and risk assessment from their bulk material counterparts. The World Health Assembly identified the assessment of health impacts of new technologies, work processes, and products as one of the activities under the Global Plan of Action on Workers' Health adopted in 2007, and the WHO Global Network of Collaborating Centers in Occupational Health has selected nanomaterials as a key focus of its activity.

The WHO developed these guidelines with the aim of protecting workers from the potential risks of nanomaterials. The recommendations are intended to help policy-makers and professionals in the field of occupational health and safety in making decisions about protection against the potential risks of nanomaterials. These guidelines are also intended to support workers and employers. However, the guidelines are not intended as a handbook or manual for safe handling of nanomaterials in the workplace because this requires addressing more general occupational hygiene issues beyond the scope of these guidelines.

Inhaled nanomaterials may be deposited in the respiratory tract and may cause inflammation and damage to lung cells and tissues. Certain nanomaterials may penetrate cell membranes and may cause damage to intracellular structures and cellular functions. Some nanomaterials may be pyrophoric or readily combustible, creating a risk of explosions and fires. Nanotoxicology exposures to nanomaterials may occur through inhalation, dermal contact, accidental injection, and ingestion, and the risk increases with the duration of exposure and the concentrations of nanoparticles in the sample or air. Inhalation presents the greatest exposure hazard. Nanomaterials suspended in a solution or slurry pose a lesser hazard; however, sonication, shaking, stirring, pouring, or spraying can result in inhalation exposure. Nanoparticles that are fixed within a matrix pose the least hazard as long as no mechanical disruption, such as grinding, cutting, or burning, occurs.

10.6 SUMMARY AND CONCLUSION

Materials and their medical applications are emerging trends, and various types of materials are synthesized for different kinds of medical applications. This chapter discusses various types of material-based products and how these products are made at a large scale in the industry. Material-based products and the names of the manufacturers in different parts of the world are explained in a detailed manner. The names and portfolios of the companies that make and invest in the production of material-based products for medical applications are discussed. The global market, investments, and market trends for material-based products and their manufacturers are also discussed in great detail. In the end, future trends and business opportunities are also discussed to understand the market direction of material-based products. The increased production of nanomaterials and their use in consumer products also produce an impact on the health of front-line workers and researchers who are exposed to various types of nanomaterials on daily basis. The WHO has classified these nanomaterials with diameters less than 100 nanometers, which usually pose health hazards to people. It's highly recommended that nanomaterials must be thoroughly tested using in vitro and other methods, and especially, long-term implications of nanomaterials must be examined in animal models before being used for clinical trials.

REFERENCES

Ali KP. 2021. https://patft.uspto.gov.
Bawa R. Regulating nanomedicine–can the FDA handle it? *Curr. Drug Del.* 2011;8(3):227–234. [PubMed] [Google Scholar]• Highlights the ongoing question of regulatory authorities and nanomedicine.
Bawa R. FDA and nanotech: Baby steps lead to regulatory uncertainty. In: Bagchi D, Bagchi M, Moriyama H, Shahidi F, editors. *Bio-Nanotechnology: A Revolution in Food, Biomedical and Health Sciences.* John Wiley & Sons, Ltd; Chichester, UK: 2013. pp. 720–732. [Google Scholar].
Binns and Kinmont. 2022. https://patft.uspto.gov.
Bobo D, Robinson KJ, Islam J, Thurecht KJ, Corrie SR. Nanoparticle-based medicines: A review of FDA-approved materials and clinical trials to date. *Pharm Res.* 2016 Oct;33(10):2373–2387. doi: 10.1007/s11095-016-1958-5. Epub 2016 Jun 14. PMID: 27299311
Casi G, Neri D. Antibody–drug conjugates: Basic concepts, examples and future perspectives. *J Control Release.* 2012;161(2):422–428.
Diamantis N, Banerji U. Antibody-drug conjugates—an emerging class of cancer treatment. *Br J Cancer.* 2016;114(4):362–367.
Dobrovolskaia MA. Pre-clinical immunotoxicity studies of nanotechnology-formulated drugs: Challenges, considerations and strategy. *J Control Release.* 2015;220:571–583.
Dosta AD. 2022. https://patft.uspto.gov.
Duncan R, Sat YN. Tumour targeting by enhanced permeability and retention (EPR) effect. *Ann Oncol.* 1998;9:39.
Eifler AC, Thaxton CS. Nanoparticle therapeutics: FDA approval, clinical trials, regulatory pathways, and case study. *Methods Mol Biol.* 2011;726:325–338. doi: 10.1007/978-1-61779-052-2_21. PMID: 21424459.
El-Say KM et al. 2022. https://patft.uspto.gov.
European Medicines A. Questions and answers on biosimilar medicines (similar biological medicinal products). 2012;44:1–1. www.medicinesforeurope.com/2012/09/27/ema-questions-and-answers-on-biosimilar-medicines-similar-biological-medicinal-products/ [Google Scholar].
Frampton IC, Paul J. 2022. https://patft.uspto.gov.

Gaspar R, Aksu B, Cuine A et al. Towards a European strategy for medicines research (2014–2020): The EUFEPS position paper on Horizon 2020. *Eur. J. Pharm. Sci.* 2012;47(5):979–987. [PubMed] [Google Scholar].

Haick H, Nakhleh M. 2021. https://patft.uspto.gov.

Hamburg MA. FDA's approach to regulation of products of nanotechnology. *Science.* 2012;336(6079):299–300. [PubMed] [Google Scholar].

Kirakossian H, Tan M. 2022. https://patft.uspto.gov.

Kumar M et al. 2021. https://patft.uspto.gov.

Lee CH. 2021. https://patft.uspto.gov.

Lobb R et al. 2021. https://patft.uspto.gov.

Louie SM, Ma R, Lowry GV, Gregory KB, Apte SC, Lead JR. Transformations of nanomaterials in the environment. *Environ. Sci. Technol.* 2012;46(13):6893–6899. [PubMed] [Google Scholar].

Nanotechnology Characterization Laboratory: National Cancer Institute US National Institutes of Health; 2016 [2/16/2016]. http://ncl.cancer.gov/.

Nowack B, Ranville JF, Diamond S et al. Potential scenarios for nanomaterial release and subsequent alteration in the environment. *Environ. Toxicol. Chem.* 2012;31(1):50–59. [PubMed] [Google Scholar].

https://patft.uspto.gov.

Patton T et al. 2021. https://patft.uspto.gov.

Patton T et al. 2022. https://patft.uspto.gov.

Romero-Ortega et al. 2019. https://patft.uspto.gov.

Schellekens H, Stegemann S, Weinstein V et al. How to regulate nonbiological complex drugs (NBCD) and their follow-on versions: Points to consider. *AAPS J.* 2014;16(1):15–21. [PMC free article] [PubMed] [Google Scholar].

Schoenfisch and Reighard, 2022. https://patft.uspto.gov.

Strong RK et al. 2022. https://patft.uspto.gov.

Tinkle S, McNeil SE, Muehlebach S, Bawa R, Borchard G, Barenholz Y et al. Nanomedicines: Addressing the scientific and regulatory gap. *Ann Reports.* 2014;1313:35–56.

Vafai K, Kosari EA. 2021. https://patft.uspto.gov.

Yun et al. 2021. https://patft.uspto.gov.

Zolnik B, Potter TM, Stern ST. Detecting reactive oxygen species in primary hepatocytes treated with nanoparticles. *Methods Mol. Biol.* (Clifton, NJ) 2011;697(3):173–179. [PubMed] [Google Scholar].

11 Challenges of Materials Products Used in Medical Applications

V. Ravinayagam and B. Rabindran Jermy

11.1 INTRODUCTION

According to the WHO, cardiovascular disease (17.9 million/year) and cancer (10 million in 2020) related deaths are increasing worldwide. The cancer burden and related mortality are expected to increase to about 30 million by 2030 (Cheng et al. 2021). Chronic and associated diseases also lead to disability, impacting workforce efficiency and financial crisis (Roth et al. 2020; Vos et al. 2020). The treatment of cancer includes surgery, chemo, radio, and photodynamics. One particular treatment is effective for some cancers, but it remains incompetent for other types of cancers (for example, skin, breast, liver, and lung cancer). Surgery is an effective way to treat non-metastatic cancer, but it needs the support of additional therapies in case of metastasis. Radiotherapy is a technique that uses high-energy rays targeted to damage and kill cancer cells, but subsequently, the irradiated normal cells can also lead to the formation of secondary malignancy. Chemo also remains unselective and can affect normal tissues in addition to cancer cells. This will eventually cause unavoidable side effects. The limitations of chemotherapy also include low response rate, drug resistance, and systemic toxicity (Xie et al. 2020). Therefore, it becomes important to focus on revolutionary material products through innovative cancer therapies (Debela et al. 2021).

Nanoparticles with a large surface area with functional abilities are applied in drug delivery, multifunctional diagnostics, radio labeling, gene delivery, tumor destructor, biosensors for pathogen detection, nucleic acid probe, optical imaging, and dental and tissue engineering (Vargason, et al., 2021). Nano-engineered pharmacologically active metal oxides, micro/meso-structured silica (zeolites, mesoporous silica), polymers (polyethylene glycol, chitosan, PLGA, dentrimers), metal organic framework (MOFs), graphene oxides, mesocarbon, and quantum dots have been increasingly applied as therapeutic tools in the treatment of chronic diseases (cancer, cardiovascular, and diabetics) (Ahmed et al. 2022; Holmannova et al. 2022; Jandt and Watts, 2020). Recently, the application of FDA-approved drugs in a more efficient way by reducing the dose level and improving pharmacological properties for diseases such as COVID-19 is gaining attention worldwide (Sahoo et al. 2021; Jermy et al. 2022). Small molecule inhibitors, such as tyrosine kinase inhibitor imatinib, and 89 several such inhibitors were approved by the United States FDA. However, the therapeutic

DOI: 10.1201/9781003317715-11

efficacy was reduced, with a lower response rate and generation of drug resistance (Zhong et al. 2021). FDA also approved the cancer treatment based on immuno-therapy (immune checkpoint inhibitor), targeting antigen (cytotoxic T lymphocyte antigen 4) (Twomey and Zhang, 2021) (Figure 11.1).

Nanotechnology-driven precision-based nanomedicine therapeutics are gain-ing momentum in the medical field. The market of nanotech and smart pills is expected to grow to $125 billion and $650 million by the year 2025. Nanoparticle physico-chemical properties, such as particle size and shape, are critical to deter-mining the efficiency of treatment. Nanotherapeutics can be effective by improving the particle penetration inside the blood vessel, target specificity, and excretion, and reducing the toxicity of nanoparticles (Friedman et al. 2021). Till now, a variety of nanoplatforms has been reported for targeted drug therapies (Figure 11.2). The nano-formulation with particle size above 10 nm exhibits a high diffusion rate, facilitating lateral movement in the blood vessel. In addition, such nanoparticles can penetrate tumor cells easily by diffusing through gaps in leaky tumor vasculature endothe-lial cells and enhancing the permeability and retention effect. However, an inho-mogeneity in the leakage vessels affects the penetration and particle distributions inside the tumors (Kobayashi et al. 2014; Niora et al. 2020). The surface chemistry of nanoformulation with different functional moieties plays a vital role in target-spe-cific coordination with cancer cells. Nanocarrier physical characteristics, such as surface area, pore volume, and pore diameter, play a defining role in improving the solubility of drugs and adhesion to cancer cells. Surface coating on the nanocarrier is important, as the formulation charge (positive or negative) plays a critical role in adhesion. The nanoformulation with a positive charge effectively passes through the membrane barriers and reaches the nucleus or cytosol (Cruz-Nova et al. 2022).

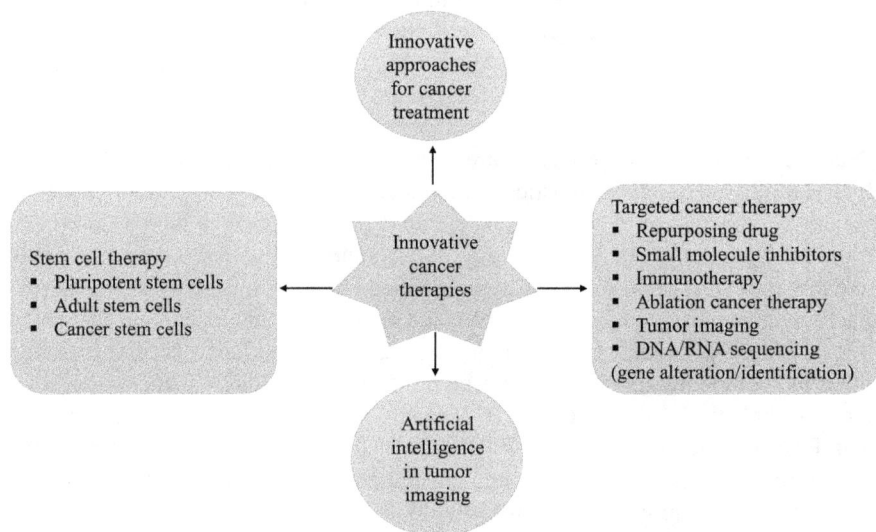

FIGURE 11.1   Innovative approaches for cancer treatment.

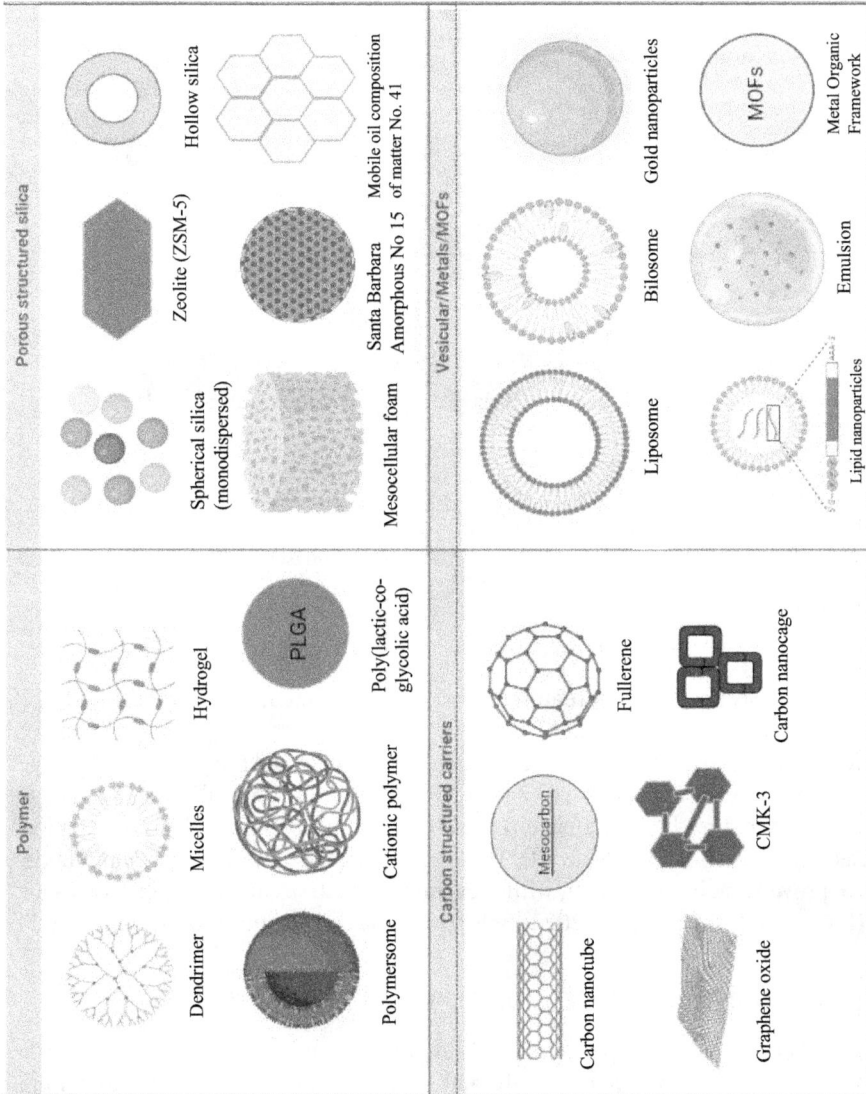

FIGURE 11.2   Different types of nanoplatforms used for targeted drug therapies.

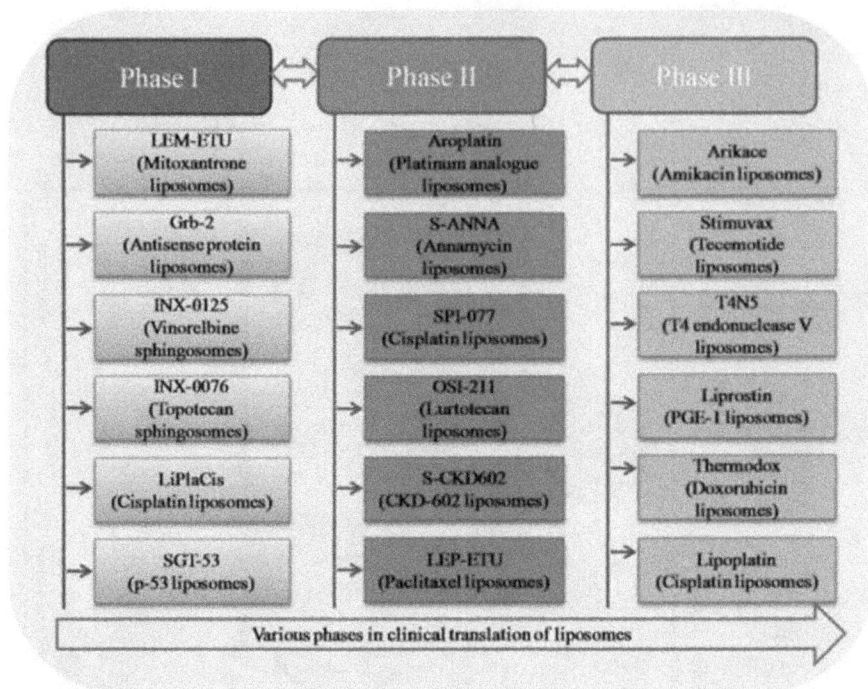

FIGURE 11.3 Liposomal formulations in various clinical phases: I, II, and III.

Source: Filipczak et al. 2020.

Further, extensive research is required to further substantiate the application of different structure nanomaterials.

Liposome, a vesicle, is generally composed of phospholipid bilayer sheets arranged in a spherical form. The outer layer is constituted by a hydrophilic head, while the inner layers contain a hydrophobic tail as part of the phospholipid. Nanoformulations, such as Doxil, DaunoXome, Onivyde, Vyxeos, AmBisome, Arikaye, and Marqibo, are FDA approved and in the market, while several formulations are in clinical stages I, II, and III (Figure 11.3) (Liu et al. 2022; Beltrán-Gracia et al. 2019; Filipczak et al. 2020).

11.2 CATIONIC POLYMER-BASED VACCINES

Pathogen bacteria, viruses, parasites, and fungi represent major health issues causing various diseases, which spread rapidly and result in high mortality (14–16 million) worldwide (Jiang et al. 2020). Recently, most of the outbreaks are caused by pathogens. The confirmed cases and deaths are continuously rising across the globe (202 countries), making this infectious spread the deadliest for mankind in modern times. In the present generation, a tremendous technological advancement is taking place in developing stimuli-responsive polymeric/silica/carbon-based materials for targeted-oriented drug therapy, diagnostic purpose, stem cell, and bioengineering (Wei et al. 2022).

Nanotherapeutics has broadened the scope for effective and efficient therapeutic approaches to deadly diseases, such as cancer, diabetes, and other metabolic disorders. In particular, targeted drug delivery can be very effective for pulmonary treatment. A pH-sensitive dexamethasone release from zinc spinel ferrite–based halloysite clay has been reported as a potential treatment for COVID-19 (Jermy et al. 2022).

Subunit vaccines have minimal side effects and are safe to use. However, it has less efficiency and less immunogenicity. Also, stimulants and adjuvants used to promote immune response are not effective to stimulate desired immune responses. To enhance the antigen transit across the mucosal barrier, different nanocarriers were reported, including polymers, silica, and liposomes (Petkar et al. 2021). Nanogels with high protein stabilization due to colloidal stability tend to assist facile cell internalization more than liposomes (Ferreira et al. 2013). The intranasal route of vaccine delivery was reported to limit the pneumococci colony formation in the nasal cavity. In order to enhance the immune response of antigens, toxin-derived mucosal adjuvants were co-administered. Though effective, such toxins are also detrimental to the central nervous system (Kong et al. 2013). In recent years, cationic-based polymers were used for developing mRNA vaccines (Park et al. 2021). The long-term adverse effect of three vaccines from Pfizer-BioNtech, AstraZeneca, and Sinopharm was investigated in the Middle Eastern region (Jordan and Saudi Arabia). The Pfizer vaccine, with the active ingredient nucleoside modified mRNA encoding COVID-19 spike protein, polyethylene glycol-2000, 1,2-distearoyl-sn-glycero-3-phosphocholine, cholesterol, (4-hydroxybutyl)azanediyl)bis(hexane-6,1-diyl)bis(2-hexyldecanoate), NaCl, monobasic potassium phosphate, KCl, dibasic sodium phosphate dihydrate, and sucrose, showed less long-term adverse effect; while Sinopharm, which is developed using inactivated virus, exhibited long-term adverse effects (Dar-Odeh et al. 2022).

11.3 THERMAL ABLATION TECHNIQUE

In cancer treatment, the thermal ablation technique is used to treat cancer cells by selective heat treatment of damaged cells with external electromagnetic waves (Rangamuwa et al. 2021). Radiowaves, microwaves, high-intense ultrasound, laser, and cryoablation are used as external sources (Yao et al. 2022; Kwak et al. 2022). The technique is convenient, as it is minimally invasive, flexible, and cost-effective (Pfannenstiel et al. 2022). However, the route of tumor heating is important for effective treatment and is challenging in thermal ablation. Ablation therapies face difficulties in limited light penetration, identification of healthy cells, and selective killing of tumor tissues (Han and Choi, 2021). Nanotechnology-driven thermal ablation has generated a lot of interest to overcome such limitations. The thermal ablation technique utilizes well-designed magnetic and gold nanoparticles in pure or nanocomposite form. The magnetic nanoparticles equipped with several functional moieties can be guided by an external source (magnetic field) and trigger heat increase with radio frequency or near-infrared light or electromagnetic field (Materón et al. 2021). The attachment of tumor functional receptors and ligands linked with hyper-branched polymers to nanoparticles can assist specific interaction with cancer cells, target specific cancer cells, heat, and destroy (Niculescu and Grumezescu, 2022). The presence of a high surface area can further allow multitasking possibilities, such as tumor imaging, labeling, and cell separation (Xuan et al. 2021). Further, such selective heat treatment prevents damage to normal cells and improves the treatment efficacy. The technique includes the following treatment steps: (i) nanoparticle attachment to cancer cells, (ii) identification of the binding characteristics through validation, and (iii) tumor cell heating using electromagnetic field (Putzer et al. 2020). However, the critical factors that need to be considered for this technique are magnetic nanoparticles toxicity, concentration, nature of biodistribution, and critical heat dose. In addition, the nanoparticle movement from the targeted site needs to be considered, along with the undesired heating of normal cells (Ashikbayeva et al. 2019). The delivery of heat with the required dose to the particular targeted cancer site is critical to upgrade lab-scale to clinical-scale requirements.

Magnetic nanoparticles (MNPs), such as super-paramagnetic iron oxide nanoparticles (SPIONs), are FDA-approved contrasting inorganic materials that have been reported for multifunctional drug delivery and diagnostic, imaging, and contrasting agents. NPs have been exhaustively used in hyperthermia. MNPs with particle sizes ranging between 1 and 100 nm have been used in thermal therapy. Spinel ferrites and iron oxide NPs, such as magnetite (Fe_3O_4) and maghemite ($\gamma\text{-}Fe_2O_3$), with high magnetic moment density are widely applied in thermal ablation. Super-paramagnetic iron oxide nanoparticles (SPIONs) are interesting properties exhibited by nanoparticles ranging between 10 and 20 nm. SPIONs magnetization to the saturation level occurs in the presence of an external magnetic field and returns to a non-metal state with the removal of an external magnetic field. SPIONs are less toxic and biocompatible. However, SPIONs (Fe_3O_4) are susceptible to oxidation and require surface modifications with ligands and antibodies. SPIONs are difficult to control and easily form aggregation (Idris et al. 2018; Dulińska-Litewka et al. 2019). Several researchers reported the removal of a template using and requiring the transformation into an inactive non-magnetic form during calcination. Indirect removal of a template using the solvent extraction technique involves the usage of a large volume of solvents and a laborious process. Spinel ferrite can be an alternative that can be explored for the thermal ablation technique. Drug delivery systems have been transformed effectively over the past seven decades. The nanotherapeutics that have been approved by FDA are shown in Figure 11.4. Precision-based nanomedicine not only improved therapeutic efficiency but also reduced treatment costs (Park et al. 2022).

Several challenges, such as solubility, permeability, target specificity, overcoming of biological barriers, and minimization of immunogenicity, were encountered in developing a drug delivery system with different functional moieties (small molecules, proteins/peptides, antibodies, and nucleic acids). Several pathbreaking research over five generations led to the development of microneedle patches, ocular and brain drug delivery, controlled drug-release implants, pH-sensitive capsules, drug-loaded contact lenses, and wound healing (Figure 11.5). The drug modification, along with environmental stimuli polymer nanocomposite, imparted intelligence to the delivery system (Rodrigues et al. 2020; Juliana et al. 2019; Akhter et al. 2022; Liu and Wu, 2021; Salih et al. 2021). Till now, nanomedicines (up to five) related to anticancer treatment have been approved by FDA (Yang et al. 2022). Drug delivery systems in nanoparticle size can easily diffuse through the biological barriers, deposit inside the organ, and exhibit toxic effects (Patnaik et al. 2021). Though several metal oxides,

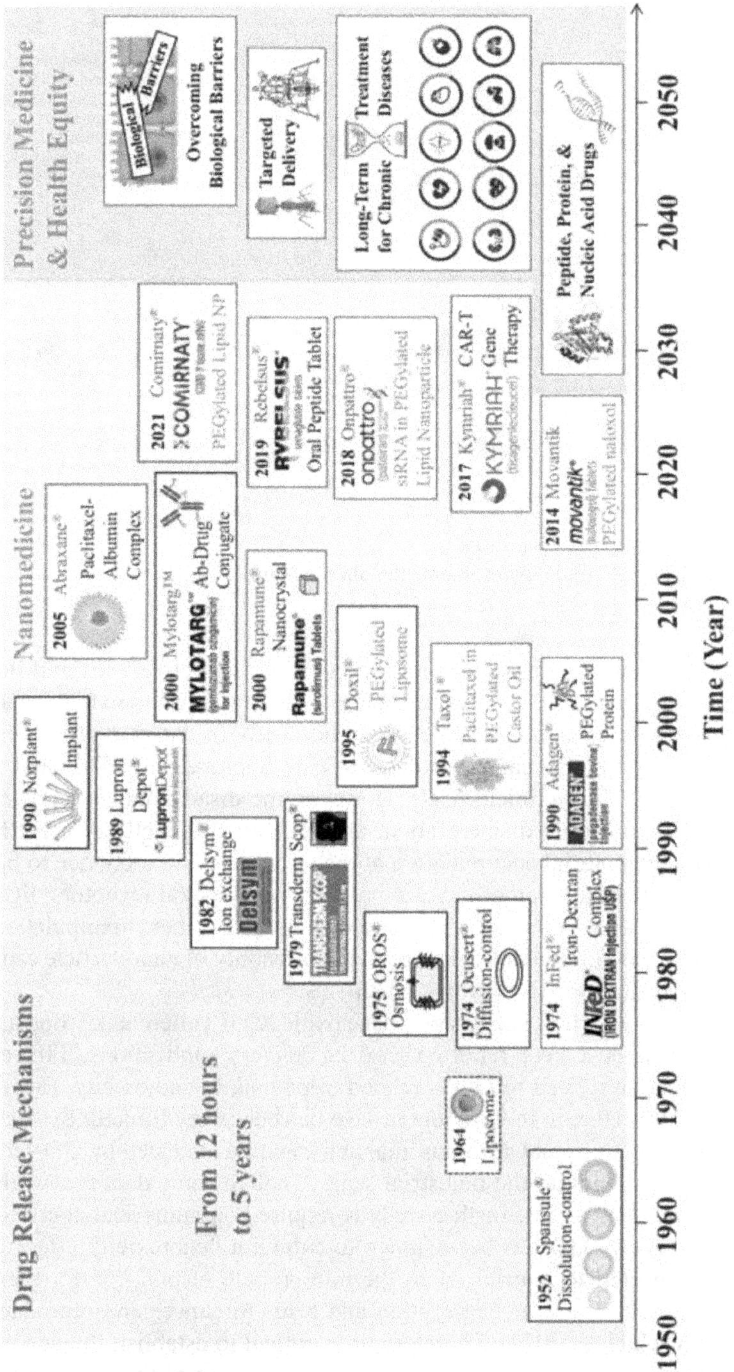

FIGURE 11.4 List of FDA-approved drug delivery systems.

Source: Park et al. 2022.

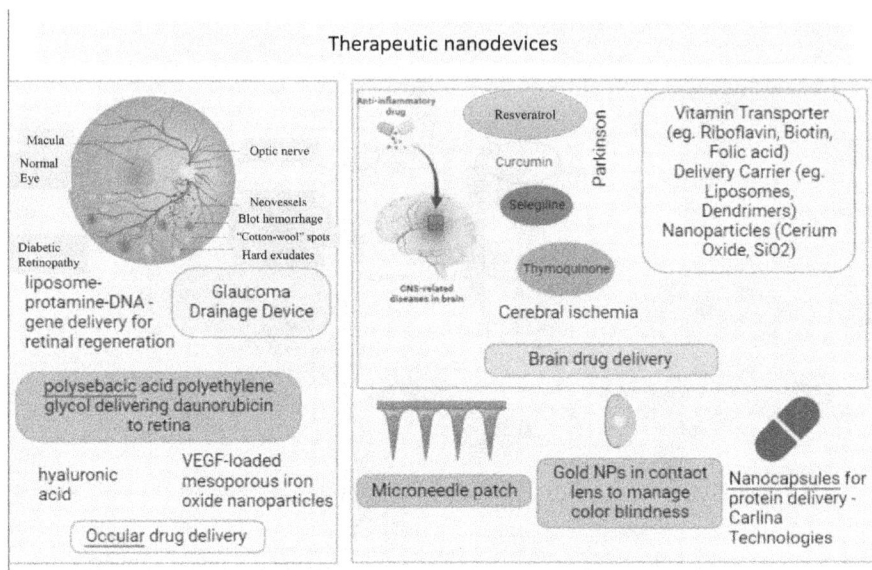

Therapeutic nanodevices

FIGURE 11.5 Challenges and advancements in nanomedicine.

such as Au, Zn, Fe, and Ti–based nanoformulations, are effective with multifunctional moieties functionalization element, such as Cu, is reported to exhibit toxicity at a high dose level (Sharma et al. 2021; Lee et al. 2016). In the case of polymeric nanoparticles, few polymeric nanoformulations were approved by FDA, and several nanocarriers are under clinical trials. However, the disadvantage of polymers includes particle aggregation, disintegration, and toxicity (Mitchell et al. 2021). It is indicated that nanomaterial accumulation at the tumor site is merely due to blood circulation and functionalization of nanoformulation with several receptors; ligands and antibodies have little influence on targeted therapy. Further, manipulation of nanoformulation with antibody or ligand exerts the possiblity of nanoparticle capture by both normal and cancer cells (Kwon et al. 2012).

Carbon-based nanocarriers, such as graphene oxide (GO), fullerene, carbon nanotube, and graphdiyne, have been reported for drug delivery applications (Tang et al. 2022). The prime issue related to GO is related to potential genotoxicity. However, the GO mutagenicity effect in in vitro and in vivo has been very limited. Systematic mammalian gene mutations and chromosomal abnormalities induced by GO need to be studied before upscaling to the industrial scale. Though some data are available related to structural aberrations, further study is required on numerical aberrations. In an exhaustive review, GO has been shown to exhibit a genotoxicity effect. The nanomaterial is reported to interfere with the microtubule responsible for the cell division process of chromosome segregation and leads to cancer and reproductive disorders (Domenech et al. 2022). Therefore, it is critical to establish the genotoxic profile of relevant nanomaterials at the initial screening stage of the industrial process. Also, the synthesis of structured mesocarbons requires expensive reagents; a multistep process; advanced instrument setup, including inert operating conditions; and high energy consumption techniques. Several rod-shaped carbon-structured replicas with superior textural features using a cost-effective technique have been reported to use a solvent deposition technique on the silica matrix (Janus et al. 2022). Similar easy and facile synthesis of carbon-based nanoplatforms needs to be optimized for further functionalization and drug loading.

Mesoporous silica with a large surface area capable of multidrug functionalization is widely used as a nanocarrier for treating chronic diseases. In general, templating agents, such as CTAB, P123, and F127, were mixed with a silica source (sodium meta silicalite, TEOS, TMOS, Ludox AS-40) in acidic or alkaline media followed by pH adjustment, filtration, and calcination to generate mesopores with unique pore morphologies, such as hexagonal MCM-41 (Borówka and Skrzypiec, 2021), hollow (Sunwoo et al. 2021), chiral (Jiang et al. 2021), cubic shapes (MCM-48, SBA-15 and SBA-16). In recent years, several literature reports have used multiple polymeric long-chain templates, trypsin (Shi et al. 2021), hard/soft templates (Haynes et al. 2020), emulsion/micelles (Cervantes-Martinez et al. 2020), and ionic liquids (Wang et al. 2021) for creating hierarchical and ordered mesoporous silica. Yang et al. (2022) have reported the synthesis of mesoporous silica films using dual templates, such as CTAB and P123. However, the synthesis of such MSNs using expensive/eco-unfriendly templates, solvents, and related chemicals without complete removal can pose high health-related hazard to humans. The design of mesoporous silica without using expensive, eco-unfriendly, and carcinogenic templates is recently gaining attention. For instance, zeolite and amorphous silica with superior surface textures have been developed using eco-friendly green metakaolin source (Arasi et al. 2021; Shu et al. 2016).

Also, for developing a porous structure, the usage of eco-friendly templates is another alternative to generating mesoporous silica. Yaya et al. (2021) have reported on mesoporous silica in the form of nanospheres using an environmentally friendly template, nanocellulose. A one-pot technique has been reported for the successful synthesis of worm-shaped mesoporous silica using hydroxyethyl cellulose as a template (Lyu et al. 2020). Mesoporous silica developed using the tannic acid template with silane functionalization is reported to act against hepatoxicity and exhibit a protective effect against liver toxicity with their innate antioxidant property (Javdani et al. 2021). MSNs with hexadecylpyridinium bromide template modified with three different functional moieties, such as amine, carboxyl, and thiol, were studied for quercetin and gemcitabine delivery. In the case of amine functionalization, there is a high quercetin-loading ability (72%) with a slow and sustained release (14%), while carboxylic acid functionalization induces high gemcitabine loading (45%) and a slow release pattern of about 15% (Zaharudin et al. 2020). Bioreducible polyethyleneimine core-shell nanostructures that are non-toxic can be upgraded as a gene and repurposing drug delivery system (Jena et al. 2022).

11.4 DENTISTRY

The nanotechnological revolution in the field of dentistry is termed as "nanodentistry". The nanoresearch market is expected to reach $125 billion by 2024 (Rambaran and Schirhagl, 2022). In dentistry, dentist treatment paradigms focus on treating tooth decay or dental cavities (dental caries) and gum disease (periodontal disease). At the time of tooth infection, the treatment involves the elimination of pathogens and the removal of carious tissues followed by the restoration of oral function. Conventional treatment strategies are effective but are compromised with several side effects, such as toxicity, drug resistance, less oral absorption, poor bioavailability, irritation, nausea, vomiting, and diarrhea (Moraes et al. 2021).

Biocompatibility and effective integration of nanoparticles with teeth and oral cavity define longevity inside the body. Therefore, in the fabrication of nanoformulation for dental applications, critical knowledge is required about nanoparticle properties, nanoformulation composition (Fadeel et al. 2015), and anatomy and physiology characteristics of the dental infection site. Minerals, hydroxyapatite, and $Ca_3(PO_4)_2$ play a major part in dental products. Metals, such as Ag, Zn, Au, TiO_2, Al, Fe_3O_4, SiO_2, and Zr, are used as pulp capping agents, for medical implants, and for related orthopedic applications. Synthetic and natural polymers, such as polyamidoamine, polymethyl methacylate, PLGA, chitosan, alginate, and pectin hyaluronic acid, are also used for different dental applications. For durability, ceramics, glasses, silicate, lithium disilicate, and leucite were used in restorative dentistry. The tooth consists of the enamel, dentin and pulp, cementum, and periodontal ligament (Olaru et al. 2021). The teeth's major composition consists of an inorganic component hydroxyapatite (HA) (96wt.%), along with organic materials (4wt.%). Hence, HA is used as an important ingredient in developing dental-related nanoproducts (Figure 11.6). The advantage of nano-engineered products includes desirable swelling capacity, variable

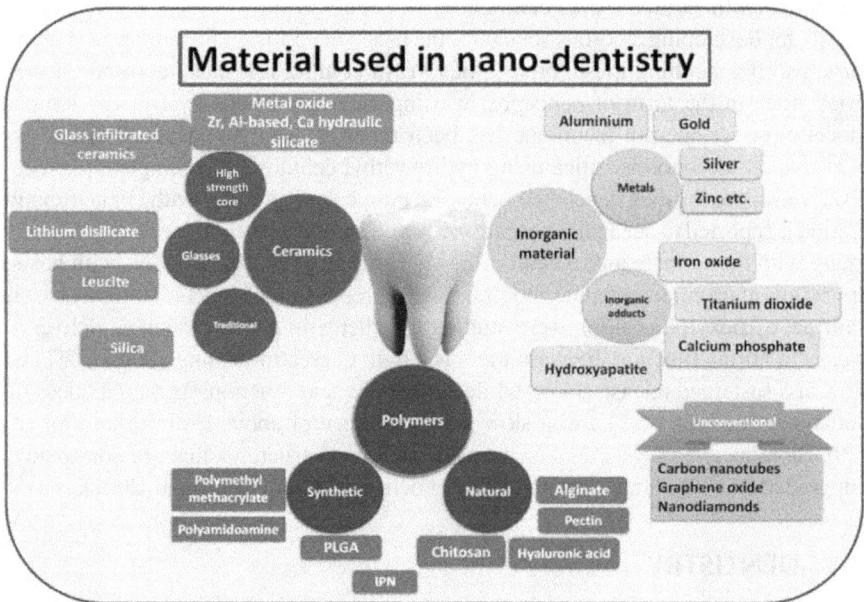

FIGURE 11.6 Overview of the materials applied in dentistry.

Source: Sreenivasalu et al. 2022.

strength and hardness, superior aesthetics, fracture resistance, durability, precision diagnostics, sustained and controlled drug release, controllable external surface and porosity, high drug loading and encapsulation, assistance in tissue regeneration, and biocompatibility (Sreenivasalu et al. 2022).

A pulp capping agent has been applied to cover the exposed part of the pulp due to traumatic injuries, infection, and dental preparation (Motwani et al. 2021). The most preferred capping agent is calcium hydroxide. Nanoparticles, such as aluminum oxide and silica nanoparticles, have been alternatively used as pulp capping agents and other dental products (Kunert and Lukomska-Szymanska, 2020). Recently, the risk assessment related to the toxicology effect (cyto and genotoxicity) of dental materials is investigated to increase the biocompatible and hazardous effect. Krause et al. (2020) have studied the bioavailability, biodistribution, and toxic effects of three different Al sources (Al_2O_3, Al^0, and $AlCl_3.6H_2O$) in in vivo study. A systematic study indicates that Al_2O_3 has different bioaccumulation and aggregation trend in the intestine compared to the other two sources. Particle size, cluster shape, composition, and shape of Al_2O_3 are reported to influence the penetration of nanoparticles across the gut-blood barrier and accumulations in organs. For instance, Al_2O_3 in the form of a rod tends to accumulate in organs than spherical-shaped Al^0 nanomaterial. The main reason for such retainment is attributed to the shape of nanoparticles (rod vs spherical) that cause ineffective excretion. A similar trend occurs with SiO_2 nanoparticles, where spherical-shaped SiO_2 excretes within 2–24 h, while even after 7 days, rod-shaped silica persists in the organ (Zhao et al. 2017). In the case of aluminum nanoparticles Al^0, a nanolayer of aluminum oxide between 2 and 5 nm at the external surface as a shell assists facile protein corona formation. Nanoparticles derived from $AlCl_3.6H_2O$ and Al^0 showed a similar solubility property. However, a completely oxidized form of Al_2O_3 exhibits complexity in protein corona formation and, thereby, influences bioavailability and tissue retention (Sieg et al. 2018). A higher proportion (2–8 fold) of nanoparticles derived from $AlCl_3.6H_2O$ was taken up by the tissue, mainly attributed to ion permeability rather than particle size effect. The study found that Al_2O_3 with a low mass fraction property accumulates in a higher proportion in organs than Al^0, while ions of $AlCl_3.6H_2O$ have a greater ability to cross the intestinal barrier.

The biocompatible effect of Al_2O_3 and SiO_2 with particle sizes of 13 nm and 12 nm were studied by evaluating the cytotoxicity (WST-8 assay) and genotoxicity using a rapid apoptosis assay Hoechst/PI apoptosis. Al_2O_3 and SiO_2 exhibited a large zeta potential of −16.8 and −9.9 mV. NP aggregation and internalization in vesicles and nuclei have been observed, resulting in a genotoxic effect from Al_2O_3. Based on TEM analysis, nanosized-particle penetration occurs through the nuclei pore and induces both cytotoxicity and genotoxicity (Hashimoto and Imazato, 2015). Phthalocyanine aluminum dye (sensitizer) has been used in photodynamic therapy in modern dentistry. In the case of caries, the fluorescent property of the dye is activated due to the presence of disease-pathogenic bacteria at the tooth-enamel microcracks. Such a property of the dye is advantageous for early diagnosis of microcracks in the tooth enamel (Zolotareva et al. 2018).

Silver nanoparticles (AgNPs) have been extensively studied and known for centuries as an additive to biomaterial to inhibit bacterial growth and treat endodontic biofilms, infections, and caries in dentistry. The release of Ag in cationic form, along with its oxidation potential, is the main reason for its antimicrobial properties (Oncu et al. 2021; Talapko et al. 2020). Titanium and titanium-based alloys are excellent biocompatible materials with versatile applications in medical implants, including orthopedic and dentistry (Quinn et al. 2020; Haugen and Chen, 2022). However, titanium alloy releases the cytotoxic ion vanadium and aluminum into the surrounding tissue after implantation, leading to serious complications, such as neurological disorders; therefore, the application of zeolite may control the release of these ions by acting as a barrier (Bedi et al. 2009; Willis et al. 2021). The drafting of antibiotics, metals, and biocompatible polymers has been developed to modify the surface of the titanium alloy to restrict bacteria colonization (Esteban et al. 2021). However, despite the antiseptic precautions applied in clinical and surgical settings, peri-implantitis can be developed after implantation, causing reoperation, osteomyelitis, implant failure, and even death (Rinke et al. 2020). As bacteria colonize and adhere to the surface forming a biofilm, several studies reported different approaches to prevent biofilm formation on the implant's surface, including organic and inorganic antibacterial agents and the incorporation of antibiotic-loaded coating (Yu et al. 2021). In addition, the application of nanomaterials with particle sizes below 10 nm in dentistry requires strict adherence to ethical and regulatory practices. A cautious approach is needed to evaluate the adverse effect of such nanoparticles. The prospected growth of nanoparticles needs to be supported with extensive in vitro and in vivo studies.

The infusion of nanotechnology in tissue engineering is shifting the role of nanocomposites as mere additives to advanced biomimicking scaffolds replicating various biological structures. Silica-ceramic-based bioactive glass is being applied in bone tissue engineering (Al-Harbi et al. 2021). In dental enamel, HA, polyatomic ion (carbonate), natural mineral fluoride, and metal, such as magnesium, are used as heteroionic substituents. In the case of biomimetic mineralization derived from histogenesis, a three-dimensional-structured scaffold has been generated by attracting calcium or phosphate ion components for the precipitation of HA via the de novo process (Ramírez-Rodríguez et al. 2021). Glycoprotein, such as laminin-1, has been widely applied as a biomimetic component. In orthodontic implants, HA, the calcium salt of phosphoric acid (tricalcium phosphate), and an amorphous mixture of calcium phosphate are commonly used to increase bone density. Protein isoforms, such as amelogenins, structural protein (collagen), and designed synthetic peptides (oligopeptide P11–4), are commonly used for biomimetic mineralization in dentistry (Dawasaz et al. 2022).

11.5 CONCLUSIONS

The treatment strategy in healthcare is continuously evolving for the benefit of mankind. The nanotechnology-based therapeutic approach offers a better scope to treat chronic diseases and dental applications. Liposome-based drugs are FDA-approved and available in the market, while nanoformulations based on drug delivery systems are already in the market. One of the main challenges in nanotherapeutics is acquiring in-depth knowledge about nanoparticle physico-chemical properties, such as particle size and shape, which determines the efficiency of treatment. In cancer tumors, inhomogeneity in the leakage vessels affects the penetration and particle distribution inside the tumors. Surface coating on the nanocarrier is important, as the formulation charge (positive or negative) plays a critical role in the adhesion and diffusion of membrane barriers and the ability to reach the nucleus or cytosol. Thermal ablation is one of the effective treatments against cancer, where magnetic nanoparticle toxicity concentration needs to be considered, along with the nature of biodistribution and critical heat doses. The delivery of heat with the required dose to the particular targeted cancer site is critical to upgrade the ablation technique from lab-scale to clinical-scale requirements. Several pathbreaking research over five generations led to the development of microneedle patches, controlled drug-release implants, pH-sensitive capsules, drug-loaded contact lenses, and wound healing. However, the disadvantages of polymers include particle aggregation, disintegration, and toxicity. It has been indicated that nanomaterial accumulation at the tumor site is merely due to blood circulation and functionalization of nanoformulation with several receptors; ligands and antibodies have little influence on targeted therapy. Several carbon-based nanocarriers, such as graphene oxide (GO), fullerene, carbon nanotube, and graphdiyne, have been reported for drug delivery applications. However, such carbon-based materials exhibit genotoxicity. Bioreducible polymer-based core-shell nanostructures that are non-toxic can be upgraded as a gene and repurposing drug delivery system. In densitry, the particle size, cluster shape, composition, and shape of nanoparticles are reported to influence the penetration of nanoparticles across the gut-blood barrier and accumulations in organs.

REFERENCES

Ahmed, H., Gomte, S.S., Prabakaran, A., Agrawal, M. and Alexander, A., 2022. Biomedical applications of mesoporous silica nanoparticles as a drug delivery carrier. *Journal of Drug Delivery Science and Technology*, p. 103729.

Akhter, M.H., Ahmad, I., Alshahrani, M.Y., Al-Harbi, A.I., Khalilullah, H., Afzal, O., Altamimi, A.S., Najib Ullah, S.N.M., Ojha, A. and Karim, S., 2022. Drug delivery challenges and current progress in nanocarrier-based ocular therapeutic system. *Gels*, 8(2), p. 82.

Al-Harbi, N., Mohammed, H., Al-Hadeethi, Y., Bakry, A.S., Umar, A., Hussein, M.A., Abbassy, M.A., Vaidya, K.G., Al Berakdar, G., Mkawi, E.M. and Nune, M., 2021. Silica-based bioactive glasses and their applications in hard tissue regeneration: A review. *Pharmaceuticals*, 14(2), p. 75.

Arasi, M.A., Salem, A. and Salem, S., 2021. Production of mesoporous and thermally stable silica powder from low grade kaolin based on eco-friendly template free route via acidification of appropriate zeolite compound for removal of cationic dye from wastewater. *Sustainable Chemistry and Pharmacy*, 19, p. 100366.

Ashikbayeva, Z., Tosi, D., Balmassov, D., Schena, E., Saccomandi, P. and Inglezakis, V., 2019. Application of nanoparticles and nanomaterials in thermal ablation therapy of cancer. *Nanomaterials*, 9(9), p. 1195.

Bedi, R.S., Beving, D.E., Zanello, L.P. and Yan, Y., 2009. Biocompatibility of corrosion-resistant zeolite coatings for titanium alloy biomedical implants. *Acta Biomaterialia*, 5(8), pp. 3265–3271.

Beltrán-Gracia, E., López-Camacho, A., Higuera-Ciapara, I., Velázquez-Fernández, J.B. and Vallejo-Cardona, A.A., 2019. Nanomedicine review: Clinical developments in liposomal applications. *Cancer Nanotechnology*, 10(1), pp. 1–40.

Borówka, A. and Skrzypiec, K., 2021. Effects of temperature on the structure of mesoporous silica materials templated with cationic surfactants in a nonhydrothermal short-term synthesis route. *Journal of Solid State Chemistry*, 299, p. 122183.

Cervantes-Martinez, C.V., Stébé, M.J., Emo, M., Lebeau, B. and Blin, J.L., 2020. Hierarchical mesoporous silica templated by the combination of fine emulsion and micelles. *Microporous and Mesoporous Materials*, 305, p. 110376.

Cheng, Z., Li, M., Dey, R. and Chen, Y., 2021. Nanomaterials for cancer therapy: Current progress and perspectives. *Journal of Hematology & Oncology*, 14(1), pp. 1–27.

Cruz-Nova, P., Ancira-Cortez, A., Ferro-Flores, G., Ocampo-García, B. and Gibbens-Bandala, B., 2022. Controlled-release nanosystems with a dual function of targeted therapy and radiotherapy in colorectal cancer. *Pharmaceutics*, 14(5), p. 1095.

Dar-Odeh, N., Abu-Hammad, O., Qasem, F., Jambi, S., Alhodhodi, A., Othman, A., Abu-Hammad, A., Al-Shorman, H., Ryalat, S. and Abu-Hammad, S., 2022. Long-term adverse events of three COVID-19 vaccines as reported by vaccinated physicians and dentists, a study from Jordan and Saudi Arabia. *Human Vaccines & Immunotherapeutics*, 18(1), p. 2039017.

Dawasaz, A.A., Togoo, R.A., Mahmood, Z., Azlina, A. and Thirumulu Ponnuraj, K., 2022. Effectiveness of self-assembling peptide (P11–4) in dental hard tissue conditions: A comprehensive review. *Polymers*, 14(4), p. 792.

Debela, D.T., Muzazu, S.G., Heraro, K.D., Ndalama, M.T., Mesele, B.W., Haile, D.C., Kitui, S.K. and Manyazewal, T., 2021. New approaches and procedures for cancer treatment: Current perspectives. *SAGE Open Medicine*, 9, p. 20503121211034366.

Domenech, J., Rodríguez-Garraus, A., López de Cerain, A., Azqueta, A. and Catalán, J., 2022. Genotoxicity of graphene-based materials. *Nanomaterials*, 12(11), p. 1795.

Dulińska-Litewka, J., Łazarczyk, A., Hałubiec, P., Szafrański, O., Karnas, K. and Karewicz, A., 2019. Superparamagnetic iron oxide nanoparticles—Current and prospective medical applications. *Materials*, 12(4), p. 617.

Esteban, J., Vallet-Regí, M. and Aguilera-Correa, J.J., 2021. Antibiotics-and heavy metals-based titanium alloy surface modifications for local prosthetic joint infections. *Antibiotics*, 10(10), p. 1270.

Fadeel, B., Fornara, A., Toprak, M.S. and Bhattacharya, K., 2015. Keeping it real: The importance of material characterization in nanotoxicology. *Biochemical and Biophysical Research Communications*, 468(3), pp. 498–503.

Ferreira, S.A., Gama, F.M. and Vilanova, M., 2013. Polymeric nanogels as vaccine delivery systems. *Nanomedicine: Nanotechnology, Biology and Medicine*, 9(2), pp. 159–173.

Filipczak, N., Pan, J., Yalamarty, S.S.K. and Torchilin, V.P., 2020. Recent advancements in liposome technology. *Advanced Drug Delivery Reviews*, 156, pp. 4–22.

Friedman, N., Dagan, A., Elia, J., Merims, S. and Benny, O., 2021. Physical properties of gold nanoparticles affect skin penetration via hair follicles. *Nanomedicine: Nanotechnology, Biology and Medicine*, 36, p. 102414.

Han, H.S. and Choi, K.Y., 2021. Advances in nanomaterial-mediated photothermal cancer therapies: Toward clinical applications. *Biomedicines*, 9(3), p. 305.

Hashimoto, M. and Imazato, S., 2015. Cytotoxic and genotoxic characterization of aluminum and silicon oxide nanoparticles in macrophages. *Dental Materials*, 31(5), pp. 556–564.

Haugen, H.J. and Chen, H., 2022. Is there a better biomaterial for dental implants than titanium?—A review and meta-study analysis. *Journal of Functional Biomaterials*, 13(2), p. 46.

Haynes, T., Bougnouch, O., Dubois, V. and Hermans, S., 2020. Preparation of mesoporous silica nanocapsules with a high specific surface area by hard and soft dual templating approach: Application to biomass valorization catalysis. *Microporous and Mesoporous Materials*, 306, p. 110400.

Holmannova, D., Borsky, P., Svadlakova, T., Borska, L. and Fiala, Z., 2022. Carbon nanoparticles and their biomedical applications. *Applied Sciences*, 12(15), p. 7865.

Idris, M.I., Zaloga, J., Detsch, R., Roether, J.A., Unterweger, H., Alexiou, C. and Boccaccini, A.R., 2018. Surface modification of SPIONs in PHBV microspheres for biomedical applications. *Scientific Reports*, 8(1), pp. 1–11.

Jandt, K.D. and Watts, D.C., 2020. Nanotechnology in dentistry: Present and future perspectives on dental nanomaterials. *Dental Materials*, 36(11), pp. 1365–1378.

Janus, R., Natkański, P., Wądrzyk, M., Lewandowski, M., Michalik, M. and Kuśtrowski, P., 2022. Deposition of poly (furfuryl alcohol) in mesoporous silica template controlled by solvent polarity: A cornerstone of facile and versatile synthesis of high-quality CMK-type carbon replicas. Nanocasting of SBA-15, SBA-16, and KIT-6. *Carbon*, 195, pp. 292–307.

Javdani, H., Etemad, L., Moshiri, M., Zarban, A. and Hanafi-Bojd, M.Y., 2021. Effect of tannic acid-templated mesoporous silica nanoparticles on iron-induced oxidative stress and liver toxicity in rats. *Toxicology Reports*, 8, pp. 1721–1728.

Jena, H., Ahmadi, Z., Kumar, P. and Dhawan, G., 2022. Bioreducible polyethylenimine core–shell nanostructures as efficient and non-toxic gene and drug delivery vectors. *Bioorganic & Medicinal Chemistry*, 69, p. 116886.

Jermy, B.R., Ravinayagam, V., Almohazey, D., Alamoudi, W.A., Dafalla, H., Akhtar, S. and Tanimu, G., 2022. PEGylated green halloysite/spinel ferrite nanocomposites for pH sensitive delivery of dexamethasone: A potential pulmonary drug delivery treatment option for COVID-19. *Applied Clay Science*, 216, p. 106333.

Jiang, C., Yao, X., Zhao, Y., Wu, J., Huang, P., Pan, C., Liu, S. and Pan, C., 2020. Comparative review of respiratory diseases caused by coronaviruses and influenza A viruses during epidemic season. *Microbes and Infection*, 22(6–7), pp. 236–244.

Jiang, X., Cui, M., Zhang, W., Xie, L. and Xu, L., 2021. Design of chiral mesoporous silica nanorods using ursodeoxycholic acid/chenodeoxycholic acid and CTAB as templates for chiral-selective release of achiral drugs. *Materials Letters*, 285, p. 129144.

Juliana, F.R., Kesse, S., Boakye-Yiadom, K.O., Veroniaina, H., Wang, H. and Sun, M., 2019. Promising approach in the treatment of glaucoma using nanotechnology and nanomedicine-based systems. *Molecules*, 24(20), p. 3805.

Kobayashi, H., Watanabe, R. and Choyke, P.L., 2014. Improving conventional enhanced permeability and retention (EPR) effects; What is the appropriate target? *Theranostics*, 4(1), p. 81.

Kong, I.G., Sato, A., Yuki, Y., Nochi, T., Takahashi, H., Sawada, S., Mejima, M., Kurokawa, S., Okada, K., Sato, S. and Briles, D.E., 2013. Nanogel-based PspA intranasal vaccine prevents invasive disease and nasal colonization by Streptococcus pneumoniae. *Infection and Immunity*, 81(5), pp. 1625–1634.

Krause, B.C., Kriegel, F.L., Rosenkranz, D., Dreiack, N., Tentschert, J., Jungnickel, H., Jalili, P., Fessard, V., Laux, P. and Luch, A., 2020. Aluminum and aluminum oxide nanomaterials uptake after oral exposure-a comparative study. *Scientific Reports*, 10(1), pp. 1–10.

Kunert, M. and Lukomska-Szymanska, M., 2020. Bio-inductive materials in direct and indirect pulp capping—a review article. *Materials*, 13(5), p. 1204.

Kwak, K., Yu, B., Lewandowski, R.J. and Kim, D.H., 2022. Recent progress in cryoablation cancer therapy and nanoparticles mediated cryoablation. *Theranostics*, 12(5), p. 2175.

Kwon, I.K., Lee, S.C., Han, B. and Park, K., 2012. Analysis on the current status of targeted drug delivery to tumors. *Journal of Controlled Release*, 164(2), pp. 108–114.

Lee, I.C., Ko, J.W., Park, S.H., Shin, N.R., Shin, I.S., Moon, C., Kim, J.H., Kim, H.C. and Kim, J.C., 2016. Comparative toxicity and biodistribution assessments in rats following subchronic oral exposure to copper nanoparticles and microparticles. *Particle and Fibre Toxicology*, 13(1), pp. 1–16.

Liu, P., Chen, G. and Zhang, J., 2022. A review of liposomes as a drug delivery system: Current status of approved products, regulatory environments, and future perspectives. *Molecules*, 27(4), p. 1372.

Liu, Y. and Wu, N., 2021. Progress of nanotechnology in diabetic retinopathy treatment. *International Journal of Nanomedicine*, 16, p. 1391.

Lyu, R., Zhang, C., Xia, T., Chen, S., Wang, Z., Luo, X., Wang, L., Wang, Y., Yu, J. and Wang, C., 2020. Efficient adsorption of methylene blue by mesoporous silica prepared using sol-gel method employing hydroxyethyl cellulose as a template. *Colloids and Surfaces A: Physicochemical and Engineering Aspects*, 606, p. 125425.

Materón, E.M., Miyazaki, C.M., Carr, O., Joshi, N., Picciani, P.H., Dalmaschio, C.J., Davis, F. and Shimizu, F.M., 2021. Magnetic nanoparticles in biomedical applications: A review. *Applied Surface Science Advances*, 6, p. 100163.

Mitchell, M.J., Billingsley, M.M., Haley, R.M., Wechsler, M.E., Peppas, N.A. and Langer, R., 2021. Engineering precision nanoparticles for drug delivery. *Nature Reviews Drug Discovery*, 20(2), pp. 101–124.

Moraes, G., Zambom, C. and Siqueira, W.L., 2021. Nanoparticles in dentistry: A comprehensive review. *Pharmaceuticals*, 14(8), p. 752.

Motwani, N., Ikhar, A., Nikhade, P., Chandak, M., Rathi, S., Dugar, M. and Rajnekar, R., 2021. Premixed bioceramics: A novel pulp capping agent. *Journal of Conservative Dentistry: JCD*, 24(2), p. 124.

Niculescu, A.G. and Grumezescu, A.M., 2022. Novel tumor-targeting nanoparticles for cancer treatment—a review. *International Journal of Molecular Sciences*, 23(9), p. 5253.

Niora, M., Pedersbæk, D., Münter, R., Weywadt, M.F.D.V., Farhangibarooji, Y., Andresen, T.L., Simonsen, J.B. and Jauffred, L., 2020. Head-to-head comparison of the penetration efficiency of lipid-based nanoparticles into tumor spheroids. *Acs Omega*, 5(33), pp. 21162–21171.

Olaru, M., Sachelarie, L. and Calin, G., 2021. Hard dental tissues regeneration—approaches and challenges. *Materials*, 14(10), p. 2558.

Oncu, A., Huang, Y., Amasya, G., Sevimay, F.S., Orhan, K. and Celikten, B., 2021. Silver nanoparticles in endodontics: Recent developments and applications. *Restorative Dentistry & Endodontics*, 46(3).

Park, K.S., Otte, A. and Park, H., 2022. Perspective on drug delivery in 2050. *Journal of Controlled Release: Official Journal of the Controlled Release Society*, 344, pp. 157–159.

Park, K.S., Sun, X., Aikins, M.E. and Moon, J.J., 2021. Non-viral COVID-19 vaccine delivery systems. *Advanced Drug Delivery Reviews*, 169, pp. 137–151.

Patnaik, S., Gorain, B., Padhi, S., Choudhury, H., Gabr, G.A., Md, S., Mishra, D.K. and Kesharwani, P., 2021. Recent update of toxicity aspects of nanoparticulate systems for drug delivery. *European Journal of Pharmaceutics and Biopharmaceutics*, 161, pp. 100–119.

Petkar, K.C., Patil, S.M., Chavhan, S.S., Kaneko, K., Sawant, K.K., Kunda, N.K. and Saleem, I.Y., 2021. An overview of nanocarrier-based adjuvants for vaccine delivery. *Pharmaceutics*, 13(4), p. 455.

Pfannenstiel, A., Iannuccilli, J., Cornelis, F.H., Dupuy, D.E., Beard, W.L. and Prakash, P., 2022. Shaping the future of microwave tumor ablation: A new direction in precision and control of device performance. *International Journal of Hyperthermia*, 39(1), pp. 664–674.

Putzer, D., Schullian, P., Eberle, G. and Bale, R.J., 2020. Thermal ablation—an option in curative treatment of HCC. *Memo-Magazine of European Medical Oncology*, 13(2), pp. 207–211.

Quinn, J., McFadden, R., Chan, C.W. and Carson, L., 2020. Titanium for orthopedic applications: An overview of surface modification to improve biocompatibility and prevent bacterial biofilm formation. *IScience*, 23(11), p. 101745.

Rambaran, T. and Schirhagl, R., 2022. Nanotechnology from lab to industry–a look at current trends. *Nanoscale Advances*, 4(18), pp. 3664–3675.

Ramírez-Rodríguez, G.B., Pereira, A.R., Herrmann, M., Hansmann, J., Delgado-López, J.M., Sprio, S., Tampieri, A. and Sandri, M., 2021. Biomimetic mineralization promotes viability and differentiation of human mesenchymal stem cells in a perfusion bioreactor. *International Journal of Molecular Sciences*, 22(3), p. 1447.

Rangamuwa, K., Leong, T., Weeden, C., Asselin-Labat, M.L., Bozinovski, S., Christie, M., John, T., Antippa, P., Irving, L. and Steinfort, D., 2021. Thermal ablation in non-small cell lung cancer: A review of treatment modalities and the evidence for combination with immune checkpoint inhibitors. *Translational Lung Cancer Research*, 10(6), p. 2842.

Rinke, S., Nordlohne, M., Leha, A., Renvert, S., Schmalz, G. and Ziebolz, D., 2020. Risk indicators for mucositis and peri-implantitis: Results from a practice-based cross-sectional study. *Journal of Periodontal & Implant Science*, 50(3), p. 183.

Rodrigues, F.S., Campos, A., Martins, J., Ambrosio, A.F. and Campos, E.J., 2020. Emerging trends in nanomedicine for improving ocular drug delivery: Light-responsive nanoparticles, mesoporous silica nanoparticles, and contact lenses. *ACS Biomaterials Science & Engineering*, 6(12), pp. 6587–6597.

Roth, G.A., Mensah, G.A., Johnson, C.O., Addolorato, G., Ammirati, E., Baddour, L.M., Barengo, N.C., Beaton, A.Z., Benjamin, E.J., Benziger, C.P. and Bonny, A., 2020. Global burden of cardiovascular diseases and risk factors, 1990–2019: Update from the GBD 2019 study. *Journal of the American College of Cardiology*, 76(25), pp. 2982–3021.

Sahoo, B.M., Ravi Kumar, B.V.V., Sruti, J., Mahapatra, M.K., Banik, B.K. and Borah, P., 2021. Drug repurposing strategy (DRS): Emerging approach to identify potential therapeutics for treatment of novel coronavirus infection. *Frontiers in Molecular Biosciences*, 8, p. 628144.

Salih, A.E., Elsherif, M., Alam, F., Yetisen, A.K. and Butt, H., 2021. Gold nanocomposite contact lenses for color blindness management. *ACS Nano*, 15(3), pp. 4870–4880.

Sharma, S., Parveen, R. and Chatterji, B.P., 2021. Toxicology of nanoparticles in drug delivery. *Current Pathobiology Reports*, pp. 1–12.

Shi, X., Zhang, P., Wu, L., Zhao, X., Jiang, J., Li, J. and Yang, B., 2021. Trypsin templated biomimetic large mesoporous silica performs favorable advantages in delivering poorly water-soluble drug. *Materials Science and Engineering: B*, 271, p. 115252.

Shu, Z., Li, T., Zhou, J., Chen, Y., Sheng, Z., Wang, Y. and Yuan, X., 2016. Mesoporous silica derived from kaolin: Specific surface area enlargement via a new zeolite-involved template-free strategy. *Applied Clay Science*, 123, pp. 76–82.

Sieg, H., Braeuning, C., Kunz, B.M., Daher, H., Kästner, C., Krause, B.C., Meyer, T., Jalili, P., Hogeveen, K., Böhmert, L. and Lichtenstein, D., 2018. Uptake and molecular impact of aluminum-containing nanomaterials on human intestinal caco-2 cells. *Nanotoxicology*, 12(9), pp. 992–1013.

Sreenivasalu, P.K.P., Dora, C.P., Swami, R., Jasthi, V.C., Shiroorkar, P.N., Nagaraja, S., Asdaq, S.M.B. and Anwer, M.K., 2022. Nanomaterials in dentistry: Current applications and future scope. *Nanomaterials*, 12(10), p. 1676.

Sunwoo, Y., Karunakaran, G. and Cho, E.B., 2021. Hollow mesoporous silica nanospheres using pentablock copolymer micelle templates. *Ceramics International*, 47(10), pp. 13351–13362.

Talapko, J., Matijević, T., Juzbašić, M., Antolović-Požgain, A. and Škrlec, I., 2020. Antibacterial activity of silver and its application in dentistry, cardiology and dermatology. *Microorganisms*, 8(9), p. 1400.

Tang, L., Li, J., Pan, T., Yin, Y., Mei, Y., Xiao, Q., Wang, R., Yan, Z. and Wang, W., 2022. Versatile carbon nanoplatforms for cancer treatment and diagnosis: Strategies, applications and future perspectives. *Theranostics*, 12(5), p. 2290.

Twomey, J.D. and Zhang, B., 2021. Cancer immunotherapy update: FDA-approved checkpoint inhibitors and companion diagnostics. *The AAPS Journal*, 23(2), pp. 1–11.

Vargason, A.M., Anselmo, A.C. and Mitragotri, S., 2021. The evolution of commercial drug delivery technologies. *Nature Biomedical Engineering*, 5(9), pp. 951–967.

Vos, T., Lim, S.S., Abbafati, C., Abbas, K.M., Abbasi, M., Abbasifard, M., Abbasi-Kangevari, M., Abbastabar, H., Abd-Allah, F., Abdelalim, A. and Abdollahi, M., 2020. Global burden of 369 diseases and injuries in 204 countries and territories, 1990–2019: A systematic analysis for the Global Burden of Disease Study 2019. *The Lancet*, 396(10258), pp. 1204–1222.

Wang, J., Zhang, C., Bai, Y., Li, Q. and Yang, X., 2021. Synthesis of mesoporous silica with ionic liquid surfactant as template. *Materials Letters*, 291, p. 129556.

Wei, H., Cui, J., Lin, K., Xie, J. and Wang, X., 2022. Recent advances in smart stimuli-responsive biomaterials for bone therapeutics and regeneration. *Bone Research*, 10(1), pp. 1–19.

Willis, J., Li, S., Crean, S.J. and Barrak, F.N., 2021. Is titanium alloy Ti-6Al-4 V cytotoxic to gingival fibroblasts—A systematic review. *Clinical and Experimental Dental Research*, 7(6), pp. 1037–1044.

Xie, Y.H., Chen, Y.X. and Fang, J.Y., 2020. Comprehensive review of targeted therapy for colorectal cancer. *Signal Transduction and Targeted Therapy*, 5(1), pp. 1–30.

Xuan, Y., Guan, M. and Zhang, S., 2021. Tumor immunotherapy and multi-mode therapies mediated by medical imaging of nanoprobes. *Theranostics*, 11(15), p. 7360.

Yang, J., Wang, X., Wang, B., Park, K., Wooley, K. and Zhang, S., 2022. Challenging the fundamental conjectures in nanoparticle drug delivery for chemotherapy treatment of solid cancers. *Advanced Drug Delivery Reviews*, p. 114525.

Yang, Y., Li, J., Yuan, H., Carlini, R. and Liu, X., 2022. The synthesis of mesoporous silica film using multi-templates directing and the effects of inorganic acids. *Materials Chemistry and Physics*, 280, p. 125808.

Yao, J., Liu, B., Wang, X., Yu, J., Cheng, Z., Han, Z., Liu, F., Zheng, R., Cheng, W., Wei, Q. and Yu, S., 2022. Long-term efficacy of microwave ablation in the treatment of subcapsular hepatocellular carcinomas of≤ 3 cm in diameter: A multicenter, propensity score-matched study. *International Journal of Hyperthermia*, 39(1), pp. 209–216.

Yaya, L., Cong, Y., Lianping, S., Qiuyang, C., Shitao, Y. and Lu, L., 2021. Rough-surface hydroxyl-group-rich hollow mesoporous silica nanospheres with nanocellulose as a template to improve the oxidation stability of bio-oil. *Biomass and Bioenergy*, 154, p. 106243.

Yu, X., Liao, X. and Chen, H., 2021. Antibiotic-loaded MMT/PLL-based coating on the surface of endosseous implants to suppress bacterial infections. *International Journal of Nanomedicine*, 16, p. 2983.

Zaharudin, N.S., Isa, E.D.M., Ahmad, H., Rahman, M.B.A. and Jumbri, K., 2020. Functionalized mesoporous silica nanoparticles templated by pyridinium ionic liquid for hydrophilic and hydrophobic drug release application. *Journal of Saudi Chemical Society*, 24(3), pp. 289–302.

Zhao, Y., Wang, Y., Ran, F., Cui, Y., Liu, C., Zhao, Q., Gao, Y., Wang, D. and Wang, S., 2017. A comparison between sphere and rod nanoparticles regarding their in vivo biological behavior and pharmacokinetics. *Scientific Reports*, 7(1), pp. 1–11.

Zhong, L., Li, Y., Xiong, L., Wang, W., Wu, M., Yuan, T., Yang, W., Tian, C., Miao, Z., Wang, T. and Yang, S., 2021. Small molecules in targeted cancer therapy: Advances, challenges, and future perspectives. *Signal Transduction and Targeted Therapy*, 6(1), pp. 1–48.

Zolotareva, J.O., Farrakhova, D.S. and Loschenov, V.B., 2018. Aluminium phthalocyanine nanoparticles application for fluorescent diagnostics and photodynamic therapy in dentistry. *KnE Energy*, pp. 568–577.

12 Research Trends in Materials Synthesis and Medical Applications

Muhammad Nawaz, Faiza Qureshi, Hira Fatima Abbas, and Tooba Mahboob

12.1 INTRODUCTION

The physicochemical attributes of fine particles differ versus nanoparticles (NPs) with alike compositions. Nanotechnology has been branded a substantial research discipline lately with a wide range of synthetic variations, strategies, and customization models at the level of size, shape, and structure, along with dimensions ranging from 1 to 100 nm (Figure 12.1). Exceptional chemical and physical attributes are offered by oxide NPs by reason of their size and their corner surface sites possessing higher density (Sagadevan et al., 2022). Additionally, developing nanotechnology has explicitly unlocked huge opportunities for the design and preparation of nanomaterials and the investigation and customization of their exclusive optical, physico-chemical, magnetic, electric, and mechanical characteristics, and employing the outcome in nano and biotechnology, as well as the amalgamation of the two. The frontiers making use of nanotechnology are skincare, drugs, manufacturing, integrated circuit technology, nutrition, environment, automation, optics, catalysts, drug delivery systems, genetics, biotherapeutics, ceramics, materials, light emitters, imaging, physical sciences, electromagnetics, electron transistors, water treatment plants, solar energy conversion, high-energy propellants and fuel cells, biochips, sensors, and more (Colvin et al., 1994; Wang, 1991). At the same time, nanotechnology has grown to be a prevalent need in several health structures (namely, regulation, prevention, diagnosis, monitoring, and therapeutics) and has grown too swiftly as a result of significantly better results (Atul et al., 2010; Ozak et al., 2013).

Nano and biomaterials have major usage in combating infectious diseases, which adds up to approximately 16.2% of total mortalities per year, as well as an inconsistent number of deaths (WHO, 2014). Infectious diseases remain a load and stress on the worldwide financial system. The absence of scrutiny, inadequate control, and sub-average prevention protocols have led to confusion in the antibiotic therapeutic regime, and this confusion becomes chaotic with drug resistance to traditional therapeutic treatments (Boucher et al., 2009).

For each treatment and infection, substantial research has been employed in discovering correlated molecular traits and additional biomarkers, such as toxins,

DOI: 10.1201/9781003317715-12

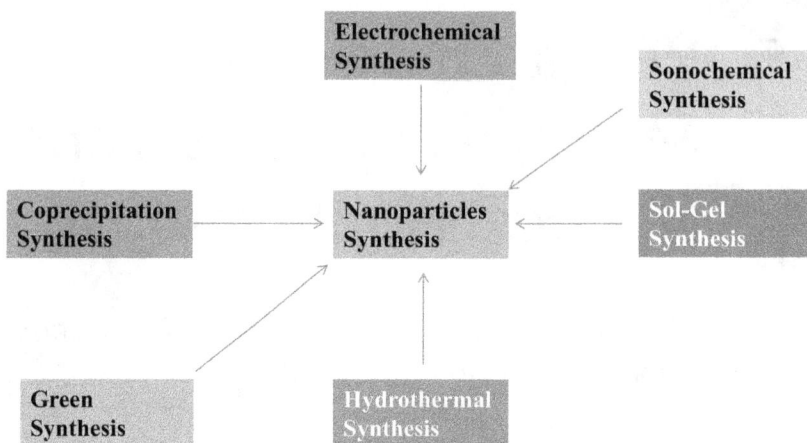

FIGURE 12.1 Demonstrating the different methods for the synthesis of nanoparticles.

antigens, or nucleic acids. Disease-initiating pathogens have a complicated and extensive range, with some having continued asymptomatic incubation periods and diagnosis of disease becomes tricky (Kaittanis et al., 2010). Molecular medicine has supplied more information about disease mechanisms and has provided a collection of investigative resources that may support reducing clinical confusion. Among these resources is nanotechnology, which brings groundbreaking molecular differentiation tools and point-of-care investigative findings. These innovative tools can be cohesive with a variety of techniques and systems resulting in enhanced and multidimensional techniques (Mcglennen, 2001). This has been achieved at a remarkable time when the outbreak of diseases is already a major health concern and is eating into regional economies, interrupting daily activities, and causing high treatment costs and higher mortalities. Even the rebirth of certain infections that were considered to be eradicated was observed with resistant species as a huge setback (V. Kyriacou et al., 2004).

Nanomedicine has proved to prevail over various shortcomings of typical therapies by the integration of nanoparticles that enabled modification of physico-chemical properties vs bulk materials. Main attributes, like subspace density, charge, structure, and proportions between surface and volume, are all worth manipulating. NPs can be tweaked to integrate with target receptors via surface properties or manipulate particle size, as well as targeted delivery of active dosage via drug-loaded NPs can be achieved. This allows selectivity as well as the possibility of lower dosages, fewer side effects, as well as a cost- and time-effective treatment plan. Primarily, nanomedicine was used to enhance the treatment of tumors (Barenholz, 2012). Presently, progressive and sophisticated trends have been made in the continuation of nanomedicine toward increasingly demanding research areas of diagnosis and treatment of a multitude of additional diseases. However, the quantity of nanotherapeutics presently authorized by the Food and Drug Administration (FDA) or in trial stages is very modest when compared to the vast amount of investigations published (Ventola, 2017; Bobo et al., 2016). Nanomedicines authorized by the FDA mostly consist of liposomes, polymers, micelles, polymer-conjugated proteins, and nanocrystals. Twelve of these treatments are listed to have nanoparticle metals, such as hydroxyapatite, calcium phosphate, and iron oxide (Ventola, 2017; Bobo et al., 2016). Out of six iron oxide NP (IONP) drugs authorized as a remedy for iron deficiency, only two (Ferumoxytol and Resovist) are available in the market (Yi-Xiang, 2015).

Regardless of the limited quantity of marketable products, metal oxide NPs (MONPs) have been researched with applications in various disciplines, from semiconductors to biomedicine (for medicinal or diagnostic objectives) (Ventola, 2017; Bobo et al., 2016). One case of biomedical use is antimicrobial action. Microbial infections are on top of the very dangerous threats to the population, including infections resulting from bacteria, viruses, protozoans, and fungi (Aderibigbe, 2017). Even though there remain several FDA-approved antimicrobial drugs, the development of microbe resistance toward drugs outweighs the current therapeutics; hence, an impending need to discover and design novel active molecules against microbial infections. There are many findings that explored the antimicrobial activity of MONPs.

12.2 SYNTHESIS OF NANOPARTICLES

12.2.1 SOL-GEL SYNTHESIS

The sol-gel method is a two-stage procedure consisting of the initial phase of the hydroxylation of the initial reactants in a liquid state, followed by its condensation, which derives a sol of NPs. A 3D metal oxide framework, identified as wet gel, thereof, is achieved by sustained condensation and inorganic polymerization methods. Supplementary thermal tampering can be affected to obtain a final crystalline state. Reaction circumstances, such as heat, solvent, pH, agitation, and the type of precursors chosen, make up the structure and attributes of the gel, which impacts their reaction kinetics and growth. Maghemite nanoparticles, in the size range of 6–15 nm, have been effortlessly acquired by treating the gels precisely at 673 K. This method offers certain benefits, such as the construction of customized NPs of a predesigned structure, pure amorphous phases, particle size regulation, controlled structure, and the homogeneity of the products, also a comparatively less heat requirement for processing the raw material. The sol-gel method has also been employed to implant iron oxide NPs onto appropriate matrices to use them for different purposes as multitasking products (Ramimoghadam et al., 2014; Sodipo and Aziz, 2016; Laurent et al., 2010). For instance, Solinas et al. (Solinas et al., 2001) have combined maghemite nanoparticles onto an inert and heat-resistant silica matrix by selecting more surface of evaporation to volume ratio in the second phase of gelation, resulting in iron oxide NPs due to the high porosity of silica. To produce magnetite, an increased proportion between surface and volume for evaporation as well as low temperature must be considered.

12.2.2 COPRECIPITATION SYNTHESIS

Magnetic iron oxide NPs are essentially produced by a wet chemical coprecipitation process, which happens to be additionally efficient versus other processes. The simple mechanism involves reacting an aqueous solution of ferrous and ferric salts together with an alkali provided with sufficient incubation time for the simultaneous precipitation of the magnetite, maghemite, and ferrous hydroxide polymorphs of iron oxides. The synthesis can be altered to achieve the different phases of iron oxide by altering the pH of the solution. Magnetite is produced under basic conditions using an Fe^{2+}/Fe^{3+} ratio equaling to 2:1 (Ramimoghadam et al., 2014). Since magnetite is extremely vulnerable to the co-occurrence of oxygen, it is readily converted to maghemite; therefore, the production of magnetite is ideal under non-oxidizing environments. Magnetite oxidation occurs when the iron ions desorb from the magnetite surface, creating positively charged vacancies in order to balance the structure's charge, transforming into maghemite. The distribution of Fe^{2+} and Fe^{3+} ions in the spinel structure is the main distinction that distinguishes the magnetite and maghemite forms of iron oxide, where the latter is unique in its crystal structure with the occurrence of positively charged positions in the octahedral sites. It is significant in nanoscience that the synthesis method brings an outcome over the ordering of the vacancies, resulting in symmetry lowering and the formation of superstructures (Cornell and Schwertmann, 2003; Glasgow et al., 2016). The fundamental advantage of this method is the allowance to scale up the product. However, a key drawback of this method is in achieving a broad particle size distribution, as crystal growth follows kinetic factors, such as pH, temperature, precursor, reaction rate, and the Fe^{2+}/Fe^{3+} ratio (Ramimoghadam et al., 2014). Consequently, the optimal reaction environment and precursors must be designated to yield the desired shape in defined NPs with the designed morphology. It was described by Babes et al. that the Fe^{2+}/Fe^{3+} ratio is crucial to improving the size of the particles (Babes et al., 1999).

12.2.3 HYDROTHERMAL SYNTHESIS

Hydrothermal synthesis encompasses the usage of autoclaves preserved at high-pressure and temperature environments. The reactions proceed within a closed chamber, preferably an autoclave. Like the coprecipitation method, the particle size of the prepared NPs is affected and controlled by the nucleation and growth rate. It is a recognized detail that if the nucleation phase is quicker than the growth phase at higher temperatures, the obtained nanoparticles would be with reduced sizes during the growth phase, notwithstanding grain growth, when increasing the reaction times (Sodipo and Aziz, 2016). Iron oxide NPs with sizes 4–27 nm were synthesized effortlessly using this method (Ramimoghadam et al., 2014). In this method, the morphology of the NPs can be tweaked by adjusting process parameters, such as reaction time, heat, pressure, and the concentration of the solutions, solvent, and complexing agents (Laurent et al., 2010). The hydrothermal technique combined with microwave synthesis has successfully yielded superparamagnetic iron oxide nanoparticles at the manufacturing scale.

12.2.4 ELECTROCHEMICAL SYNTHESIS

The very latest synthetic approach for the iron oxide nanoparticles and mostly the magnetite and maghemite polymorphs is the electrochemical method. The simplest method offers particle size regulation and no excessive reaction requirements, except that the temperature used is not higher than the electrolyte's boiling point. As the electronic flow and potential are the variable parameters in the electrochemical process, kinetic control and thermodynamic control can be determined during the synthesis. While the method is simple, as the reactions occur at room temperature, the necessary nucleation sites and progress are not accomplished, resulting in randomly ordered NPs or amorphous products (Zeng et al., 2017). More aspects were put forward by Cabrera et al. (Cabrera et al., 2007), who focused on an easy electrochemical synthesis of iron oxide NPs. The distance pervasive between the electrodes is one overriding aspect, as it regulates the transmission kinetics of hydroxyl ions for their relocation from the cathode to the anode, producing iron hydroxide. When the distance is increased, the required pH to produce iron hydroxide is not available due to the deficient number of hydroxyl ions that would not have reached the anode. The optimum distance between the anode and cathode was found to be 5 cm or less. The current density is one more aspect to be focused on as the magnetite precipitate volume grows with an increase in the current density. A larger current density guarantees the opening of additional active sites to expedite the reaction and formation of a precipitate (Cabrera et al., 2007).

12.2.5 SONOCHEMICAL SYNTHESIS

The sonochemical method makes use of ultrasonography to procedure different phases of the precursor and prominently monodisperse NPs by reason of quick and rapid cooling practiced in the procedure. At high heat, the salt precursors are changed to nanoparticles as a hot spot is created with the rapid collapse of sonically induced voids. This method successfully produces iron oxide NPS with exceptional properties. Vijaykumar et al. (2000) recommend that particles of 10 nm with a superparamagnetic attribute were produced through sonochemical means. The process was further enhanced by altering the surfactants and precursors used to improve the magnetic properties of the obtained NPs. The sonochemical method permits the preparation of monodisperse NPs with several morphological attributes but still does not allow for industrial scale-up (Sodipo and Aziz, 2016; Laurent et al., 2010; Nawaz et al., 2022).

12.2.6 GREEN SYNTHESIS

Recent ecological trends have favored this synthetic approach for the synthesis of iron oxide NPs, principally being environmentally supportive and the production of safe NPs among all methods reported here. Countless organic origins—for example, plants (Devi et al., 2019), fungi (Chatterjee et al., 2020), bacteria (Fatemi et al., 2018; Jubran et al., 2020), viruses, and algae (Salem et al., 2019)—have been widely used for the production of iron oxide NPs in a variety of morphologies. Such cases have resulted in more stable particles, as biomaterials play the role of reducing, capping, and stabilizing agents. All types of green synthesis require two vital steps, bioreduction and biosorption, wherein metal ions change into their stable forms, followed by the consequent adhering of these metal ions onto the surfaces of living organisms to form stable complexes (Priya et al., 2021; Lakshminarayanan et al., 2021). Several other bio-extracts from plants can be used to prepare the nanoparticles with diverse sizes and morphology. Additionally, microorganisms, such as bacteria and fungi, can be employed to prepare the nanoparticles (Priya et al., 2021).

12.2.7 NANOMATERIALS AGAINST BACTERIAL INFECTIONS

To reiterate, one-dimensional nanoscale materials exhibit distinctive physicochemical properties, as opposed to their regular form (Wang et al., 2017a), which helps them work well against disease-causing pathogens. These features comprise their easiness of synthesis; biocompatibility (Nawaz et al., 2018, 2022; Faiza et al., 2020, 2022); controlled delivery by factors such as pH, light, and heat (Nawaz et al., 2018; Wang et al., 2017a); and improvement in drug dissolution and performance (Huh and Kwon, 2011). Nanomaterials are considered important in drug delivery because of their small size and wide surface area, providing them with competitive advantages over regular medications in the treatment of infectious diseases. Also, the customization of NPs made of Zn, Ce, Cu, Se, Au, Ag, Ti, Cd, Al, Mg, Ni, Cd, and supermagnetic is also applied (Slavin et al., 2017; Hemeg, 2017). Nanomaterials, such as ZnO, Ag, Au, TiO_2, Fe_2O_3, and CuO, are considered effective against different strains of bacteria (Slavin et al., 2017; Hemeg, 2017). The potency of many antibiotics is limited due to poor membrane transport (Andrade et al., 2013), while nanoparticles enriched with drugs go through the host cell, expediting the intracellular delivery of drugs by endocytosis (Wang et al., 2017a). The membrane permeation of protein-based drugs may be accomplished via the interaction of lipids at the surface using gold nanoparticles (Huang et al., 2010). Additionally, nanoparticles were used as a delivery vehicle for antimicrobial agents, and as a result, the biocidal rate was vastly enhanced (Esmaeillou et al., 2017; Zaidi et al., 2017; Hadiya et al., 2018). The benefits of using NPs as delivery carrier result from their tiny dimension and customizable size vectors, which are due to their small and controllable size; their protective action against enzymes that would otherwise destroy antimicrobial compounds; their capacity to efficiently transport antibiotics; and their ability to accommodate various therapeutics onto a single carrier (Esmaeillou et al., 2017; Zaidi et al., 2017; Hadiya et al., 2018).

12.2.8 COPPER OXIDE NANOPARTICLES

The antimicrobial potential of copper oxide nanoparticles (CuO NPs) against animal as well as plant pathogens has been reported in previous studies. CuO NPs disable the synthesis of multidrug resistance biofilms and, hence, demonstrate the possibility to act as an antimicrobial coating agent/product (Lewis Oscar et al., 2015). In other studies, Cu-NPs have been reported to obstruct the growth of multidrug-resistant strains, such as MRSA and *P. aeruginosa* (Zhang et al., 2014). The activity of Cu-NPs against microbes is similar to that of silver nanoparticles, but also, copper oxide nanoparticles are cost-effective. The mechanism involved in copper oxide nanoparticles antibacterial activity relies on the production of ROS that frequently prompts the degradation of DNA, which proves the particle-specific activity of copper oxide nanoparticles despite releasing metallic ions. The influence of CuO-NPs on the expression of intracellular protein and bacterial denitrification has been investigated in previous studies. The metabolic functions (nitrogen metabolism, active transform, electron transfer) of bacteria are influenced by the entrance of copper oxide nanoparticles (Su et al., 2015). A number of metals can be used in conjugation with nanoparticles, such as gallium. The phagosomal maturation of infected macrophages with *Mycobacterium tuberculosis* has been facilitated by gallium nanoparticles, thus, resulting in the growth inhibition of pathogens (Choi et al., 2017).

12.2.9 IRON OXIDE NANOPARTICLES

Iron oxide (Fe_2O_3) nanoparticles are also important and can be synthesized using different methods (Babes et al., 1999; Berry and Curtis, 2003). The mode of action of these NPs against bacteria involves dissolving metal ions and generating reactive oxygen species (ROS) (Wang et al., 2017b). The superparamagnetic IONPs can interact with microbial cells by diffusing through the membrane and disturbing the electron migration (El-Zowalaty et al., 2015). IONPs can harm macromolecules as well, like DNA and proteins, by the generation of ROS (Leuba et al., 2013). Pan et al. reported a reduction of graphene oxide (rGO)–IONP by chemically depositing Fe^{2+}/Fe^{3+} ions on rGO nanosheets in aqueous ammonia. The in vivo results confirmed a high antibacterial rate as hydroxyl radicals were generated that caused physico-chemical damage, consequently inactivating MRSA (Pan et al., 2016).

12.2.10 ZINC OXIDE NANOPARTICLES

Zinc oxide has been prepared via a variety of techniques, from green chemistry to microwave synthesis (Salem et al., 2015; Nagvenkar et al., 2016), and used mostly for antimicrobial purposes, against free-living bacteria, and also for inhibition of biofilm growth (Hsueh et al., 2015; Sarwar et al., 2016). The bactericidal action of these NPs depends on two important steps; the dissolved metal ions leading to the formation of reactive oxygen species (Nagvenkar et al., 2016; Sarwar et al., 2016). ZnO emits cations, which, by surface adsorption or by entering the cell, interact with structural moieties in proteins and nucleic acids to restrict enzymatic action and the regular physiological processes (Yu et al., 2014). A few researchers also observed that Zn^{+2} doesn't have adequate efficiency against microbes, instigating doubt on the proposed mechanism of dissolved metal ions (Aydin Sevinç and Hanley, 2010). DNA damage, protein leakage, membrane depolarization, and fluidity were observed in *Vibrio cholera* when nano-ZnO was used, causing substantial oxidative stress (Sarwar et al., 2016). Ehsan and Sajjad showed that nano-ZnO loaded with an antibiotic agent demonstrated effective antibacterial action versus *S. aureus, Proteus, Acinetobacter, P. aeruginosa*, and *E. coli*, which had developed drug resistance against the loaded agents, but the presence of a nanocarrier improved the action (Ehsan and Sajjad, 2017). The literature also describes that these NPs produce ROS in the absence of light as well owing to the surface structure of the NPs. The various morphologies serve as enzyme inhibitors, nanopyramids being extremely successful (Lakshmi Prasanna and Vijayaraghavan, 2015). When compared to Au and IONPs, the effect of nano-ZnO versus MDR gram-positive and gram-negative pathogens are less toxic toward mammalian cells at concentrations used (Aswathanarayan and Vittal, 2017).

12.2.11 Silver Nanoparticles

A green method for the preparation of silver nanoparticles (AgNPs) has recently shown tremendous potential against various pathogens through the use of plants as well as microbes (Ribeiro et al., 2018). To date, in accordance with all the evidence, silver nanoparticles are likely the most encouraging nanoparticles belonging to the inorganic group that could be utilized to combat bacterial infections (Natan and Banin, 2017).

Limited strategies have been developed to examine how silver nanoparticles induce cell death, which particularly involves disrupted cell walls, production of ROS, inactivated respiratory enzymes, and also the multiplication of cell components. The integration of silver nanoparticles in the cell membrane results in increased permeability of the cell membrane. The charge of the cell wall is modified by the adsorption of silver nanoparticles, consequently turning the membrane porous, hence more permeable. ATP formation and DNA replication were affected extensively by the interaction of silver nanoparticles by the formation of ROS. Whereby the compelled mechanism behind the antibacterial potential is yet to be determined. All the gathered information shows a very limited bactericidal mechanism of silver nanoparticles, which may determine the uncommon resistance of bacteria against silver. However, silver nanoparticles amazingly were established as more successful against *P. aeruginosa* and MRSA bacteria, as compared to commercially available genatimicin and vanomycin (Saeb et al., 2014).

The potential of silver nanoparticles targeting ampicillin-resistant *E. coli*, erythromycin-resistant *S. pyogenes*, and multidrug-resistant *P. aeruginosa* has been predicted by Lara and team (Lara et al., 2010). It was revealed that the upregulation of antioxidant genes and ATPase pumps, AgNPs, were equipped for bacterial growth inhibition, which includes *E. coli* and *S. aureus* (Nagy et al., 2011). Hydrofiber® dressings having silver and nanocrystalline silver are convincing agents targeting antibiotic-resistant bacteria, which mainly count VRE, MRSA, and *S. marcescens* by preventing biofilm production on the surface of biomaterials (Percival et al., 2007). The bactericidal activities of silver nanoparticles immobilized on the nanoscale silicate palette (AgNP/NSPs) have been indicated by Su and associates. AgNP/NSPs inhibited the growth of *E. coli* and MRSA by the production of ROS (Su et al., 2011).

The antibacterial activity of antimicrobial peptides has been significantly enhanced by the coupling of antimicrobial peptides with silver nanoparticles. Among antimicrobial peptides, one of which is extensively used is Polymyxin B, as it has antibacterial activity by interfacing endotoxin LPS within the external layer of gram-negative bacteria (Lambadi et al., 2015). The growth of biofilms containing bacteria has been inhibited by silver nanoparticles functionalized with Polymyxin and eradicates endotoxins completely from the solution (Lambadi et al., 2015). The restricted action of antimicrobial peptides with silver nanoparticles resulted in improved activity against microbial in contrast with free antimicrobial peptides, and furthermore, the toxicity of silver nanoparticles has been reduced by coupling with antimicrobial peptides. Lately, a study was conducted on silver nanoparticles, which depicts a framework comprising a cysteine having antimicrobial peptides combined with silver nanoparticles. As a consequence of coupling cysteine with silver nanoparticles, the Ag-S bond showed enhanced stability and antimicrobial potential in comparison with a combination utilizing electrostatic interference (Pal et al., 2016).

12.2.12 Gold Nanoparticles

Gold metal is recognized as passive and safe but not so when it turns to Au^{+1} and Au^{+2} (Merchant, 1998). AuNPs can be obtained by either chemically reducing Au salts or by green synthesis making use of bio-extracts. Among all methods, chemical synthesis by the reduction of chloroauric acid using citrate is considered the most utilized method (Fernandes and Baptista, 2017). A few investigations have tended to the capability of utilizing AuNPs as antibacterial specialists, yet some contention actually exists (Shamaila et al., 2016). Positively charged as well as aquaphobic-enhanced gold NPs were demonstrated to be viable against a wide range of pathogens, including MRSA. These gold-NPs showed higher safety toward mammalian cells (biocompatibility) and vastly lower resistance developed against the drug. Galic acid–covered gold NPs have additionally been discovered to be effective against gram-negative and gram-positive microbes (Kim et al., 2017). One-pot preparation of cinnamaldehyde immobilized on gold NPs was achieved with efficient in vivo and in vitro biofilm suppression of over 80% against gram-positive bacteria (methicillin-sensitive and methicillin-resistant strains of *S. aureus*, MSSA, and MRSA, respectively) and gram-negative (*E. coli* and *P. aeruginosa*) (Ramasamy et al., 2017). Likewise, the combination of gold NPs and ultrathin graphitic carbon nitride was reported as exhibiting significant bactericidal potential against MDR and a highly potent in eradicating existing MDR-biofilms and inhibiting the development of further biofilms in vitro (Wang et al., 2017b). In a similar manner, a combination of existing antibiotics with AuNPs—for example, vancomycin and methicillin—builds their innate activity against MDR strains (Lai et al., 2015; Payne et al., 2016). As of late, Payne and teammates established a single-step synthesis of kanamycin-coated gold-NPs with high antimicrobial action against bacteria, including kanamycin-resistant strains. A huge decrease in the MIC among the different microbial strains tried for Kan-gold NPs was noticed by researchers when contrasted with the free medication. This increased adequacy was due to the interruption of the bacterial envelope, leading to the spillage of the cytoplasmic substance and subsequent cell demise (Payne et al., 2016). AuNPs with bacterial exopolysaccharide (EPS) were synthesized by Pradeepa and colleagues, and were functionalized with antibiotics (four quinolones). Noteworthy bactericidal actions against MDR bacteria were observed by authors when compared with free medications. Among all tested bacteria, *E. coli* was the most vulnerable MDR bacteria, and *K. pneumoniae* and *S. aureus* were closely behind (Pradeepa et al., 2016). Lately, Yang and coworkers demonstrated the impact of small molecule (6-aminopenicillanic corrosive, APA) coated gold NPs to combat MDR bacteria (Yang et al., 2017). AuNPs were loaded on to electrospun filaments of poly(ε-caprolactone) (PCL)/gelatin to transport agents that prevented wound disease that is caused by MDR bacteria and exhibited a reduction in MDR bacterial contamination in vitro and in vivo (Yang et al., 2017).

12.2.13 NANOPARTICLES IN DENTAL RESTORATIONS

Adhesives are used as the restoration material in minimal intervention dentistry (MID) (Pradeepa et al., 2016). The most common adhesive is dentin (Sofan et al., 2017) but with a slight issue of coming off after some time as the adhesion between surfaces destabilizes (Ferracane, 2017). The reason for this is the collagenous, hydrophilic nature of dentin as well as the hydrolytic degradation of the polymeric covalent bond. Eventually, the total failure of the adhesive bond to the dentin surface occurs (Amin et al., 2022). The combination of adhesives has been tested to study the bonding to human teeth (Sun et al., 2017). A similar study with TiO_2-NPs was found to enhance biocompatibility and reduce solubility and water sorption, recommending the use of these NPs in MID (Esteban Florez et al., 2020). One more study concluded that the combination of adhesive and TiO_2-NPs result in a higher degree of conversion (DC) over conventional adhesives (Ramos-Tonello et al., 2017). The TiO_2-NPs also enhance the mechanical and physico-chemical attributes of adhesive fillers (Sturmer et al., 2021), making them potential reinforcing fillers in MID (Ibrahim et al., 2017).

Previously, TiO_2-NPs were used as a resin formed by a light-curable orthodontic composite paste to decrease enamel demineralization and provide antibacterial support for dental adhesive systems. The sheer bond strength and the adhesive remnant index for the resin with TiO_2-NPs were equivalent to those of the control resin biomineralized adhesive (Poosti et al., 2013), with a positive effect on tooth remineralization in simulated body fluids (Srinivasan et al., 2012).

Hydroxyapatite is a natural calcium phosphate formed chemically and morphologically similar to human hard tissues (Wei and Ma, 2004) and an important constituent in teeth and bones. It is the reason for rigidity and strength in dentures, and its regular dimensions are 60 nm long and 5–20 nm wide (Kuśnieruk et al., 2016). Nanoscale hydroxyapatite is competitively researched in cariology morphological and mineral resemblance to bone and teeth (Nozari et al., 2017), and its biocompatible, bioactive, and antibacterial nature (Huang et al., 2009) gives it an advantage over currently used restorative material (Cai et al., 2007).

Remineralization benefits of nanohydroxyapatite have been observed in the usage of restorative substances or toothpaste (Shahmoradi et al., 2018). A research that tested different concentrations of nanohydroxyapatite with pH-cycling conditions revealed enhanced remineralization of initial enamel caries lesions (Huang et al., 2009). Nanohydroxyapatite also constructed new layers on the demineralized enamel surface (Huang et al., 2011) and provided caries prevention (Tschoppe et al., 2011). These NPs work by constructing a fresh layer on carious teeth via the deposition of calcium and phosphate ions (Mok et al., 2021) and can also enhance dentin remineralization (Tao et al., 2019). The resulting restorations were long term, with enhanced acid neutralization and inhibition of secondary caries (Zhang et al., 2016). Also, a continuous release of calcium and phosphate ions was observed that resulted in an anticaries environment (Xie et al., 2017).

A combination of nano-Ag with agents for antimicrobial and remineralization (quaternary ammonium dimethacrylate and nano-amorphous calcium phosphate) used with adhesives could be a good option for caries prevention (Melo et al., 2013). Nanocalcium phosphate–filled dental adhesive exhibited strong bonding toward enamel and reduces cariogenic biofilm (Kulshrestha et al., 2016; Xie et al., 2019). Nanocomposite calcium fluoride NPs showed increased fluoride release, strength, and load-bearing abilities as a contender for caries-inhibiting restoration matter (Weir et al., 2012). Calcium fluoride NPs improved by increased labile fluoride concentration in the buccal liquid (Sun and Chow, 2008).

Bioceramics, such as glass, are surface-reactive biomaterial (Boccaccini et al., 2016) that mimics bone and tooth tissue after they dissolve (Ali et al., 2014). The influence of various ions on the biomedical and dental purposes of bioactive glass has been reviewed. Nanobioactive glass used in resin results in the formation of even apatite coating on the tooth surface with no side effects (Odermatt et al., 2020), seals the cavities of dentinal tubules, and reduces dentin permeability and sensitivity (Lee et al., 2007). A similar composite, when used on demineralized dentin, resulted in increased microhardness (Jang et al., 2018; Schwendicke et al., 2019).

Silica is an inorganic mineral (Yang et al., 2022) usually used as a colloid (Gaishun et al., 2002) for collagen infiltration without precipitating on the surface (Forsback et al., 2004; Deyhle et al., 2011). Calcium-silica NPs used as fillers enhanced the mechanical functions of the resin as well as used to carry ciprofloxacin hydrochloride for supportive caries prevention (Zhang et al., 2018). As reported in a research, calcium-silica mesoporous NPs reduced roughness and minimized tooth surface loss versus casein phosphopeptide–amorphous calcium phosphate, titanium fluoride, and sodium fluoride to reduce dental erosion (Canto et al., 2020). Adhesives with calcium silicate are good in acid neutralization, apatite formation, and enamel remineralization (Yang et al., 2022). Comparatively, nanohydroxyapatite permeated notably more minerals than silica NPs (Karumuri et al., 2020). Another successful combination reported was collagen penetrated with hydroxyapatite and nanosilica for the remineralization of dentin (Besinis et al., 2012). Bionanosilica from rice husks also exhibited dentin hydroxyapatite formation with additional antimicrobial activity (Aprillia et al., 2022) as well as a potential catalyst for the regeneration/repair of dental hard tissues (Chiang et al., 2014).

12.2.14 NANOPARTICLES IN SCAFFOLDS/BONE GRAFTING

Bones are natural nanodimensional matter. For grafting, in areas such as the face, buccal region, neck, ears and nose, and head, organic composites like collagen are used that are supported by some inorganic materials. Nanocrystallites have open microstructure, with nanopores that can be filled by the grafting material that allows fast cell growth. Factors to consider for ideal grafting biomaterial should be bone induction, right processibility, non-sinter, synthetic, highly porous, nanodimensional, and ability to degrade by osteoclasts (Takahashi and Nyvad, 2011).

The TiO_2 NPs are good as bone grafts, owing to their higher strength, biocompatibility, low elastic modulus, corrosion resistance, and exceptionally low weight of titanium utilized in the graft structure (Lautenschlager and Monaghan, 1993). Titanium becomes the deserving biomaterial for the aforementioned reasons and is ideal for the human body to be used as a metallic prosthesis. It also becomes the selected matter for the assembly of internal metal plates, wires, and meshes used in fracture fixtures, cranioplasty plates and meshes, cranioplasty wires, and coronary artery stents (Agnihotry et al., 2017). In addition, titanium meshes and scaffoldings, as well as prostheses, are popular in nose, eye, maxilla, mandible, and ear reconstruction techniques, and ossicular substitutions (Schmeidl et al., 2021).

Bone is a vigorous tissue that regularly renews and repairs using its inherent remodeling activity through interactions of osteoclasts and osteoblasts with signaling factors to get rid of old and injured tissue in order to construct a new bone (Ralston, 2021). Such a synergism works well for the preservation of bone balance. The restoration of bone fractures and the repair of critical bone irregularities are challenges for orthopedics, traumatologists, and maxillofacial surgeons (Chen et al., 2020a). Owing to the patient-specific needs and constraints in bone regeneration, the surgical and medical usage of synthetic bone grafts remains a very crucial update in bone regenerative therapy (Kupikowska-Stobba and Kasprzak, 2021). Modern NP-based biomaterials allow the synthesis of bone implants with properties such as osteoconduction and osteoinduction, at the same time being biocompatible and bioresorbable (Chandra and Pandey, 2020; Tahmasebi et al., 2020; Collon et al., 2021). Such material is nano-sized and bioactive, which effectively supports modern biomedical trends and biotechnology (Kumar et al., 2020; Huang et al., 2020). Nanodimension bioactive matter offers greater bone rejuvenation potential because of its unique biological conduct as compared to its bulk forms (Lyons et al., 2020). Even for orthotopic and metastatic bone tumors, several NPs, including procedures and diagnostics, were positively employed in the last couple of years (Gao et al., 2021; Ojo et al., 2020).

Biological barriers work not so well against NPs in the range of 1–100 nm, as they easily pass through, and the attributes that this size brings, such as increased surface area, surface mechanics, optics, magnetism, quantum effect, electronic, and inherent bioactivity, make NPs substantial in medical technology (Khan et al., 2019). Likewise, nanobiotechnology protocols offer increased drug dissolution and improved bioavailability and, overall, pharmacokinetic and pharmacodynamic improvements to provide a targeted approach (van der Meel et al., 2019; Mitchell et al., 2021). For the procedures of hard tissues (including also those with restricted bioavailability and high immunogenicity of autografts and allografts, and bioinaction of marketed biomaterials) (Baldwin et al., 2019), outstanding advancement has been made in the production of material for bone regeneration in the last twenty or so years. These advanced materials and applications can be classified as follows: (a) first generation, prosthetics derived by bioinert forms, like metal, alloy, synthetic polymer, and bioactive ceramic; (b) second generation, osteoconductive and osteoinductive devices made from biologically potent, bioresorbable forms, like calcium phosphates, bioactive ceramic, and polyesters; and (c) third generation, progressive and multitasking biomaterials having osteogenic potential (Fattahian et al., 2019; Jin et al., 2021). One of the nanodimensional features is the presence of conditional toxicity, and the challenge lies in achieving the right balance between the therapeutic and adverse effects. NPs can migrate into neighboring cells and tissues, as well as often cluster or drift into blood vessels, resulting in side effects (Wang et al., 2021a). The toxic or adverse effects of the NPs on humans lie in many parameters, such as morphology, size, composition, porosity, surface dynamics, as well as some secondary factors, like aggregation state and chemistry with biomolecules (Wang et al., 2020b; Tortella et al., 2020). Traditional therapy for bone grafting makes use of mostly allografts and autografts, and some combination-based substitutes with calcium phosphate (Tiomnova et al., 2021). Calcium phosphate NPs have been vastly studied as bone graft substitutes (Zhao et al., 2021) and might also be useful in targeted drug delivery to cells or tissues due to their high adsorption potential, microstructure, lattice-borne tunable attributes, and customizable biodegradation levels as needed in the application (Parent et al., 2017). Specifically beneficial biomaterial for hard tissue healing and restoration is synthetic hydroxyapatite, $Ca_{10}(PO_4)_6(OH)_2$ (Florea et al., 2020), otherwise found as a mineral in metamorphous and pyrogenic rocks and a key mineral in bones and teeth (Liang et al., 2021; Dasgupta et al., 2021).

Nanohydroxyapatite possesses additional properties than microhydroxyapatite, such as higher protein adsorption, better cell adhesion, and greater bioactivity (Lara-Ochoa et al., 2021; Liang et al., 2021). Additionally, they have a unique potential to inhibit apoptotic cell death, thus improving cell proliferation and activity in terms of bone growth (Lara-Ochoa et al., 2021), and with the bone mimicking composition, new bone growth is increased while being safe, too (Oryan et al., 2020; Wang et al., 2021a).

Bioactive glass, mainly silica has been reportedly advantageous in the production of biosubstitutes and protocols for tissue restoration (Sonatkar and Kandasubramanian, 2021). Due to their quick and stable interaction with living tissues and surface dynamics that mimic apatite formation under biological environments, bioglass became essential in biomaterial design (van Vugt et al., 2017). A high amount of SiO_2 bioglass, as much as 60%, is effective for secure binding with the bone tissue without the need for connective tissues) and also supports apatite layer generation at the bone surface and collagen (Kaur et al., 2019; Sonatkar and Kandasubramanian, 2021). Moreover, with the core bone-stimulative properties of silicon-based bioglass (Brunello et al., 2019; Srinath et al., 2020), the dissolution of bioglass has also been observed that results in the release of subsidiary ions (calcium, sodium, and phosphorous) that contribute in the repair and regeneration of bones by encouraging mineralization, starting cellular functions, and regulating the protein and gene expression related to osteogenesis and angiogenesis (Sergi et al., 2020). It has been observed that the bioactivity of silica-based bioactive glass can be further enhanced by adding other metals/ions, such as zinc (Chen et al., 2020c; Marin et al., 2021), silver (Vale et al., 2019; Mortazavi et al., 2021), magnesium (Karakuzu-Ikizler et al., 2020; de Araujo Bastos Santana et al., 2021), strontium (Araujo et al., 2021; Katunar et al., 2022), and copper (Chitra et al., 2020; Akhtach et al., 2021).

Iron oxide (Fe_2O_3) is considered important in modern biomedicine and in bone tissue engineering due to its non-toxicity/bioactivity (Friedrich et al., 2021; Fan et al., 2020). The biomedical application of iron oxide nanoparticles depends on size, reactivity, magnetism, and surface chemistry (Ramazanov et al., 2021). It has been noticed that the surface modification of iron oxide nanoparticles with therapeutic molecules (Raghubir et al., 2020) and biomolecule conjugated with macromolecule (Zarei et al., 2021; Khodaei et al., 2022) and with inorganic capping layers (Divband et al., 2020; Miola et al., 2021) paves the way toward the fabrication of accurate and efficient strategies for bone healing and regeneration as well as bone infection and cancer (Popescu et al., 2020; Dong et al., 2020).

Mesoporous silica (SiO_2) nanoparticles have received great attention due to their tunable properties for biomedical applications, such as tissue engineering (Li et al.,

2020a; Yu et al., 2021), cancer therapy (Chen et al., 2020b; Kundu et al., 2021), regenerative medicine (Hou et al., 2020; Zhang et al., 2021a), and drug/biomolecule delivery (Almáši et al., 2021; Galhano et al., 2022). It has been observed that the addition of mesoporous silica within a three-dimensional nano-network provides excellent opportunities for the selective management of bone cancer and bone infection (Zhou et al., 2022; Carvalho et al., 2020). Due to the unique properties of silica, it has been used for efficient drug loading/delivery for several drugs and biomolecules (Szewczyk et al., 2021; Yao et al., 2021; Seljak et al., 2020). The mesoporous silica-based nanocomposite was used for the delivery and release of vancomycin for the treatment of bone defects and bone infections. Furthermore, the selective management of bone cancer can be accomplished with mesoporous silica by targeting the receptors that are overexpressed in cancer cells (Hu et al., 2021).

Copper (Cu) has a very important role in the body and is involved in several functions, such as maintaining the normal function of the blood vessels, bones, nerves, immune system, and wound healing (Wang et al., 2021c; Szabo et al., 2021). It has been reported that Cu plays a significant role in bone metabolism, and its deficiency causes bone anomalies and deformities (Rondanelli et al., 2021). Furthermore, Cu deficiency causes an inhibited activity of oxidase, resulting in the increased solubility of the bone collagen stability and reduced bone strength (Gaffney-Stomberg, 2019). Due to the beneficial role of copper, it is significant to design Cu-based nanoformulations for bone healing applications (Mitra et al., 2019). It was reported that copper and its different nanoformulations possess excellent osteogenic, angiogenic, and antibacterial properties (Wang et al., 2021b; Shen et al., 2022). Furthermore, Cu-based nanoformulations are good candidates in bone tissue engineering, as they enhanced mineralization, osteoclastogenesis, osteogenesis, and angiogenesis (Bozorgi et al., 2021; Wu et al., 2021).

Silver nanoparticles (Ag NPs) are studied a lot in biomedical and industrial applications due to their useful biological activities, good electrical conductivity, catalytic activity, and optical properties (Gherasim et al., 2020; Lagashetty et al., 2020). Silver nanoparticles are of great interest in dentistry and in orthopedics, where chances of infection are more due to the implanted devices (Marques et al., 2020; Coman et al., 2021). Silver nanoparticles are also important in bone healing applications as they stimulate osteogenesis and inhibit osteoclastogenesis (He et al., 2020; Lee et al., 2021). Due to the multifunction of silver nanoparticles, they can induce an antimicrobial effect in nanostructured-based implants or devices while stimulating osteogenic activity (Zhao et al., 2020; Ramyaa et al., 2021).

Gold nanoparticles (AuNPs) have attracted attention in the research due to their nano-sized structure, biocompatibility, and optical and electroconductivity properties (Nejati et al., 2022). In modern therapy, AuNPs are used in target drug delivery, biomolecule delivery, biomedical imaging, and diagnosis (Vodyashkin et al., 2021; Li et al., 2020a]). In the bone healing application, gold nanoparticles exhibit intrinsic osteogenic effects by promoting the differentiation of pluripotent cells and biomimetic apatite formation (Zhang et al., 2021b). AuNPs inhibit osteoclastogenesis (Bai et al., 2020; Nah et al., 2020) and accelerate bone formation (Zhang et al., 2021b; Samadian et al., 2021). To understand the AuNP-mediated osteogenic differentiation, several molecular mechanisms were proposed (Shi et al., 2021; Li et al., 2021).

It was proposed that stem cells may undergo osteogenic differentiation in response to the extracellular and intracellular gold nanoparticles by means of an integrin-mediated signaling pathway (Li et al., 2021). It has been suggested that the osteogenic ability of gold nanoparticles is strongly related to their concentration (Huang et al., 2021), shape (Yuan et al., 2019), and size (Zhang et al., 2021c). The impressive functionalization of gold nanoparticles resulted in the fabrication of AuNP-based composites for bone repair and regeneration (Li et al., 2020a). Furthermore, the electrical and optical properties of gold nanoparticles have been utilized for the management of bone infections and bone cancer (Sun et al., 2021; Wang et al., 2021a).

12.2.15 Nanoparticles in Magnetic Hyperthermia Therapy and Magnetic Resonance Imaging

Nanoparticles, such as magnetic nanoparticles, are used as a contrast agent for magnetic resonance imaging and are also studied for magnetic hyperthermia therapy. The response of magnetic nanoparticles to the external magnetic field is important in cancer therapy due to its ability to deliver the drug to the target, reducing the non-specific toxicity of chemotherapeutic agents (Liao et al., 2015; Nawaz et al., 2018). Iron oxide nanoparticles are widely studied and can be easily synthesized and modified easily. Iron oxide nanoparticles are considered important due to their magnetic properties in the presence of an external magnetic field (Nunes et al., 2022; Da Silva Bruckmann et al., 2022; Swiętek et al., 2022). Conversely, iron oxide nanoparticles are associated with a drawback due to their aggregation (Rhoden et al., 2021). So to overcome this issue, surface modification with silica is very useful, as it increases stability and biocompatibility (Bruckmann et al., 2022). It was observed that the use of magnetic hyperthermia has higher sensitivity of tumor cells to heat as compared to healthy cells. The increase in local tumor tissue temperature (41–46°C) causes

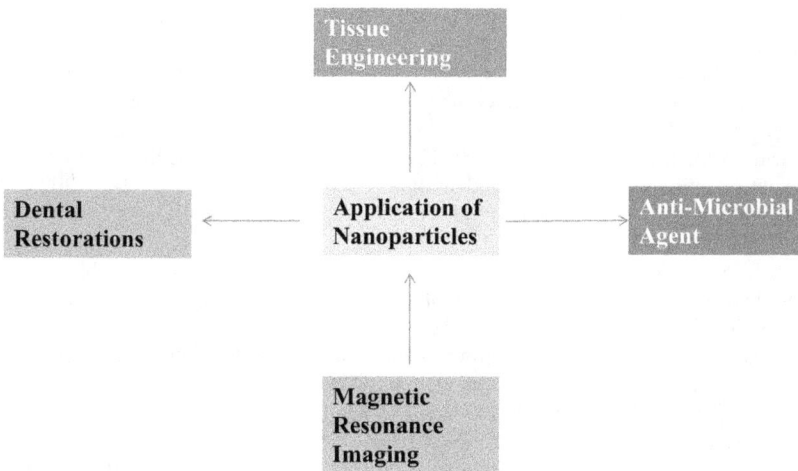

FIGURE 12.2 Biomedical applications of nanoparticles.

cell damage for different pathways as well as sensitizes cells to drug chemotherapy (Healy et al., 2022). Cell damage is supposed to occur by different pathways: it can occur through the conversion of energy to heat (Neel relaxation) or mechanical damage caused by the magnetic nanoparticle rotation in response to the external magnetic field direction (Brownian relaxation) (Wang et al., 2020a) or by the production of heat shock proteins or increase in immune response (Liao et al., 2015).

12.3 CONCLUSION

This chapter provided a summary of the different types of methods for the synthesis of nanomaterials. It also provided details on how different nanomaterials can be employed for biomedical applications. So far, we have also covered the biomedical applications of different nanomaterials as bacterial agents, dental applications, tissue engineering, and magnetic resonance imaging.

REFERENCES

Aderibigbe, B.A. Metal-based nanoparticles for the treatment of infectious diseases. *Molecules*. 2017, 22, E1370.

Agnihotry, A.; Fedorowicz, Z.; Nasser, M.; Gill, K.S. Resorbable versus titanium plates for orthognathic surgery. *Cochrane Database Syst. Rev.* 2017, 10, CD006204.

Akhtach, S.; Tabia, Z.; El Mabrouk, K.; Bricha, M.; Belkhou, R. A comprehensive study on copper incorporated bio-glass matrix for its potential antimicrobial applications. *Ceram. Int.* 2021, 47, 424–433.

Ali, S.; Farooq, I.; Iqbal, K. A review of the effect of various ions on the properties and the clinical applications of novel bioactive glasses in medicine and dentistry. *Saudi Dent. J.* 2014, 26, 1–5.

Almáši, M.; Matiašová, A.A.; Šuleková, M.; Beňová, E.; Ševc, J.; Váhovská, L.; Lisnichuk, M.; Girman, V.; Zeleňáková, A.; Hudák, A.; et al. In vivo study of light-driven naproxen release from gated mesoporous silica drug delivery system. *Sci. Rep.* 2021, 11, 20191.

Amin, F.; Fareed, M.A.; Zafar, M.S.; Khurshid, Z.; Palma, P.J.; Kumar, N. Degradation and stabilization of resin-dentine interfaces in polymeric dental adhesives: An updated review. *Coatings*. 2022, 12, 1094.

Andrade, F.; Rafael, D.; Videira, M.; Ferreira, D.; Sosnik, A.; Sarmento, B. Nanotechnology and pulmonary delivery to overcome resistance in infectious diseases. *Adv. Drug Deliv. Rev.* 2013, 65, 1816–1827.

Aprillia, I.; Alinda, S.D.; Suprastiwi, E. Efficacy of rice husk nanosilica as a caries treatment (dentin hydroxyapatite and antimicrobial analysis). *Eur J Dent.* 2022, 16(4), 875–879. doi: 10.1055/s-0041-1741373. Epub 2022 Jun 21. PMID: 35728609; PMCID: PMC9683886.

Araujo, M.; Silva, A.; Cabal, B.; Bartolomé, J.; Mello-Castanho, S. In vitro bioactivity and antibacterial capacity of 45S5 Bioglass®-based compositions containing alumina and strontium. *J. Mater. Res. Technol.* 2021, 13, 154–161.

Aswathanarayan, J.B.; Vittal, R.R. Antimicrobial, biofilm inhibitory and anti-infective activity of metallic nanoparticles against pathogens *MRSA* and *Pseudomonas aeruginosa* PA01. *Pharm. Nanotechnol.* 2017, 5, 148–153.

Atul, R.I.; Thakare, S.R.; Khati, N.T.; Wankhade, A.V.; Burghate, D.K. Green synthesis of selenium nanoparticles under ambient condition. *Chalcogenide Lett.* 2010, 7, 485–489.

Aydin Sevinç, B.; Hanley, L. Antibacterial activity of dental composites containing zinc oxide nanoparticles. *J. Biomed. Mater. Res. B Appl. Biomater.* 2010, 94, 22–31.

Babes, L.; Denizot, B.; Tanguy, G.; Le Jeune, J.J.; Jallet, P. Synthesis of iron oxide nanoparticles used as MRI contrast agents: A parametric study. *J. Colloid Interface Sci.* 1999, 212, 474–482.

Bai, X.; Gao, Y.; Zhang, M.; Chang, Y.N.; Chen, K.; Li, J.; Zhang, J.; Liang, Y.; Kong, J.; Wang, Y.; et al. Carboxylated gold nanoparticles inhibit bone erosion by disturbing the acidification of an osteoclast absorption microenvironment. *Nanoscale.* 2020, 12, 3871–3878.

Baldwin, P.; Li, D.J.; Auston, D.A.; Mir, H.S.; Yoon, R.S.; Koval, K.J. Autograft, allograft, and bone graft substitutes: Clinical evidence and indications for use in the setting of orthopaedic trauma surgery. *J. Orthop. Trauma.* 2019, 33, 203–213.

Barenholz, Y.C. Doxil®-the first FDA-approved nano-drug: Lessons learned. *J Control Release.* 2012, 160(2), 117–134.

Berry, C.C.; Curtis, A.S.G. Functionalisation of magnetic nanoparticles for applications in biomedicine. *J. Phys. D. Appl. Phys.* 2003, 36, R198–R206.

Besinis, A.; van Noort, R.; Martin, N. Infiltration of demineralized dentin with silica and hydroxyapatite nanoparticles. *Dent. Mater.* 2012, 28, 1012–1023.

Bobo, D.; Robinson, K.J.; Islam, J.; Thurecht, K.J.; Corrie, S.R. Nanoparticle-based medicines: A review of FDA-approved materials and clinical trials to date. *Pharmaceutical Research.* 2016, 33(10), 2373–2387.

Boccaccini, A.R.; Brauer, D.S.; Hupa, L. *Bioactive Glasses: Fundamentals, Technology and Applications*; Royal Society of Chemistry: London, UK, 2016.

Boucher, H.W.; Talbot, G.H.; Bradley, J.S.; Edwards, J.E.; Gilbert, D.; Rice, L.B.; et al. Bad bugs, no drugs: No eskape! An update from the infectious diseases society of America. *Clin Infect Dis.* 2009, 48(1), 1–12.

Bozorgi, A.; Mozafari, M.; Khazaei, M.; Soleimani, M.; Jamalpoor, Z. Fabrication, characterization, and optimization of a novel copper-incorporated chitosan/gelatin-based scaffold for bone tissue engineering applications. *BioImpacts.* 2021, 11.

Bruckmann, F.D.S.; Rossato Viana, A.; Tonel, M.Z.; Fagan, S.B.; Garcia, W.J.D.S.; Oliveira, A.H.D.; Rhoden, C.R.B. Influence of magnetite incorporation into chitosan on the adsorption of the methotrexate and in vitro cytotoxicity. *Environ. Sci. Pollut. Res.* 2022, 29, 70413–70434.

Brunello, G.; Elsayed, H.; Biasetto, L. Bioactive glass and silicate-based ceramic coatings on metallic implants: Open challenge or outdated topic? *Materials.* 2019, 12, 2929.

Cabrera, L.; Gutierrez, S.; Menendez, N.; Morales, M.; Herrasti, P. Magnetite nanoparticles: Electrochemical synthesis and characterization. *Electrochimica Acta.* 2007, 53, 3436–3441.

Cai, Y.; Liu, Y.; Yan, W.; Hu, Q.; Tao, J.; Zhang, M.; Shi, Z.; Tang, R. Role of hydroxyapatite nanoparticle size in bone cell proliferation. *J. Mater. Chem.* 2007, 17, 3780–3787.

Canto, F.M.T.; Alexandria, A.K.; Justino, I.B.; Rocha, G.M.; Cabral, L.M.; Ferreira, R.D.S.; Pithon, M.M.; Maia, L.C. The use of a new calcium mesoporous silica nanoparticle versus calcium and/or fluoride products in reducing the progression of dental erosion. *J. Appl. Oral Sci.* 2020, 28.

Carvalho, G.C.; Sábio, R.M.; de Cássia Ribeiro, T.; Monteiro, A.S.; Pereira, D.V.; Ribeiro, S.J.L.; Chorilli, M. Highlights in mesoporous silica nanoparticles as a multifunctional controlled drug delivery nanoplatform for infectious diseases treatment. *Pharm. Res.* 2020, 37, 191.

Chandra, G.; Pandey, A. Biodegradable bone implants in orthopedic applications: A review. *Biocybern. Biomed. Eng.* 2020, 40, 596–610.

Chatterjee, S.; Mahanty, S.; Das, P.; Chaudhuri, P.; Das, S. Biofabrication of iron oxide nanoparticles using manglicolous fungus Aspergillus niger BSC-1 and removal of Cr (VI) from aqueous solution. *Chem. Eng. J.* 2020, 385, 123790.

Chen, J.; Ashames, A.; Buabeid, M.A.; Fahelelbom, K.M.; Ijaz, M.; Murtaza, G. Nanocomposites drug delivery systems for the healing of bone fractures. *Int. J. Pharm.* 2020a, 585, 119477.

Chen, M.; Hu, J.; Wang, L.; Li, Y.; Zhu, C.; Chen, C.; Shi, M.; Ju, Z.; Cao, X.; Zhang, Z. Targeted and redox-responsive drug delivery systems based on carbonic anhydrase IX-decorated mesoporous silica nanoparticles for cancer therapy. *Sci. Rep.* 2020b, 10, 14447.

Chen, Y.H.; Tseng, S.P.; Wu, S.M.; Shih, C.J. Structure-dependence of anti-methicillin-resistant Staphylococcus aureus (MRSA) activity on ZnO-containing bioglass. *J. Alloys Compd.* 2020c, 848, 156487.

Chiang, Y.-C.; Lin, H.-P.; Chang, H.-H.; Cheng, Y.-W.; Tang, H.-Y.; Yen, W.-C.; Lin, P.-Y.; Chang, K.-W.; Lin, C.-P. A mesoporous silica biomaterial for dental biomimetic crystallization. *ACS Nano.* 2014, 8, 12502–12513.

Chitra, S.; Bargavi, P.; Balasubramaniam, M.; Chandran, R.R.; Balakumar, S. Impact of copper on in-vitro biomineralization, drug release efficacy and antimicrobial properties of bioactive glasses. *Mater. Sci. Eng. C.* 2020, 109, 110598.

Choi, S-R.; Britigan, B.E.; Moran, D.M.; Narayanasamy, P. Gallium nanoparticles facilitate phagosome maturation and inhibit growth of virulent *Mycobacterium tuberculosis* in macrophages. *PLoS One.* 2017; 12(5), e0177987.

Collon, K.; Gallo, M.C.; Lieberman, J.R. Musculoskeletal tissue engineering: Regional gene therapy for bone repair. *Biomaterials.* 2021, 275, 120901.

Colvin, V.L.; Schlamp, M.C.; Alivisatos, A.P. Light emitting diodes made from cadmium selenide nanocrystals and a semiconducting polymer. *Nature.* 1994, 370, 354–357.

Coman, A.N.; Mare, A.; Tanase, C.; Bud, E.; Rusu, A. Silver-deposited nanoparticles on the titanium nanotubes surface as a promising antibacterial material into implants. *Metals.* 2021, 11, 92.

Cornell, R.M.; Schwertmann, U. *The Iron Oxides: Structure, Properties, Reactions, Occurrences and Uses*, 2nd ed.; VCH: Weinheim, Germany, 2003.

Dasgupta, S.; Mondal, S.; Ray, S.; Singh, Y.; Maji, K. Hydroxyapatite-collagen nanoparticles reinforced polyanhydride based injectable paste for bone substitution: Effect of dopant addition in vitro. *J. Biomater. Sci. Polym. Ed.* 2021, 32, 1312–1336.

Da Silva Bruckmann, F.; Ledur, C.M.; Da Silva, I.Z.; Dotto, G.L.; Rhoden, C.R.B. A DFT theoretical and experimental study about tetracycline adsorption onto magnetic graphene oxide. *J Mol. Liq.* 2022, 353, 118837.

de Araujo Bastos Santana, L.; Oliveira Junior, P.H.; Damia, C.; dos Santos Tavares, D.; dos Santos, E.A. Bioactivity in SBF versus trace element effects: The isolated role of Mg2+ and Zn2+ in osteoblast behavior. *Mater. Sci. Eng. C.* 2021, 118, 111320.

Devi, H.S.; Boda, M.A.; Shah, M.A.; Parveen, S.; Wani, A.H. Green synthesis of iron oxide nanoparticles using Platanus orientalis leaf extract for antifungal activity. *Green Process. Synth.* 2019, 8, 38–45.

Deyhle, H.; Bunk, O.; Müller, B. Nanostructure of healthy and caries-affected human teeth. *Nanomed. Nanotechnol. Biol. Med.* 2011, 7, 694–701.

Divband, B.; Gharehaghaji, N.; Atashi, Z. High transverse relaxivity and anticancer agent loading/release characteristics of porous calcium phosphate coated iron oxide nanoparticles. *Biointerface Res. Appl. Chem.* 2020, 11, 10402–10411.

Dong, S.; Chen, Y.; Yu, L.; Lin, K.; Wang, X. Magnetic hyperthermia–synergistic H_2O_2 self-sufficient catalytic suppression of osteosarcoma with enhanced bone-regeneration bioactivity by 3D-printing composite scaffolds. *Adv. Funct. Mater.* 2020, 30, 1907071.

Ehsan, S.; Sajjad, M. Bioinspired synthesis of zinc oxide nanoparticle and its combined efficacy with different antibiotics against multidrug resistant bacteria. *J. Biomater. Nanobiotechnol.* 2017, 8, 159–175.

El-Zowalaty, M.E.; Al-Ali, S.H.H.; Husseiny, M.I.; Geilich, B.M.; Webster, T.J.; Hussein, M.Z. The ability of streptomycin-loaded chitosan-coated magnetic nanocomposites to possess antimicrobial and antituberculosis activities. *Int. J. Nanomed.* 2015, 10, 3269–3274.

Esmaeillou, M.; Zarrini, G.; Rezaee, M.A.; Mojarrad, J.S.; Bahadori, A. Vancomycin capped with silver nanoparticles as an antibacterial agent against multi-drug resistance bacteria. *Adv. Pharm. Bull.* 2017, 7, 479–483.

Esteban Florez, F.L.; Kraemer, H.; Hiers, R.D.; Sacramento, C.M.; Rondinone, A.J.; Silvério, K.G.; Khajotia, S.S. Sorption, solubility and cytotoxicity of novel antibacterial nanofilled dental adhesive resins. *Sci Rep.* 2020, 10(1), 13503. doi: 10.1038/s41598-020-70487-z. PMID: 32782299; PMCID: PMC7421579.

Faiza, Q.; Nawaz, M.; Mohammad, A.A.; Firdos, A.K.; Mahmoud, M.B.; Samar, A.A.; Rayyanah, A.; Alok, K.P.; Veeranoot, N.; Maria de, L.P.; Polrat, W. Synthesis of M-Ag$_3$PO$_4$, (M = Se, Ag, Ta) nanoparticles and their antibacterial and cytotoxicity study. *I. J. Mol. Sci.* 2022, 23(19), 11403.

Faiza, Q.; Nawaz, M.; Rehman, S.; Sarah, A.A.; Sumaira, S.; Veeranoot, N.; Muhammad, T. Synthesis and characterization of cadmium-bismuth microspheres for the catalytic and photocatalytic degradation of organic pollutants, with antibacterial, antioxidant and cytotoxicity assay. *J. Photochem. Photobiol. B: Biol.* 2020, 202, 111723.

Fan, D.; Wang, Q.; Zhu, T.; Wang, H.; Liu, B.; Wang, Y.; Liu, Z.; Liu, X.; Fan, D.; Wang, X. Recent advances of magnetic nanomaterials in bone tissue repair. *Front. Chem.* 2020, 8, 745.

Fatemi, M.; Mollania, N.; Momeni-Moghaddam, M.; Sadeghifar, F. Extracellular biosynthesis of magnetic iron oxide nanoparticles by Bacillus cereus strain HMH1: Characterization and in vitro cytotoxicity analysis on MCF-7 and 3T3 cell lines. *J. Biotechnol.* 2018, 270, 1–11.

Fattahian, H.; Mansouri, K.; Mansouri, N. Biomaterials, substitutes, and tissue engineering in bone repair: Current and future concepts. *Comp. Clin. Pathol.* 2019, 28, 879–891.

Fernandes, A.R.; Baptista, P.V. Gene silencing using multifunctionalized gold nanoparticles for cancer therapy. *Methods Mol. Biol.* 2017, 1530, 319–336.

Ferracane, J.L. Models of caries formation around dental composite restorations. *J. Dent. Res.* 2017, 96, 364–371.

Florea, D.A.; Chircov, C.; Grumezescu, A.M. Hydroxyapatite particles-directing the cellular activity in bone regeneration processes: An up-to-date review. *Appl. Sci.* 2020, 10, 3483.

Forsback, A.P.; Areva, S.; Salonen, J. Mineralization of dentin induced by treatment with bio-active glass S53P4 in vitro. *Acta Odontol. Scand.* 2004, 62, 14–20.

Friedrich, R.P.; Cicha, I.; Alexiou, C. Iron oxide nanoparticles in regenerative medicine and tissue engineering. *Nanomaterials.* 2021, 11, 2337.

Gaffney-Stomberg, E. The impact of trace minerals on bone metabolism. *Biol. Trace Elem. Res.* 2019, 188, 26–34.

Gaishun, V.; Tulenkova, O.; Melnichenko, I.; Baryshnin, S.; Potapenok, Y.; Xlebokazov, A.; Strek, W. Preparation and properties of colloidal nanosize silica dioxide for polishing of monocrystalline silicon wafers. *Mater. Sci.* 2002, 20, 19–22.

Galhano, J.; Marcelo, G.A.; Duarte, M.P.; Oliveira, E. Ofloxacin@Doxorubicin-Epirubicin functionalized MCM-41 mesoporous silica–based nanocarriers as synergistic drug delivery tools for cancer related bacterial infections. *Bioorg. Chem.* 2022, 118, 105470.

Gao, X.; Li, L.; Cai, X.; Huang, Q.; Xiao, J.; Cheng, Y. Targeting nanoparticles for diagnosis and therapy of bone tumors: Opportunities and challenges. *Biomaterials.* 2021, 265, 120404.

Gherasim, O.; Puiu, R.A.; Bîrca, A.C.; Burdus, el, A.-C.; Grumezescu, A.M. An Updated review on silver nanoparticles in biomedicine. *Nanomaterials.* 2020, 10, 2318.

Glasgow, W.; Fellows, B.; Qi, B.; Darroudi, T.; Kitchens, C.; Ye, L.; Crawford, T.M.; Mefford, O.T. Continuous synthesis of iron oxide (Fe$_3$O$_4$) nanoparticles via thermal decomposition. *Particuology.* 2016, 26, 47–53.

Hadiya, S.; Liu, X.; Abd El-Hammed, W.; Elsabahy, M.; Aly, S.A. Levofloxacin-loaded nano-particles decrease emergence of fluoroquinolone resistance in *Escherichia coli. Microb. Drug Resist.* 2018, 24(8), 1098–1107.

He, W.; Zheng, Y.; Feng, Q.; Elkhooly, T.A.; Liu, X.; Yang, X.; Wang, Y.; Xie, Y. Silver nano-particles stimulate osteogenesis of human mesenchymal stem cells through activation of autophagy. *Nanomed. Nanotechnol. Biol. Med.* 2020, 15, 337–353.

Healy, S.; Bakuzis, A.F.; Goodwill, P.W.; Attaluri, A.; Bulte, J.W.; Ivkov, R. Clinical magnetic hyperthermia requires integrated magnetic particle imaging. *Wiley Interdiscip. Rev. Nanomed. Nanobiotechnol.* 2022, 14, e1779.

Hemeg, H.A. Nanomaterials for alternative antibacterial therapy. *Int. J. Nanomed.* 2017, 12, 8211–8225.

Hou, Y.T.; Wu, K.C.W.; Lee, C.Y. Development of glycyrrhizin-conjugated, chitosan-coated, lysine-embedded mesoporous silica nanoparticles for hepatocyte-targeted liver tissue regeneration. *Materialia.* 2020, 9, 100568.

Hsueh, Y.H.; Ke, W.J.; Hsieh, C.T.; Lin, K.S.; Tzou, D.Y.; Chiang, C.L. ZnO nanoparticles affect bacillus subtilis cell growth and biofilm formation. *PLoS One.* 2015, 10, e0128457.

Hu, H.; Yang, W.; Liang, Z.; Zhou, Z.; Song, Q.; Liu, W.; Deng, X.; Zhu, J.; Xing, X.; Zhong, B.; et al. Amplification of oxidative stress with lycorine and gold-based nanocomposites for synergistic cascade cancer therapy. *J. Nanobiotechnol.* 2021, 19, 221.

Huang, C.; Dong, J.; Zhang, Y.; Chai, S.; Wang, X.; Kang, S.; Yu, D.; Wang, P.; Jiang, Q. Gold Nanoparticles-loaded polyvinylpyrrolidone/ethylcellulose coaxial electrospun nanofibers with enhanced osteogenic capability for bone tissue regeneration. *Mater. Des.* 2021, 212, 110240.

Huang, H.; Feng, W.; Chen, Y.; Shi, J. Inorganic nanoparticles in clinical trials and translations. *Nano Today.* 2020, 35, 100972.

Huang, S.; Gao, S.; Cheng, L.; Yu, H. Remineralization potential of nano-hydroxyapatite on initial enamel lesions: An in vitro study. *Caries Res.* 2011, 45, 460–468.

Huang, S.; Gao, S.; Yu, H. Effect of nano-hydroxyapatite concentration on remineralization of initial enamel lesion in vitro. *Biomed. Mater.* 2009, 4, 034104.

Huang, Y.; Yu, F.; Park, Y.; Wang, J.; Shin, M.; Chung, H.; et al. Co-administration of protein drugs with gold nanoparticles to enable percutaneous delivery. *Biomaterials.* 2010, 31, 9086–9091.

Huh, A.J.; Kwon, Y.J. "Nanoantibiotics": A new paradigm for treating infectious diseases using nanomaterials in the antibiotics resistant era. *J. Control. Release.* 2011, 156, 128–145.

Ibrahim, M.A.; Meera, P.B.; Neo, J.; Fawzy, A.S. Characterization of Chitosan/TiO$_2$ nanopowder modified glass-ionomer cement for restorative dental applications. *J. Esthet. Restor. Dent.* 2017, 29, 146–156.

Jang, J.-H.; Lee, M.G.; Ferracane, J.L.; Davis, H.; Bae, H.E.; Choi, D.; Kim, D.-S. Effect of bioactive glass-containing resin composite on dentin remineralization. *J. Dent.* 2018, 75, 58–64.

Jin, S.; Xia, X.; Huang, J.; Yuan, C.; Zuo, Y.; Li, Y.; Li, J. Recent advances in PLGA-based biomaterials for bone tissue regeneration. *Acta Biomater.* 2021, 127, 56–79.

Jubran, A.; Al-Zamely, O.M.; Al-Ammar, M.H. A study of iron oxide nanoparticles synthesis by using bacteria. *Int. J. Pharm. Qual. Assur.* 2020, 11, 88–92.

Kaittanis, C.; Santra, S.; Perez, J.M. Emerging nanotechnology-based strategies for the identification of microbial pathogenesis. *Adv. Drug Deliv. Rev.* 2010, 62, 408–423.

Karakuzu-Ikizler, B.; Terzio glu, P.; Basaran-Elalmis, Y.; Tekerek, B.S.; Yücel, S. Role of magnesium and aluminum substitution on the structural properties and bioactivity of bioglasses synthesized from biogenic silica. *Bioact. Mater.* 2020, 5, 66–73.

Karumuri, S.; Mandava, J.; Pamidimukkala, S.; Uppalapati, L.V.; Konagala, R.K.; Dasari, L. Efficacy of hydroxyapatite and silica nanoparticles on erosive lesions remineralization. *J. Conserv. Dent. JCD.* 2020, 23, 265.

Katunar, M.R.; Pastore, J.I.; Cisilino, A.; Merlo, J.; Alonso, L.S.; Baca, M.; Haddad, K.; Cere, S.; Ballarre, J. Early sseointegration of strontium-doped coatings on titanium implants in an osteoporotic rat model. *Surf. Coat. Technol.* 2022, 433, 128159.

Kaur, G.; Kumar, V.; Baino, F.; Mauro, J.; Pickrell, G.; Evans, I.; Bretcanu, O. Mechanical properties of bioactive glasses, ceramics, glass-ceramics and composites: State-of-the-art review and future challenges. *Mater. Sci. Eng. C.* 2019, 104, 109895.

Khan, I.; Saeed, K.; Khan, I. Nanoparticles: Properties, applications and toxicities. *Arab. J. Chem.* 2019, 12, 908–931.

Khodaei, A.; Jahanmard, F.; Madaah Hosseini, H.R.; Bagheri, R.; Dabbagh, A.; Weinans, H.; Amin Yavari, S. Controlled temperature-mediated curcumin release from magneto-thermal nanocarriers to kill bone tumors. *Bioact. Mater.* 2022, 11, 107–117.

Kim, D.; Kim, M.; Shinde, S.; Sung, J.; Ghodake, G. Cytotoxicity and antibacterial assessment of gallic acid capped gold nanoparticles synthesized at ambient temperature. *Coll. Surfaces B Biointerfaces.* 2017, 149, 162–167.

Kulshrestha, S.; Khan, S.; Hasan, S.; Khan, M.E.; Misba, L.; Khan, A.U. Calcium fluoride nanoparticles induced suppression of Streptococcus mutans biofilm: An in vitro and in vivo approach. *Appl. Microbiol. Biotechnol.* 2016, 100, 1901–1914.

Kumar, P.; Saini, M.; Dehiya, B.S.; Sindhu, A.; Kumar, V.; Kumar, R.; Lamberti, L.; Pruncu, C.I.; Thakur, R. Comprehensive survey on nanobiomaterials for bone tissue engineering applications. *Nanomaterials.* 2020, 10, 2019.

Kundu, M.; Sadhukhan, P.; Ghosh, N.; Ghosh, S.; Chatterjee, S.; Das, J.; Brahmachari, G.; Sil, P.C. In vivo therapeutic evaluation of a novel bis-lawsone derivative against tumor following delivery using mesoporous silica nanoparticle based redox-responsive drug delivery system. *Mater. Sci. Eng. C.* 2021, 126, 112142.

Kupikowska-Stobba, B.; Kasprzak, M. Fabrication of nanoparticles for bone regeneration: New insight into applications of nanoemulsion technology. *J. Mater. Chem. B.* 2021, 9, 5221–5244.

Kuśnieruk, S.; Wojnarowicz, J.; Chodara, A.; Chudoba, T.; Gierlotka, S.; Lojkowski, W. Influence of hydrothermal synthesis parameters on the properties of hydroxyapatite nanoparticles. *Beilstein J. Nanotechnol.* 2016, 7, 1586–1601.

Kyriacou, V.; Brownlow, W.J.; Xu, X.-H.N. Using nanoparticle optics assay for direct observation of the function of antimicrobial agents in single live bacterial cells. *Biochemistry.* 2004, 43, 140–147.

Lagashetty, A.; Ganiger, S.K.P.; Reddy, S. Green synthesis, characterization and antibacterial study of Ag-Au bimetallic nanocomposite using tea powder extract. *Biointerface Res. Appl. Chem.* 2020, 11, 8087–8095.

Lai, H.Z.; Chen, W.Y.; Wu, C.Y.; Chen, Y.C. Potent antibacterial nanoparticles for pathogenic bacteria. *ACS Appl. Mater. Interfaces.* 2015, 7, 2046–2054.

Lakshminarayanan, S.; Shereen, M.F.; Niraimathi, K.L.; Brindha, P.; Arumugam, A. One-pot green synthesis of iron oxide nanoparticles from Bauhinia tomentosa: Characterization and application towards synthesis of 1, 3 diolein. *Sci. Rep.* 2021, 11, 8643.

Lakshmi Prasanna, V.; Vijayaraghavan, R. Insight into the mechanism of antibacterial activity of ZnO: Surface defects mediated reactive oxygen species even in the dark. *Langmuir.* 2015, 31, 9155–9162.

Lambadi, P.R.; Sharma, T.K.; Kumar, P.; Vasnani, P.; Thalluri, S.M.; Bisht, N.; et al. Facile biofunctionalization of silver nanoparticles for enhanced antibacterial properties, endotoxin removal, and biofilm control. *Int. J. Nanomed.* 2015, 10, 2155–2171.

Lara, H.H.; Ayala-Núñez, N.V.; Ixtepan Turrent, L.; del, C.; Rodríguez Padilla, C. Bactericidal effect of silver nanoparticles against multidrug-resistant bacteria. *World J. Microbiol. Biotechnol.* 2010, 26, 615–621.

Lara-Ochoa, S.; Ortega-Lara, W.; Guerrero-Beltrán, C.E. Hydroxyapatite Nanoparticles in drug delivery: Physicochemistry and applications. *Pharmaceutics.* 2021, 13, 1642.

Laurent, S.; Forge, D.; Port, M.; Roch, A.; Robic, C.; Elst, L.V.; Muller, R.N. Magnetic iron oxide nanoparticles: Synthesis, stabilization, vectorization, physicochemical characterizations, and biological applications. *Chem. Rev.* 2010, 110, 2574.

Lautenschlager, E.P.; Monaghan, P. Titanium and titanium alloys as dental materials. *Int. Dent. J.* 1993, 43, 245–253.

Lee, B.-S.; Kang, S.-H.; Wang, Y.-L.; Lin, F.-H.; Lin, C.-P. In vitro study of dentinal tubule occlusion with sol-gel DP-bioglass for treatment of dentin hypersensitivity. *Dent. Mater. J.* 2007, 26, 52–61.

Lee, D.; Ko, W.K.; Kim, S.J.; Han, I.B.; Hong, J.B.; Sheen, S.H.; Sohn, S. Inhibitory effects of gold and silver nanoparticles on the differentiation into osteoclasts in vitro. *Pharmaceutics.* 2021, 13, 462.

Leuba, K.D.; Durmus, N.G.; Taylor, E.N.; Webster, T.J. Short communication: Carboxylate functionalized superparamagnetic iron oxide nanoparticles (SPION) for the reduction of *S. aureus* growth post biofilm formation. *Int. J. Nanomedicine.* 2013, 8, 731–736.

Lewis Oscar, F.; MubarakAli, D.; Nithya, C.; Priyanka, R.; Gopinath, V.; Alharbi, N.S.; et al. One pot synthesis and anti-biofilm potential of copper nanoparticles (CuNPs) against clinical strains of Pseudomonas aeruginosa. *Biofouling.* 2015, 31, 379–391.

Li, H.; Pan, S.; Xia, P.; Chang, Y.; Fu, C.; Kong, W.; Yu, Z.; Wang, K.; Yang, X.; Qi, Z. Advances in the application of gold nanoparticles in bone tissue engineering. *J. Biol. Eng.* 2020a, 14, 14.

Li, L.; Zhang, Y.; Wang, M.; Zhou, J.; Zhang, Q.; Yang, W.; Li, Y.; Yan, F. Gold nanoparticles combined human-defensin 3 gene-modified human periodontal ligament cells alleviate periodontal destruction via the p38 MAPK pathway. *Front. Bioeng. Biotechnol.* 2021, 9, 35.

Liang, W.; Ding, P.; Li, G.; Lu, E.; Zhao, Z. Hydroxyapatite nanoparticles facilitate osteoblast differentiation and bone formation within sagittal suture during expansion in rats [corrigendum]. *Drug Des. Dev. Ther.* 2021, 15, 3617–3618.

Liao, S.H.; Liu, C.H.; Bastakoti, B.P.; Suzuki, N.; Chang, Y.; Yamauchi, Y.; Lin, F.L.; Wu, K.C. Functionalized magnetic iron oxide/alginate core-shell nanoparticles for targeting hyperthermia. *Int. J. Nanomed.* 2015, 10, 3315.

Lyons, J.G.; Plantz, M.A.; Hsu, W.K.; Hsu, E.L.; Minardi, S. Nanostructured biomaterials for bone regeneration. *Front. Bioeng. Biotechnol.* 2020, 8, 922.

Marin, C.P.; Crovace, M.C.; Zanotto, E.D. Competent F18 bioglass-Biosilicate® bone graft scaffold substitutes. *J. Eur. Ceram. Soc.* 2021, 41, 7910–7920.

Marques, L.; Martinez, G.; Guidelli, É.; Tamashiro, J.; Segato, R.; Payão, S.L.M.; Baffa, O.; Kinoshita, A. Performance on bone regeneration of a silver nanoparticle delivery system based on natural rubber membrane NRL-AgNP. *Coatings.* 2020, 10, 323.

Mcglennen, R.C. Miniaturization technologies for molecular diagnostics. *Clin. Chem.* 2001, 47, 393–402.

Melo, M.A.; Cheng, L.; Weir, M.D.; Hsia, R.C.; Rodrigues, L.K.; Xu, H.H. Novel dental adhesive containing antibacterial agents and calcium phosphate nanoparticles. *J. Biomed. Mater. Res. B Appl. Biomater.* 2013, 101, 620–629.

Merchant, B. Gold, the noble metal and the paradoxes of its toxicology. *Biologicals.* 1998, 26, 49–59.

Miola, M.; Bellare, A.; Gerbaldo, R.; Laviano, F.; Vernè, E. Synthesis and characterization of magnetic and antibacterial nanoparticles as filler in acrylic cements for bone cancer and comorbidities therapy. *Ceram. Int.* 2021, 47, 17633–17643.

Mitchell, M.J.; Billingsley, M.M.; Haley, R.M.; Wechsler, M.E.; Peppas, N.A.; Langer, R. Engineering precision nanoparticles for drug delivery. *Nat. Rev. Drug Discov.* 2021, 20, 101–124.

Mitra, D.; Li, M.; Kang, E.T.; Neoh, K.G. Transparent copper-based antibacterial coatings with enhanced efficacy against Pseudomonas aeruginosa. *ACS Appl. Mater. Interfaces.* 2019, 11, 73–83.

Mok, Z.H.; Mylonas, P.; Austin, R.; Proctor, G.; Pitts, N.; Thanou, M. Calcium phosphate nanoparticles for potential application as enamel remineralising agent tested on hydroxyapatite discs. *Nanoscale.* 2021, 13, 20002–20012.

Mortazavi, S.; Rahsepar, M.; Hosseinzadeh, S. Modification of mesoporous structure of silver-doped bioactive glass with antibacterial properties for bone tissue applications. *Ceram. Int.* 2021, 48, 8276–8285.

Nagvenkar, A.P.; Deokar, A.; Perelshtein, I.; Gedanken, A. A one-step sonochemical synthesis of stable ZnO–PVA nanocolloid as a potential biocidal agent. *J. Mater. Chem. B*. 2016, 4, 2124–2132.

Nagy, A.; Harrison, A.; Dutta, P.K. Silver nanoparticles embedded in zeolite membranes: Release of silver ions and mechanism of antibacterial action. *Int. J. Nanomed.* 2011, 6, 1833–1852.

Nah, H.; Lee, D.; Lee, J.S.; Lee, S.J.; Heo, D.N.; Lee, Y.H.; Bang, J.B.; Hwang, Y.S.; Moon, H.J.; Kwon, I.K. Strategy to inhibit effective differentiation of RANKL-induced osteoclasts using vitamin D-conjugated gold nanoparticles. *Appl. Surf. Sci.* 2020, 527, 146765.

Natan, M.; Banin, E. From nano to micro: Using nanotechnology to combat microorganisms and their multidrug resistance. *FEMS Microbiol. Rev.* 2017, 41, 302–322.

Nawaz, M.; Mohammad, A.A.; Alejandro, P.P.; Soleiman, H.; Faiza, Q.; Anwar, U.-H.; Abbas, S.H.; Muhammad, T. Sonochemical synthesis of $ZnCo_2O_4/Ag_3PO_4$ heterojunction photocatalysts for the degradation of organic pollutants and pathogens: A combined experimental and computational study. *New J Chem*, 2022, 46(29), 14030–14042.

Nawaz, M.; Slimani, Y.; Ercan, I.; Michele, K.L.; Ernandes T.T.N.; Chariya K.; Abdelhamid, E. Magnetic and pH-responsive magnetic nanocarriers. In *Stimuli Responsive Polymeric Nanocarriers for Drug Delivery Applications: Advanced Nanocarriers for Therapeutics*, 1st ed., vol. 2, Abdel Salam Hamdy Makhlouf, Nedal Y. Abu-Thabit eds.; Woodhead Publishing: Sawston, October 2018, pp. 37–85.

Nejati, K.; Dadashpour, M.; Gharibi, T.; Mellatyar, H.; Akbarzadeh, A. Biomedical applications of functionalized gold nanoparticles: A review. *J. Clust. Sci.* 2022, 33, 1–16.

Nozari, A.; Ajami, S.; Rafiei, A.; Niazi, E. Impact of nano hydroxyapatite, nano silver fluoride and sodium fluoride varnish on primary teeth enamel remineralization: An in vitro study. *J. Clin. Diagn. Res. JCDR*. 2017, 11, ZC97.

Nunes, F.B.; Da Silva Bruckmann, F.; Da Rosa Salles, T.; Rhoden, C.B.R. Study of phenobarbital removal from the aqueous solutions employing magnetite-functionalized chitosan. *Environ. Sci. Pollut. Res.* 2022, 1–14.

Odermatt, R.; Par, M.; Mohn, D.; Wiedemeier, D.B.; Attin, T.; Tauböck, T.T. Bioactivity and physico-chemical properties of dental composites functionalized with nano- vs. micro-sized bioactive glass. *J. Clin. Med.* 2020, 9, 772.

Ojo, O.A.; Olayide, I.I.; Akalabu, M.C.; Ajiboye, B.O.; Ojo, A.B.; Oyinloye, B.E.; Ramalingam, M. Nanoparticles and their biomedical applications. *Biointerface Res. Appl. Chem.* 2020, 11, 8431–8445.

Oryan, A.; Hassanajili, S.; Sahvieh, S.; Azarpira, N. Effectiveness of mesenchymal stem cell-seeded onto the 3D polylactic acid/polycaprolactone/hydroxyapatite scaffold on the radius bone defect in rat. *Life Sci.* 2020, 257, 118038.

Ozak, S.T.; Ozkan, P. Nanotechnology and dentistry. *Eur. J. Dent.* 2013, 7, 145–151.

Pal, I.; Brahmkhatri, V.P.; Bera, S.; Bhattacharyya, D.; Quirishi, Y.; Bhunia, A.; et al. Enhanced stability and activity of an antimicrobial peptide in conjugation with silver nanoparticle. *J. Colloid Interface Sci.* 2016, 483, 385–393.

Pan, W.Y.; Huang, C.C.; Lin, T.T.; Hu, H.Y.; Lin, W.C.; Li, M.J.; et al. Synergistic antibacterial effects of localized heat and oxidative stress caused by hydroxyl radicals mediated by graphene/iron oxide-based nanocomposites. *Nanomed. Nanotechnol. Biol. Med.* 2016, 12, 431–438.

Parent, M.; Baradari, H.; Champion, E.; Damia, C.; Viana-Trecant, M. Design of calcium phosphate ceramics for drug delivery applications in bone diseases: A review of the parameters affecting the loading and release of the therapeutic substance. *J. Control. Release*. 2017, 252, 1–17.

Payne, J.N.; Waghwani, H.K.; Connor, M.G.; Hamilton, W.; Tockstein, S.; Moolani, H.; et al. Novel synthesis of kanamycin conjugated gold nanoparticles with potent antibacterial activity. *Front. Microbiol.* 2016, 7, 607.

Percival, S.L.; Bowler, P.G.; Dolman, J. Antimicrobial activity of silver-containing dressings on wound microorganisms using an *in vitro* biofilm model. *Int. Wound J.* 2007, 4, 186–191.

Poosti, M.; Ramazanzadeh, B.; Zebarjad, M.; Javadzadeh, P.; Naderinasab, M.; Shakeri, M.T. Shear bond strength and antibacterial effects of orthodontic composite containing Titanium dioxide (TiO_2) nanoparticles. *Eur. J. Orthod.* 2013, 35, 676–679.

Popescu, R.C.; Straticiuc, M.; Mustăciosu, C.; Temelie, M.; Truşcă, R.; Vasile, B.Ş.; Boldeiu, A.; Mirea, D.; Andrei, R.F.; Cenuşă, C.; et al. Enhanced internalization of nanoparticles following ionizing radiation leads to mitotic catastrophe in MG-63 human osteosarcoma cells. *Int. J. Mol. Sci.* 2020, 21, 7220.

Priya, N.; Kaur, K.; Sidhu, A.K. Green synthesis: An eco-friendly route for the synthesis of iron oxide nanoparticles. *Front. Nanotechnol.* 2021, 3, 655062.

Raghubir, M.; Rahman, C.N.; Fang, J.; Matsui, H.; Mahajan, S.S. Osteosarcoma growth suppression by riluzole delivery via iron oxide nanocage in nude mice. *Oncol. Rep.* 2020, 43, 169–176.

Ralston, S.H. Bone structure and metabolism. *Medicine.* 2021, 49, 567–571.

Ramasamy, M.; Lee, J.H.; Lee, J. Direct one-pot synthesis of cinnamaldehyde immobilized on gold nanoparticles and their antibiofilm properties. *Coll. Surfaces B Biointerfaces.* 2017, 160, 639–648.

Ramazanov, M.; Karimova, A.; Shirinova, H. Magnetism for drug delivery, MRI and hyperthermia applications: A review. *Biointerface Res. Appl. Chem.* 2021, 11, 8654–8668.

Ramimoghadam, D.; Bagheri, S.; Hamid, S.B.A. Progress in electrochemical synthesis of magnetic iron oxide nanoparticles. *J. Magn. Magn. Mater.* 2014, 368, 207–229.

Ramos-Tonello, C.M.; Lisboa-Filho, P.N.; Arruda, L.B.; Tokuhara, C.K.; Oliveira, R.C.; Furuse, A.Y.; Rubo, J.H.; Borges, A.F.S. Titanium dioxide nanotubes addition to self-adhesive resin cement: Effect on physical and biological properties. *Dent. Mater.* 2017, 33, 866–875.

Ramyaa Shri, K.; Subitha, P.; Narasimhan, S.; Murugesan, R.; Narayan, S. Fabrication of dexamethasone-silver nanoparticles entrapped dendrimer collagen matrix nanoparticles for dental applications. *Biointerface Res. Appl. Chem.* 2021, 11, 14935–14955.

Rhoden, C.R.B.; da Silva Bruckmann, F.; da Rosa Salles, T.; Junior, C.G.K.; Mortari, S.R. Study from the influence of magnetite onto removal of hydrochlorothiazide from aqueous solutions applying magnetic graphene oxide. *J. Water Process Eng.* 2021, 43, 102262.

Ribeiro, A.P.C.; Anbu, S.; Alegria, E.C.B.A.; Fernandes, A.R.; Baptista, P.V.; Mendes, R.; et al. Evaluation of cell toxicity and DNA and protein binding of green synthesized silver nanoparticles. *Biomed. Pharmacother.* 2018, 101, 137–144.

Rondanelli, M.; Faliva, M.A.; Infantino, V.; Gasparri, C.; Iannello, G.; Perna, S.; Riva, A.; Petrangolini, G.; Tartara, A.; Peroni, G. Copper as dietary supplement for bone metabolism: A review. *Nutrients.* 2021, 13, 2246.

Saeb, A.T.M.; Alshammari, A.S.; Al-brahim, H.; Al-rubeaan, K.A. Production of silver nanoparticles with strong and stable antimicrobial activity against highly pathogenic and multidrug resistant bacteria. *Sci. World J.* 2014, 2, 704708.

Sagadevan, S.; Imteyaz, S.; Murugan, B.; Anita, L.J.; Sridewi, N.; Weldegebrieal, G.; Fatimah, I.; Oh, W.A. Comprehensive review on green synthesis of titanium dioxide nanoparticles and their diverse biomedical applications. *Green Process. Synth.* 2022, 11, 44–63.

Salem, D.M.; Ismail, M.M.; Aly-Eldeen, M.A. Biogenic synthesis and antimicrobial potency of iron oxide (Fe_3O_4) nanoparticles using algae harvested from the Mediterranean Sea, Egypt. *Egypt. J. Aquat. Res.* 2019, 45, 197–204.

Salem, W.; Leitner, D.R.; Zingl, F.G.; Schratter, G.; Prassl, R.; Goessler, W.; et al. Antibacterial activity of silver and zinc nanoparticles against *Vibrio cholerae* and enterotoxic *Escherichia coli*. *Int. J. Med. Microbiol.* 2015, 305, 85–95.

Samadian, H.; Khastar, H.; Ehterami, A.; Salehi, M. Bioengineered 3D nanocomposite based on gold nanoparticles and gelatin nanofibers for bone regeneration: In vitro and in vivo study. *Sci. Rep.* 2021, 11, 13877.

Sarwar, S.; Chakraborti, S.; Bera, S.; Sheikh, I.A.; Hoque, K.M.; Chakrabarti, P. The antimicrobial activity of ZnO nanoparticles against *Vibrio cholerae*: Variation in response depends on biotype. *Nanomedicine Nanotechnology, Biol. Med.* 2016, 12, 1499–1509.

Schmeidl, K.; Janiszewska-Olszowska, J.; Grocholewicz, K. Clinical features and physical properties of gummetal orthodontic wire in comparison with dissimilar archwires: A critical review. *BioMed Res. Int.* 2021, 2021, 6611979.

Schwendicke, F.; Al-Abdi, A.; Moscardó, A.P.; Cascales, A.F.; Sauro, S. Remineralization effects of conventional and experimental ion-releasing materials in chemically or bacterially-induced dentin caries lesions. *Dent. Mater.* 2019, 35, 772–779.

Seljak, K.B.; Kocbek, P.; Gašperlin, M. Mesoporous silica nanoparticles as delivery carriers: An overview of drug loading techniques. *J. Drug Deliv. Sci. Technol.* 2020, 59, 101906.

Sergi, R.; Bellucci, D.; Cannillo, V. A review of bioactive glass/natural polymer composites: State of the art. *Materials.* 2020, 13, 5560.

Shahmoradi, M.; Rohanizadeh, R.; Sonvico, F.; Ghadiri, M.; Swain, M. Synthesis of stabilized hydroxyapatite nanosuspensions for enamel caries remineralization. *Aust. Dent. J.* 2018, 63, 356–364.

Shamaila, S.; Zafar, N.; Riaz, S.; Sharif, R.; Nazir, J.; Naseem, S. Gold nanoparticles: An efficient antimicrobial agent against enteric bacterial human pathogen. *Nanomaterials.* 2016, 6(4), 71.

Shen, Q.; Qi, Y.; Kong, Y.; Bao, H.; Wang, Y.; Dong, A.; Wu, H.; Xu, Y. Advances in copper-based biomaterials with antibacterial and osteogenic properties for bone tissue engineering. *Front. Bioeng. Biotechnol.* 2022, 9, 795425.

Shi, Y.; Han, X.; Pan, S.; Wu, Y.; Jiang, Y.; Lin, J.; Chen, Y.; Jin, H. Gold nanomaterials and bone/cartilage tissue engineering: Biomedical applications and molecular mechanisms. *Front. Chem.* 2021, 9, 546.

Slavin, Y.N.; Asnis, J.; Hafeli, U.O.; Bach, H. Metal nanoparticles: Understanding the mechanisms behind antibacterial activity. *J. Nanobiotechnology.* 2017, 15, 65.

Sodipo, B.K.; Aziz, A.A. Recent advances in synthesis and surface modification of superparamagnetic iron oxide nanoparticles with silica. *J. Magn. Magn. Mater.* 2016, 416, 275–291.

Sofan, E.; Sofan, A.; Palaia, G.; Tenore, G.; Romeo, U.; Migliau, G. Classification review of dental adhesive systems: From the IV generation to the universal type. *Ann. Stomatol.* 2017, 8, 1–17.

Solinas, S.; Piccaluga, G.; Morales, M.; Serna, C. Sol-gel formation of γ-Fe$_2$O$_3$/SiO$_2$ nanocomposites. *Acta Mater.* 2001, 49, 2805–2811.

Sonatkar, J.; Kandasubramanian, B. Bioactive glass with biocompatible polymers for bone applications. *Eur. Polym. J.* 2021, 160, 110801.

Srinath, P.; Abdul Azeem, P.; Venugopal Reddy, K. Review on calcium silicate-based bioceramics in bone tissue engineering. *Int. J. Appl. Ceram. Technol.* 2020, 17, 2450–2464.

Srinivasan, S.; Jayasree, R.; Chennazhi, K.P.; Nair, S.V.; Jayakumar, R. Biocompatible alginate/nano bioactive glass ceramic composite scaffolds for periodontal tissue regeneration. *Carbohydr. Polym.* 2012, 87, 274–283.

Sturmer, M.; Garcia, I.M.; Souza, V.S.; Visioli, F.; Scholten, J.D.; Samuel, S.M.W.; Leitune, V.C.B.; Collares, F.M. Titanium dioxide nanotubes with triazine-methacrylate monomer to improve physicochemical and biological properties of adhesives. *Dent. Mater.* 2021, 37, 223–235.

Su, H.-L.; Lin, S.-H.; Wei, J.-C.; Pao, I.-C.; Chiao, S.-H.; Huang, C.-C.; et al. Novel nanohybrids of silver particles on clay platelets for inhibiting silver-resistant bacteria. *PLoS One.* 2011, 6, e21125.

Su, Y.; Zheng, X.; Chen, Y.; Li, M.; Liu, K. Alteration of intracellular protein expressions as a key mechanism of the deterioration of bacterial denitrification caused by copper oxide nanoparticles. *Sci. Rep.* 2015, 5, 15824.

Sun, J.; Petersen, E.J.; Watson, S.S.; Sims, C.M.; Kassman, A.; Frukhtbeyn, S.; Skrtic, D.; Ok, M.T.; Jacobs, D.S.; Reipa, V.; et al. Biophysical characterization of functionalized titania nanoparticles and their application in dental adhesives. *Acta Biomater.* 2017, 53, 585–597.

Sun, J.; Xing, F.; Braun, J.; Traub, F.; Rommens, P.M.; Xiang, Z.; Ritz, U. Progress of phototherapy applications in the treatment of bone cancer. *Int. J. Mol. Sci.* 2021, 22, 1354.

Sun, L.; Chow, L.C. Preparation and properties of nano-sized calcium fluoride for dental applications. *Dent. Mater.* 2008, 24, 111–116.

Swiętek, M.; Ma, Y.H.; Wu, N.P.; Paruzel, A.; Tokarz, W.; Horák, D. Tannic acid coating augments glioblastoma cellular uptake of magnetic nanoparticles with antioxidant effects. *Nanomaterials.* 2022, 12, 1310.

Szabo, R.; Bodolea, C.; Mocan, T. Iron, copper, and zinc homeostasis: Physiology, physiopathology, and nanomediated applications. *Nanomaterials.* 2021, 11, 2985.

Szewczyk, A.; Skwira, A.; Konopacka, A.; Sadej, R.; Prokopowicz, M. Mesoporous silica-bioglass composite pellets as bone drug delivery system with mineralization potential. *Int. J. Mol. Sci.* 2021, 22, 4708.

Tahmasebi, E.; Alam, M.; Yazdanian, M.; Tebyanian, H.; Yazdanian, A.; Seifalian, A.; Mosaddad, S.A. Current biocompatible materials in oral regeneration: A comprehensive overview of composite materials. *J. Mater. Res. Technol.* 2020, 9, 11731–11755.

Takahashi, N.; Nyvad, B. The role of bacteria in the caries process: Ecological perspectives. *J. Dent. Res.* 2011, 90, 294–303.

Tao, S.; He, L.; Xu, H.H.; Weir, M.D.; Fan, M.; Yu, Z.; Zhang, M.; Zhou, X.; Liang, K.; Li, J. Dentin remineralization via adhesive containing amorphous calcium phosphate nanoparticles in a biofilm-challenged environment. *J. Dent.* 2019, 89, 103193.

Tiomnova, O.T.; Coelho, F.; Pellizaro, T.A.G.; Enrique, J.; Chanfrau, R.; de Oliveira Capote, T.S.; Basmaji, P.; Pantoja, Y.V.; Guastaldi, A.C. Preparation of scaffolds of amorphous calcium phosphate and bacterial cellulose for use in tissue regeneration by freeze-drying process. *Biointerface Res. Appl. Chem.* 2021, 11, 7357–7367.

Tortella, G.R.; Rubilar, O.; Durán, N.; Diez, M.C.; Martínez, M.; Parada, J.; Seabra, A.B. Silver nanoparticles: Toxicity in model organisms as an overview of its hazard for human health and the environment. *J. Hazard. Mater.* 2020, 390, 121974.

Tschoppe, P.; Zandim, D.L.; Martus, P.; Kielbassa, A.M. Enamel and dentine remineralization by nano-hydroxyapatite toothpastes. *J. Dent.* 2011, 39, 430–437.

Vale, A.C.; Pereira, P.R.; Barbosa, A.M.; Torrado, E.; Alves, N.M. Optimization of silver-containing bioglass nanoparticles envisaging biomedical applications. *Mater. Sci. Eng. C.* 2019, 94, 161–168.

van der Meel, R.; Sulheim, E.; Shi, Y.; Kiessling, F.; Mulder, W.J.M.; Lammers, T. Smart cancer nanomedicine. *Nat. Nanotechnol.* 2019, 14, 1007–1017.

van Vugt, T.A.; Geurts, J.A.P.; Arts, J.J.; Lindfors, N.C. Biomaterials in treatment of orthopedic infections. In *Management of Periprosthetic Joint Infections (PJIs)*; Woodhead Publishing (Elsevier): Duxford, UK, 2017, pp. 41–68.

Ventola, C.L. Progress in nanomedicine: Approved and investigational nanodrugs progress in nanomedicine. *J Clin Pharm Ther.* 2017, 42(12), 742–755.

Vijayakumar, R.; Koltypin, Y.; Felner, I.; Gedanken, A. Sonochemical synthesis and characterization of pure nanometer-sized Fe3O4 particles. *Mater. Sci. Eng. A.* 2000, 286, 101–105.

Vodyashkin, A.A.; Rizk, M.G.; Kezimana, P.; Kirichuk, A.A.; Stanishevskiy, Y.M. Application of gold nanoparticle-based materials in cancer therapy and diagnostics. *Chem. Engineering.* 2021, 5, 69.

Wang, C.; Zhao, N.; Huang, Y.; He, R.; Xu, S.; Yuan, W. Coordination of injectable self-healing hydrogel with Mn-Zn ferrite@ mesoporous silica nanospheres for tumor MR imaging and efficient synergistic magnetothermal-chemo-chemodynamic therapy. *Chem. Eng. Technol.* 2020a, 401, 126100.

Wang, K.; Cheng, W.; Ding, Z.; Xu, G.; Zheng, X.; Li, M.; Lu, G.; Lu, Q. Injectable silk/hydroxyapatite nanocomposite hydrogels with vascularization capacity for bone regeneration. *J. Mater. Sci. Technol.* 2021a, 63, 172–181.

Wang, L.; Hu, C.; Shao, L. The antimicrobial activity of nanoparticles: Present situation and prospects for the future. *Int. J. Nanomed.* 2017a, 12, 1227–1249.

Wang, L.; Huang, F.; Cai, G.; Yao, L.; Zhang, H.; Lin, J. An electrochemical aptasensor using coaxial capillary with magnetic nanoparticle, urease catalysis and PCB electrode for rapid and sensitive detection of *Escherichia coli* O157:H7. *Nanotheranostics.* 2017b, 1, 403–414.

Wang, N.; Dheen, S.T.; Fuh, J.Y.H.; Kumar, A.S. A review of multi-functional ceramic nanoparticles in 3D printed bone tissue engineering. *Bioprinting.* 2021b, 23, e00146.

Wang, N.; Fuh, J.Y.H.; Dheen, S.T.; Senthil Kumar, A. Functions and applications of metallic and metallic oxide nanoparticles in orthopedic implants and scaffolds. *J. Biomed. Mater. Res.-Part B Appl. Biomater.* 2021c, 109, 160–179.

Wang, N.; Maskomani, S.; Meenashisundaram, G.K.; Fuh, J.Y.H.; Dheen, S.T.; Anantharajan, S.K. A study of titanium and magnesium particle-induced oxidative stress and toxicity to human osteoblasts. *Mater. Sci. Eng. C Mater. Biol. Appl.* 2020b, 117, 111285.

Wang, Y.H.N. Nanometer-sized semiconductor clusters: Materials synthesis, quantum size effects, and photophysical properties. *J. Phys. Chem.* 1991, 95, 525–532.

Wei, G.; Ma, P.X. Structure and properties of nano-hydroxyapatite/polymer composite scaffolds for bone tissue engineering. *Biomaterials.* 2004, 25, 4749–4757.

Weir, M.D.; Moreau, J.L.; Levine, E.D.; Strassler, H.E.; Chow, L.C.; Xu, H.H. Nanocomposite containing CaF2 nanoparticles: Thermal cycling, wear and long-term water-aging. *Dent. Mater.* 2012, 28, 642–652.

WHO. *The top 10 causes of death.* Fact sheet N_310. 2014. www.who.int/mediacentre/factsheets/fs310/en.

Wu, H.; Yang, S.; Xiao, J.; Ouyang, Z.; Yang, M.; Zhang, M.; Zhao, D.; Huang, Q. Facile synthesis of multi-functional nanocomposites by precise loading of Cu^{2+} onto MgO nano-particles for enhanced osteoblast differentiation, inhibited osteoclast formation and effective bacterial killing. *Mater. Sci. Eng. C.* 2021, 130, 112442.

Xie, X.; Wang, L.; Xing, D.; Qi, M.; Li, X.; Sun, J.; Melo, M.A.S.; Weir, M.D.; Oates, T.W.; Bai, Y.; et al. Novel rechargeable calcium phosphate nanoparticle-filled dental cement. *Dent. Mater. J.* 2019, 38, 1–10.

Xie, X.-J.; Xing, D.; Wang, L.; Zhou, H.; Weir, M.D.; Bai, Y.-X.; Xu, H.H. Novel rechargeable calcium phosphate nanoparticle containing orthodontic cement. *Int. J. Oral Sci.* 2017, 9, 24–32.

Yang, S.-Y.; Han, A.R.; Kim, K.-M.; Kwon, J.-S. Acid neutralizing and remineralizing orthodontic adhesive containing hydrated calcium silicate. *J. Dent.* 2022, 123, 104204.

Yang, X.; Yang, J.; Wang, L.; Ran, B.; Jia, Y.; Zhang, L.; et al. Pharmaceutical intermediate-modified gold nanoparticles: Against multidrug-resistant bacteria and wound-healing application via an electrospun scaffold. *ACS Nano.* 2017, 11, 5737–5745.

Yao, C.; Zhu, M.; Han, X.; Xu, Q.; Dai, M.; Nie, T.; Liu, X. A bone-targeting enoxacin delivery system to eradicate staphylococcus Aureus-related implantation infections and bone loss. *Front. Bioeng. Biotechnol.* 2021, 9, 749910.

Yi-Xiang, W. Current status of superparamagnetic iron oxide contrast agents for liver magnetic resonance imaging. *World J. Gastroenterol.* 2015, 21(47), 13400–13402.

Yu, J.; Zhang, W.; Li, Y.; Wang, G.; Yang, L.; Jin, J.; et al. Synthesis, characterization, antimicrobial activity and mechanism of a novel hydroxyapatite whisker/nano zinc oxide biomaterial. *Biomed. Mater.* 2014, 10, 015001.

Yu, Y.; Yu, X.; Tian, D.; Yu, A.; Wan, Y. Thermo-responsive chitosan/silk fibroin/amino-functionalized mesoporous silica hydrogels with strong and elastic characteristics for bone tissue engineering. *Int. J. Biol. Macromol.* 2021, 182, 1746–1758.

Yuan, L.; Qi, X.; Qin, G.; Liu, Q.; Zhang, F.; Song, Y.; Deng, J. Effects of gold nanostructures on differentiation of mesenchymal stem cells. *Colloids Surf. B Biointerfaces*. 2019, 184, 110494.

Zaidi, S.; Misba, L.; Khan, A.U. Nano-therapeutics: A revolution in infection control in post antibiotic era. *Nanomed. Nanotechnol. Biol. Med.* 2017, 13, 2281–2301.

Zarei, S.; Sadighian, S.; Rostamizadeh, K.; Khalkhali, M. Theragnostic magnetic core-shell nanoparticle as versatile nanoplatform for magnetic resonance imaging and drug delivery. *Biointerface Res. Appl. Chem.* 2021, 11, 13276–13289.

Zeng, P.; Zhao, Y.; Lin, Y.; Wang, X.; Li, J.; Wang, W.; Fang, Z. Enhancement of Electrochemical performance by the oxygen vacancies in hematite as anode material for lithium-ion batteries. *Nanoscale Res. Lett.* 2017, 12, 13.

Zhang, B.; Ding, Z.; Dong, J.; Lin, F.; Xue, Z.; Xu, J. Macrophage-mediated degradable gelatin-coated mesoporous silica nanoparticles carrying pirfenidone for the treatment of rat spinal cord injury. *Nanomed. Nanotechnol. Biol. Med.* 2021a, 37, 102420.

Zhang, L.; Weir, M.D.; Chow, L.C.; Antonucci, J.M.; Chen, J.; Xu, H.H. Novel rechargeable calcium phosphate dental nanocomposite. *Dent. Mater.* 2016, 32, 285–293.

Zhang, Y.; Huang, C.; Chang, J. Ca-doped mesoporous SiO_2/dental resin composites with enhanced mechanical properties, bioactivity and antibacterial properties. *J. Mater. Chem. B.* 2018, 6, 477–486.

Zhang, Y.; Wang, P.; Mao, H.; Zhang, Y.; Zheng, L.; Yu, P.; Guo, Z.; Li, L.; Jiang, Q. PEGylated gold nanoparticles promote osteogenic differentiation in in vitro and in vivo systems. *Mater. Des.* 2021b, 197, 109231.

Zhang, Y.; Wang, P.; Wang, Y.; Li, J.; Qiao, D.; Chen, R.; Yang, W.; Yan, F. Gold nanoparticles promote the bone regeneration of periodontal ligament stem cell sheets through activation of autophagy. *Int. J. Nanomed.* 2021c, 16, 61–73.

Zhang, Y.; Zhu, P.; Li, G.; Zhao, T.; Fu, X.; Sun, R.; et al. Facile preparation of monodisperse, impurity-free, and antioxidation copper nanoparticles on a large scale for application in conductive ink. *ACS Appl. Mater. Interfaces*. 2014, 6, 560–567.

Zhao, R.; Yang, R.; Cooper, P.R.; Khurshid, Z.; Shavandi, A.; Ratnayake, J. Bone grafts and substitutes in dentistry: A review of current trends and developments. *Molecules*. 2021, 26, 3007.

Zhao, Y.; Liu, J.; Zhang, M.; He, J.; Zheng, B.; Liu, F.; Zhao, Z.; Liu, Y. Use of silver nanoparticle–gelatin/alginate scaffold to repair skull defects. *Coatings*. 2020, 10, 948.; 476.

Zhou, S.; Zhong, Q.; Wang, Y.; Hu, P.; Zhong, W.; Huang, C.B.; Yu, Z.Q.; Ding, C.D.; Liu, H.; Fu, J. Chemically engineered mesoporous silica nanoparticles-based intelligent delivery systems for theranostic applications in multiple cancerous/noncancerous diseases. *Coord. Chem. Rev.* 2022, 452, 214309.

Index

For Product Safety Concerns and Information please contact our EU
representative GPSR@taylorandfrancis.com
Taylor & Francis Verlag GmbH, Kaufingerstraße 24, 80331 München, Germany

www.ingramcontent.com/pod-product-compliance
Lightning Source LLC
Chambersburg PA
CBHW060351220326
41598CB00023B/2885